Tired Thyroid

From Hyper to Hypo to Healing
Breaking the TSH Rule

Barbara S. Lougheed

DISCLAIMER

The author is a thyroid patient herself, not a doctor or medical professional. This book summarizes her research findings on various thyroid-related topics. It is her interpretation of numerous research studies and personal observations, and was written to share information with others who may have similar problems. It is not medical advice and should not be used to diagnose or treat any condition or disease. It is not exhaustive and cannot possibly cover all conditions. It is the patient's responsibility to consult a doctor for any diagnosis, treatment, and medication or supplement changes. Any information followed without a doctor's advice is done at the patient's own risk.

The author and publisher are not liable or responsible for any loss, damage, or injury alleged to be caused directly or indirectly by the information contained in this book. This book is not a substitute for medical counseling.

DEDICATION

This book is dedicated to my husband Marty, whose support (and editing skills!) allowed me to write this book. When I would sometimes lose focus, he would set me straight. He was the perfect sounding board, and allowed me to bounce umpteen ideas off of him during this process. If it weren't for him, this book would have been of much lower quality because I don't even realize I speak in medical jargon. His questions, criticisms, and suggestions led to numerous rewrites, in an effort to better explain difficult concepts, and to clarify confusing points.

CONTENTS

PART III: Where Do We Go From Here?

ACKNOWLEDGMENTS

I would like to acknowledge the following people:

CC, whose faith in me led me to launch TiredThyroid.com,
Dr. Z, who *insisted* I write this book,
JR, whose critiques improved my writing,
JMM, who helped me with difficult charts,
the patients who contributed their stories for case studies,
and all the patients on internet forums who made me realize
how complicated thyroid physiology really is!

1

Introduction

If I don't speak up, who will?

Who are you to write a book like this? What are your credentials?

Who *am* I? I'm a hypothyroid patient who did not feel well following mainstream medical protocols that my doctors practiced, so I turned to the internet for information, and found even more questionable protocols being pushed by fellow thyroid patients. I did not know anything about thyroid physiology when I started this journey, but common sense made me question some highly dogmatic (opinionated) statements from both sides. Because I had the time, a computer, and a deep desire to learn the truth (it would benefit me!), I set out to find the truth. I researched every dogmatic statement made by either side to ascertain the truth. I read hundreds of medical journal articles and thousands of posts on thyroid patient forums. I learned a lot of terminology by reading patient forums, where discussions revolve around TSH, T4, T3, rT3, cortisol and ferritin. I then used the keywords to query medical journals using Google Scholar, and read till my eyes would glaze over from information overload. Eventually, the facts revealed themselves, and they rarely supported either side's view. I believe that anyone who can read, who has access to a computer, who has a basic knowledge of biology, chemistry, math, and statistics, would come to the same conclusions I have. The biology, chemistry, and math I learned in public high school were more than enough to understand the material. I did not learn statistics until college, but a basic understanding of ratios and percentages (which I learned in elementary school) is essential, because math can be used to quantify and compare results. Math is a wonderful tool because it can clarify concepts and reveal conceptual flaws. Sometimes things will literally "not add up." An analytical aptitude (excelling in writing science lab reports and making charts and graphs) was also helpful. When I took Biology in the 9th grade, spreadsheet software did not exist, all calculations were computed manually, and data was hand-plotted on graph paper. This book could not have been written without the luxury of word processing and spreadsheet computer software. Medical terminology seemed foreign at first, but with internet search engines, any topic can be learned, if someone takes the time to look it up.

I was actually asked to write this book by a highly successful M.D. who is board certified in his specialty. He found my TiredThyroid.com website while searching for information that might help his wife, who is hypothyroid. He contacted me and insisted that I write a book. I initially dismissed the idea, because I'm not a doctor, and thought I had nothing to write about that wasn't already on the website. But he was insistent, and made me promise him that I would write a book. As I mulled the idea over, I realized I could create a useful reference book—one that I'd wished I'd had when I started this journey. It is my hope that the information in this book prevents patients from making the same mistakes I did.

No, I do not have a medical degree or any medical credentials, nor do I pretend to, but this book is not about teaching someone to do their own thyroidectomy or any medical procedure, which I concede requires years of study and hands-on training. The simple question I was trying to answer was: what is the optimal thyroid hormone replacement dose for a hypothyroid patient? I believed the answer to that question could be found if I understood thyroid physiology. Patients on thyroid forums often ask whether some of their other ailments could be thyroid-related, such as osteoporosis, insulin resistance, etc. There are multiple studies on all these related topics, so I researched them too, and they became chapters of their own.

Why did you write the book?

When I realized just how much misinformation was out there about thyroid physiology, I felt like I had stepped in a pile of dog poop. Should I say anything? Or just wash my shoes off, not say a word, and move on? Obviously, I decided to speak up, or you wouldn't be reading this book. This book is a compilation of everything I have learned about thyroid physiology over the past six years, which is longer than it takes to earn a Ph.D. It is also considerably longer than the six weeks of endocrinology and reproduction that is offered in some medical school curriculums. The actual time medical schools devote to thyroid physiology may not amount to more than a few days, because diabetes, the reproductive system, cancer, infertility, and pregnancy are also covered in that six week block. I wrote this book because I felt that others could benefit from what I've learned. But even with several years of study, I still don't know everything about the endocrine system, because it is *so* complex. Some will not agree with what I've written, and I am certainly not immune to harsh criticism. It seemed appropriate to address some of these remarks in an introduction to the book.

You have no medical background and have no right to be so judgmental.

True, but *why* isn't the medical profession aware of all the issues I have highlighted in the case studies? Are the medical school textbooks not covering the material? Who writes the textbooks? Why don't they understand the basics of thyroid physiology? Who determines what material *is* covered? I don't know the answers to any of these questions, but my goal in writing this book was to create a textbook of sorts that explains thyroid physiology in more detail than I believe is currently understood by anyone in the medical profession (doctors, nurses, etc.), or by patients, and family members of patients. I hope the result is some much needed change in thyroid treatment for patients.

The word "judgmental" can be applied to both doctors and patients. Many patients are exasperated that they can't get the prescription thyroid hormones that they need, and then become incensed at doctors, who are only following what they were taught in medical school. But doctors who are not hypothyroid have no idea what patients go through, and are sometimes rudely dismissive of valid health concerns that *are* caused by low thyroid levels, like weight gain, hair loss, fatigue, and depression. Again, it is my hope that this book will provide the proof to doctors that patients' concerns are real, medically based, and treatable.

Anybody can make up a case study. Doctors didn't really say those things.

Unfortunately, they did say those things. Or that's what the patients recall their doctors said to them. Really, I could not make this stuff up. That's why I felt these stories needed to be told. Thyroid patients need to know that they're not alone; that every thyroid patient suffers from all the misinformation out there. The five case studies are the medical biographies of four real people (plus me) who were generous enough to share their stories with me for this book. I learned so much when looking for research references to explain the medical issues they dealt with. And yes, I really did read every reference included in this book. For every reference listed, there are dozens more I read that didn't quite make the point as well, so they weren't included. Intensive research supports the concepts presented in this book, which are based on actual thyroid physiology. Hopefully, these case studies will be as instructive to others as they were to me.

I read another book/website that says the exact opposite of what you say, and people are getting well on those protocols, so you must be wrong.

These kinds of generalizations are part of the problem, which is applying the concept of "if it worked for me, then it must work for everyone." Unfortunately, we are not all carbon copies of each other, and there are myriad genetic variations in the endocrine system so that what works for one person may be an absolute disaster for another. Specifically, these other protocols did not work for me. There are horror stories from patients following doctor's protocols, *and* horror stories from patients following other patient protocols. In my opinion, neither side has the advantage here, for the reason I just mentioned—neither side is recognizing that patients are all biochemically individual and that no one treatment works for everyone. Prescriptions need to be custom tailored to the individual.

If a protocol works for someone, they feel well, and all lab values in a Comprehensive Metabolic Profile and Complete Blood Count are fine, then I would say they may have found their optimal dose, and should stick with it. On the other hand, if multiple lab values are testing high and exceed the reference ranges, like SHBG, fasting blood glucose, ALT, alkaline phosphatase, etc., then perhaps this "ideal dose" is causing damage to the body at a level that can't be seen by the naked eye. Some of these are markers for overmedication that can lead to osteoporosis and diabetes. To ignore these red flags and encourage others to follow the same protocol shows a lack of understanding of physiology, and a disregard for the health of others.

How can I use this book?

This was meant to be a reference book, so the chapters do not have to be read in any particular order. Each chapter explains one topic in detail. In fact, I would fully expect that while some chapters may be of major interest to some patients, others may never even look at those same chapters. But there should certainly be something for everyone.

The first section of this book consists of five case studies of real thyroid patients. I followed their lives throughout the years and turned the health issues they experienced into thyroid teaching points. The first chapter covers my life, a Graves' hyperthyroid patient who had radioactive iodine (RAI) treatment, who then became hypothyroid and now takes replacement thyroid hormone. The second story is of a man who suffered a blow to the head as a child, which damaged his pituitary gland. This resulted in multiple low hormone levels due to lack of pituitary stimulation (thyroid, cortisol, testosterone, growth hormone), yet he was not properly diagnosed until he was nearly 50 years old. The third story that many will identify with is of a hypothyroid 86-year-old woman with Hashimoto's disease. Doctors' rigid adherence to the TSH paradigm kept her ill for many years. They then prescribed a variety of pharmaceuticals to treat her low thyroid symptoms. The fourth story is of a young man with an iron loading condition, which eventually caused his thyroid and/or pituitary gland to underperform. The final story is of a woman with Graves' disease who refused to have radioactive iodine treatment, even though it was recommended repeatedly. She is now in remission using a combination of pharmaceutical and alternative methods. All of these are written as medical biographies, and may be easier for people to read and identify with.

The second section updates the individual topic pages on TiredThyroid.com; charts and graphs have been added where it was relevant to help explain the material, and some chapters have quite a bit of new information. There are four new chapters that are not on the website: autoimmunity and autism, reproductive problems, iodine, and thyroid physiology. I found some of the material eye-opening and hope readers will too.

The last section allowed me to summarize my thoughts. In many ways, this book reminded me of the lab reports I used to do in science classes: look at data, hypothesize, look for research that confirms or refutes the hypothesis, build charts or graphs to illustrate the points, and then draw conclusions. What alarmed me was the amount of research I found that refuted so much of the prevailing dogma, and which did not hold up to scrutiny at all. How is it possible that so much unsupported dogma is accepted as fact? Well, most doctors that patients see do not perform scientific research, and for that matter, most patients don't either. Maybe both sides just unconditionally accept what they've been told, or have read. For doctors, many believe a patient is well when their TSH is in range. (I disagree.) And for patients, many believe that 3-5 grains of desiccated thyroid will bring their health back and that synthetic levothyroxine is "crap." (I disagree.)

If someone is searching for references to discuss a controversial thyroid topic with their doctor, like TSH, then the TSH chapter in the second section is what they're looking for. Each of these chapters has multiple references from legitimate medical journals to show that prevailing dogma should be questioned. On the other hand, if someone wants to see what effect dosing by TSH has had on other patients, then I would direct them to the case studies in the first section, where it is mentioned at various points throughout each case. If nothing else, I hope this book sparks discussion and a rethinking of current treatments.

PART I:

YOU ARE NOT ALONE

1

In Search of Eyebrows

You cannot use opinions to form the facts!

I became hyperthyroid from Graves' disease and had radioactive iodine (RAI) treatment that effectively "nuked" my thyroid in 1993. I then became hypothyroid and have been on prescription thyroid medications ever since. While I had been relatively well on Synthroid for about five years after RAI, I started losing my hair and eyebrows and exhibiting other hypothyroid symptoms around 1998, after taking a prednisone pack for a back injury. I read about desiccated thyroid in a newspaper article in 2002 and changed prescriptions, thinking it would help my hair and other symptoms, but my hair never did fully return. In 2007, I joined some thyroid internet groups, hoping to find some answers, but eventually realized much of the advice given did not apply to me. I then began my own search, looking for the best thyroid hormone replacement for me, and this is the story of my journey. Hopefully, you will not make the same mistakes I did. My story starts shortly after I was born, because in hindsight, there were already signs in my childhood that indicate I was borderline hypothyroid. Maybe others will recognize themselves too.

My early years

My paternal grandmother regularly retold the story of how I would "cry, cry, cry" when I was an infant. My Mom confirmed that yes, I cried all night, slept all day, and had a red rash all over my face as an infant. Now a mother myself, I don't know how they put up with me! Was my cortisol rhythm backwards at birth? Cortisol is the hormone that keeps you awake and is normally highest in the morning (helps you wake up), and lowest at night (helps you fall asleep). I have been a night owl for as long as I can remember, and have always marveled at early risers. One study found that night owls were more prone to mental and physical health problems than early risers.[1] Interestingly, thyroid conditions lead to both mental and physical health problems.

My doctors must have thought my problems were due to a milk allergy because I was put on soy formula. In one study, children who were given soy formula as infants later had a higher incidence of autoimmune thyroid disease (such as Graves' hyperthyroidism or Hashimoto's hypothyroidism).[2]

When I was about 8 years old, I remember eating dried apricots. Shortly after, I became a little wheezy, but I didn't think much about it. It always went away after a while. Then one day, I must've exceeded my tolerable threshold of whatever was in the apricots, because I really had trouble breathing, and I made a whistling sound with each exhale. I remember telling my Mom I couldn't breathe and was actually taken to the ER (emergency room), but by the time we got there, the wheezing had diminished considerably, so I was never admitted. Whistling and wheezing are classic asthma symptoms, and it turns out that dried apricots are commonly preserved with sulfur dioxide, a known trigger for asthmatics.[3] In any case, I never ate dried apricots after that, and only many years later, when reading about allergies, did I make the connection that the sulfur dioxide in the dried apricots was the probable cause of my asthma attack. Other than that one incident, I did not wheeze or have chronic asthma, nor have I ever used an inhaler. However, I did have the typical runny nose of someone with allergies. My early health records note "allergic rhinitis."

At age 12, I had the typical sweet tooth of kids my age and frequently bought Starburst candy at the local drugstore. These are brightly colored, sweet, fruit-flavored chewy candy squares. The strawberry, orange, lemon, and cherry flavors are tinted with the food colors red 40, yellow 6, yellow 5, and blue 1. It was around this time that I developed chronic eczema on my hands over the wrist area. It turns out I'm seriously allergic/sensitive to yellow 5 food color, but I didn't know it at the time. Actually, I remember eczema on various parts of my body throughout the years: behind the knees, on the inner elbows, and now it was on my wrists. It seemed like it would move and settle in different places as the years went on. In later years, it moved up to certain knuckle joints on my fingers and then my neck. It is intermittent now, not chronic, and I can't remember when I last had an episode; but it was chronic when I was 12.

When I went to the doctor to get something for the rash on my hand, I believe I was given some sort of hydrocortisone cream to relieve the itching. I remember the itching being most intense in the middle of the night, and my Mom told me she could actually hear me scratching myself raw during the night, even while I was asleep. Cortisol, a natural inflammatory produced by our bodies, is lowest at night, and my cortisol levels must have been very low.

I noticed my legs were really dry during this time; my shins had the pattern of snake-skin or fishnet stockings. This may have been one of the first signs of my being hypo-thyroid, induced somewhat by the cortisol cream I was taking for the eczema. In hindsight, my cortisol levels may have been less than optimal to begin with, and the topical hydrocortisone cream only further suppressed my adrenals from producing their own cortisol. Cortisol is necessary for normal thyroid metabolism. A study of children with atopic dermatitis (eczema) confirms that topical steroids rapidly relieve symptoms, but are accompanied by a fall in plasma cortisol.[4]

My hearing is not perfect and I first noticed it in elementary school, when I would think someone said one thing, when they actually said another. It wasn't so much that I couldn't hear them, rather, I couldn't make out what they said—more like a lack of clarity rather than a lack of volume. An example was the eighth grade spelling bee, where the word was *cupboard*, and I spelled *covered*. Interestingly, my mother is hard-of-hearing, and so was her father, and this trait has been observed in other family lines. In fact, whenever a new thyroid forum member mentions hearing problems, other group members will jokingly pipe up with "what?" Low thyroid levels may be the cause of hearing loss. When two infants with hearing loss were diagnosed as hypothyroid, they were put on thyroid replacement and their hearing improved. One baby's hearing returned to normal, while the other's improved.[5]

I tried beer for the first time in college. The next day, I thought I had come down with a bad cold, because my throat was raw, my voice was hoarse and raspy, and I just didn't feel well. It went away in a few days, just like a cold would. The second time I drank beer confirmed to me that I have a serious allergy/sensitivity to beer. That time, I completely lost my voice for an entire week. No sound came out when I tried to talk—I truly could not speak. That was the only time that's happened, because in the same way I don't eat dried fruit like apricots anymore, I never drink beer, or any alcoholic drinks now. Beer is known to contain sulfites, so the allergy may have been along the same lines. Beer also contains hops (a flower), and others have reported allergic reactions to hops.[6]

At 25, I graduated from college and moved out of state. I was now doing my own grocery shopping and could buy whatever I wanted! A regular item in my grocery cart was something like a mint oreo cookie— it wasn't the Oreo brand and had a green filling. In hindsight, that filling must've had yellow 5 food color in it, because most artificially green products like lime gelatin or green frosting get their color from yellow 5. In any case, the eczema on my hand was pretty bad that year so I saw a dermatologist. He prescribed Lidex ointment (a topical corticosteroid), a triamcinolone injection (a long-acting synthetic corticosteroid), and erythromycin antibiotic tablets for one week. He never asked about my diet, so I continued eating the cookies and using the creams to control the itching. In hindsight, I can see how all these corticosteroids only further suppressed my own natural cortisol production, and that I may have already been borderline hypothyroid.

Later that same year, I met up with a past acquaintance when he flew into town for a seminar. I'd met him in college three years earlier, but I'd moved shortly after so we never got to know each other back then. This time we really hit it off, but I was so embarrassed about my hand. I actually have the dermatologist's report that says: *acute eczematous eruption with fissuring and crusting on the skin of the hands and fingers.* The layman's translation is *gross right hand.* This old college friend was so sweet that he never stared at my hand or asked me about it, and since my left hand was completely normal, always moved to my left side to hold my hand. And sure enough, I married him two years later, when I was 27.

Weddings tend to be stressful events, and shortly after, while on our honeymoon actually, we both came down with a nasty cold. It felt like I was coughing up a lung at times, it was so bad. Luckily, this was before strict airline security regulations on fluids, for I would've never made it home without the bottle of Robitussin I brought on board.

Our wedding was in March, but I never fully recovered and my tonsils became quite enlarged. White, rice-sized objects were lodged in the tonsils and gave off a foul smell; I would use a toothpick to dislodge them, but new ones would continue to replace them. That November, I was referred to an ENT (ear-nose-throat doctor) and on Thanksgiving week, at age 27, my tonsils were surgically removed. Anecdotally, a number of thyroid forum members have had their tonsils removed, so thyroid health must somehow be crucial to tonsil health.

Pregnancy

I was told at an annual ob-gyn exam that I should start my family before age 30. So at age 29, two months before I turned 30, I got pregnant! It was a routine pregnancy, and I had the typical symptoms: morning nausea (threw up every morning for the first trimester), ravenous hunger, swollen ankles, and my hair and skin looked the best they ever have in my life. My hair was thicker[7] and shinier than ever, and my skin was softer and smoother—I had that "pregnant glow" people talk about. Apparently thyroxine[8] (T4—a thyroid hormone), estrogen, and progesterone[9] are at their highest levels in a pregnant woman, and all have positive effects on both skin and hair.[10]

In September, my doctor and I got into an argument about my due date. They had me down on their calendar as due at the end of August, but I knew, because I had charted my ovulation 9 months earlier (charting worked!), that my due date was in September. Why did the doctor and I have different due dates? It's because pregnancy due dates are calculated with the assumption that a menstrual cycle is exactly 28 days long, or 4 weeks apart. Mine were always 5-7 weeks apart, which is actually another hypothyroid symptom. Women who are hypothyroid will usually have heavy periods more than 28 days apart (oligomenorrhea), and women that are hyperthyroid will have scant periods (hypomenorrhea) less than 28 days apart.[11] I ovulated regularly, I was just slower than normal. This particular cycle would've been 6 weeks long, which means ovulation was actually 4 weeks from the previous period, not 2 weeks, as the doctor had assumed. So the date I was expecting to deliver was considered two weeks overdue by the doctor.

August came and went and I was still pregnant, but other than being enormous, I felt as well as anyone who's nine months pregnant could feel. When I went in for my weekly visit the first week of September, I was told that I was late and that I had to come in for a stress test.

"What? Why?"

"You're past your due date and we have to make sure the baby's ok."

"But I'm not even due for another week."

"No, you were due in August."

"No, I'm due in September. Mid-September."

He looks at my chart and the wheel that calculates due dates and states again that I'm already overdue.

"So what happens if I don't have this baby soon?" I ask.

"We schedule you and induce labor. We'll have to schedule you for next Thursday if you don't go into labor before then."

"You can schedule it but I'm not showing up. I'm not going to let you induce labor when I'm not even overdue."

My husband is in the exam room with me, but doesn't say a word. He knows you do not argue with a nine months' pregnant, hormonal woman if you have any brains.

Finally, the doctor asked me when I *thought* I was due. My date was a couple of days within his two week window, which is when, for malpractice purposes I assume, they must induce labor.

Sure enough, I went into labor the following Monday, 38 weeks from conception, right on *my* due date, which was before the Thursday deadline the doctor had set. Whew!

My labor was typical, taking hours, but I remember a period when my whole body just shook, like I was having a whole body seizure I couldn't control. I remember them covering this particular symptom in the Lamaze class. I wonder now if it's not a low cortisol symptom during the long duration of labor. I was also not allowed to eat for hours, and in some ways, the shaking resembles a hypoglycemic seizure. They reassured us in class that it happens to some women, not all, it's perfectly normal, and not to become alarmed about it. Sure enough, the shaking eventually stopped but it *was* alarming not to have control over my own body.

Overall, childbirth was normal, breastfeeding was not a problem, my hair shed and regrew, and the 40 pounds I'd gained slowly came off. This meant my pituitary and hormones worked just fine. What took the longest time to heal was my left hand. What? The hospital bed, like most, had steel bars on the sides, and apparently with every contraction, I must've grabbed onto the bar and squeezed it, trying to bend steel. Hubby did say that in the beginning, when he was holding my hand, he thought I was going to break his fingers with each contraction. I could not make a fist for over 8 weeks, while all other functions "down below" healed well before that!

Graves' disease

I started allergy shots when I was 33. Testing showed I am most allergic to cats and mold, and that I have low levels of antinuclear antibodies (ANA), which are often found in those with autoimmune diseases.[12] Lupus patients tend to have high ANA antibodies, but I do not exhibit any lupus symptoms. In hindsight, this should have triggered some thyroid antibody tests, but it didn't.

Annual routine labwork later that year showed white blood cells below the reference range at 3.65 thousand/uL (3.8-10.8), and total T4 below mid-range at 43% or 7.9 mcg/dL (4.5-12.5). White blood cells (WBC) are produced in the bone marrow and a low count[13] could just be normal for me (congenital condition), reflect an infection (no), be caused by drugs I was taking (none), or indicate an autoimmune disorder (most probable for me). Subsequent labwork through the years shows my WBC count is always at the bottom of the range. WBCs are the soldiers of the immune system.

One December, when I was 34, I started exhibiting hyperthyroid symptoms. December is always a very stressful month, because like many women, I was now a mother, working full-time, and trying to squeeze all the holiday tasks into a day that was still only 24 hours long. Gotta decorate the tree, send out Christmas cards, shop for presents, wrap the presents, bake cookies, the list was endless, the days too short. Did I buy the right presents for everyone? Did I spend too much money? What if I got someone the wrong gift? All this stress led me to eat the abundant variety of yummy home-made cookies I'd baked, and I ate a *lot* of them that December. I noticed my heart was beating faster because I could hear and feel it at night, and in spite of eating the equivalent of a package of oreos each night, I was not gaining any weight. All wheat products, including cookies, contain gluten. Many with autoimmune disease find that gluten exacerbates their condition.[14]

If Christmas activities were not enough, we also closed on a construction loan to build a new, larger house that December. We had been saving for years, and there was no reason not to start building, but as anyone who owns a home knows, signing on that dotted line for a home mortgage is quite stressful—it's probably the biggest purchase of anyone's lifetime. We had not put our current starter home on the market yet, because, well, there just wasn't time to do everything! It was a big risk, signing to build the new house before our current home was sold, and I knew there was a possibility we could be stuck paying two mortgages. On the other hand, it would be just as much stress to have to move twice, find another place to rent, and to pay moving fees twice. Was I doing the right thing? What if one of us lost our jobs? How would we pay for two mortgages? That December culminated in the perfect storm of time, emotional, and financial stress, and coupled with lots of gluten, and already present ANA antibodies, blossomed into full-blown hyperthyroid Graves' disease. Stress has been implicated as a trigger in many cases of Graves' disease.[15]

Christmas came and went, and in January, with the Christmas cookies finally devoured, I started rapidly losing weight. My heart rate was constantly fast, I felt hot, and I was having problems sleeping at night. I would have a bowel movement within an hour of a meal. Always medically curious, I looked up *fast heart rate* in my family medical guide, and it talked about Graves' disease and hyperthyroidism. One of the diagnostic tests was to stretch your arms out and look closely at your hands. Was there a tremor? OMG! Yes there was! I continued to read about hyperthyroidism and vaguely remembered that I had an older female relative who had protruding eyes and a goiter (mass around her neck from an enlarged thyroid gland). Oh no, I must have Graves' disease!

Autoimmune thyroid diseases like Graves' (hyperthyroid) and Hashimoto's (hypothyroid) tend to run in families. My mother has Hashi's, and one of her aunts and a couple of her first cousins have the bulging eyes that are characteristic of Graves'. Not everyone with Graves' presents with thyroid eye disease (TED), so there may actually be other cases in the family that we just don't know about. I was fortunate and did not get TED or a goiter, so you would never guess that I have Graves' disease.

The family medical guide I'd read said that Graves' could be confirmed with a blood test, so I made an appointment with my doctor, and saw his Physician's Assistant (PA).

"I think I might be hyperthyroid and want to get tested for it. I'm hot all the time, my heart's racing, and I'm always starving even though I'm eating a lot, and not gaining any weight."

"Maybe you're pregnant," was the PA's response.

"I've *been* pregnant, this is different." So after listening to my heart, taking my temperature and observing my hand tremor, I got my referral to an endocrinologist. Pregnant? Seriously? I guess all he'd heard was "eating a lot."

My endo didn't seem much older than me and had a pleasant demeanor. I'm guessing the first thing he did was run the usual diagnostic tests for Graves', because I remember a visit where he was looking at labwork and saying, "yes, you have Graves'." I didn't know then to ask for all my medical records so only have my recollection to go on, but I do remember him saying something about my TSH (Thyroid Stimulating Hormone) being suppressed (a hyperthyroid indicator); maybe it was around .03 mIU/L. Then he explained the three options for Graves' treatment: anti-thyroid drugs, a thyroidectomy, or radioactive iodine (RAI). He gave me some literature to read that explained the choices in more detail, and I would return later for a follow-up to discuss my decision.

Before my return appointment, I went to my public library and found a book about Graves' disease that talked about the three options. Remember, this was 1993 and before everyone had internet access. A thyroidectomy seemed risky to me, because it was surgery so close to my vocal cords and it meant cutting me open. The way anti-thyroid drugs were explained, it sounded like it was a hit or miss proposition—in some people, it brought the condition under control and they could then stop the drugs; but in others, the remission was temporary, and the drugs would have to be resumed when the hyper-thyroidism returned. The drugs would also have to be taken for extended periods of time; it was not a one-dose procedure. RAI, on the other hand, was presented as a relatively simple, painless, one-time procedure. I don't remember reading any of the potential horrible side effects that I am now aware of. But based on what I read and my state at the time (exhausted from being hyper), I chose RAI. I wanted to be fixed, and fixed now! (Impatience is a hyperthyroid symptom, by the way.)

I remember two procedures at the hospital: one was for some sort of scan, and in the second procedure, I was given a pill in a plastic cup. After each procedure, I was not given any special instructions of what to do or not to do. I wasn't told to stay away from anyone and slept that night, as usual, with my husband in the same bed. I had the procedure done over my lunch break and went back to work that afternoon for the remainder of the day. At least I had my own office cubicle, so wasn't interacting with innocent bystanders. Since I didn't glow in the dark and certainly didn't feel any differently, no one would ever know I was actually radioactive.

Looking back, I did not remain hyper for very long. I became symptomatic in December, saw my doctor in January, an endocrinologist in February, and had the RAI procedure in April. My body was in overdrive for barely four months. My endocrinologist told me on my final visit that he had given me a very low dose of RAI (8 mCi)—just enough so that I wouldn't be hyper anymore. He also said my labs six weeks after the RAI showed that I had some residual function, which is what he was aiming for. And I do remember him telling me my TSH had gone up to about 20 mIU/L (a hypothyroid TSH by any standard). I was started on a Synthroid (levothyroxine) dose of 88 mcg, which was later lowered to 75 mcg, and I actually did fine for many years. I was never a hyperactive overachiever type to start with, so just returned to what was normal for me. I did not have protruding eyes before the procedure, and did not get them after either. RAI is contraindicated in anyone with thyroid eye disease, because it can make it worse. RAI also appears to have induced the eye disease in some patients.[16] It is just one of many side effects of RAI that are never mentioned.

I was very hypothyroid post-RAI and I remember one morning, when the alarm clock went off, reaching out to hit the snooze button and my arm cramped up. I've had leg cramps before, but an arm cramp? While reaching for an alarm clock? That was ridiculous! But muscle cramps and pain are not uncommon in severely hypothyroid patients.[17] As most people on thyroid medications know, it takes a full six weeks for levothyroxine (Synthroid or T4) to kick in, and week after week, my health improved till I felt back to normal.

Loss

At 36, I was nearing the end of my biological window for having any more children, so we decided to try again. It took longer this time to get pregnant, but I eventually conceived again. The typical nausea I had last time set in, but what was new was a profound fatigue I did not have the first time around. During the first pregnancy, I managed to complete a university computer programming class (during my first four months of pregnancy) with no real fatigue. I was even at the university computer lab till midnight on some nights with no problem and received an *A* for the course. This was while still working fulltime at my day job. My own thyroid supplied enough thyroid hormone for both my baby and me during the first pregnancy, but with this second pregnancy, post-RAI, I was completely dependent on my Synthroid dose of 75 mcg. What many doctors don't realize is that when a woman is pregnant, her thyroid should immediately begin producing more T4 to support the increased metabolic needs of the pregnancy. A pregnant woman on thyroid medication should have her dose increased by close to 50%.[18] I knew I was pregnant before I even missed my period and went in for testing before I was 6 weeks along. I was referred with no problem to an ob-gyn, who promptly did the typical testing, which included a thyroid TSH test. The results were sent back to the ob-gyn's office, and my lab results were filed away in my chart and not read until my next office visit 6 weeks later, when the first trimester was already over.

In the meantime, I was so tired I was terrified of dozing off while driving. I had no energy, and on workdays would go into the office conference room during the second half of my lunch hour, close the blinds, and take a nap. I was concerned something was wrong, and eventually, it was time for my 6 week office visit with the ob-gyn. My lab results were finally looked at, and "oh my, your TSH is flagged as out-of-range at 10!" Obviously, an increase in my dose was warranted. But my ob-gyn had no idea what to do, so referred me back to my primary care doctor. More than one study on pregnant hypo-thyroid women has shown an average dose increase of 50% is warranted, which means I might have done well on 112 mcg (1.5 x 75), but instead, my levothyroxine dose was raised to 88 mcg from 75 mcg. Still other studies show that an average thyroid produces 100 mcg T4 daily,[19] so 1.5 x 100 mcg would be 150 mcg. In any case, 88 mcg was not enough for me when I was pregnant. I did perk up a little, but was still quite tired. Of course, I was also older during this pregnancy (37), so an amniocentesis and sonogram were ordered.

My husband took time off from work to accompany me to my 12-week sonogram. During my first pregnancy, the sonogram was exciting and the technician took a number of pictures. Every time she moved the transducer probe, our son was in a different position; he was obviously awake and active, and there was even a picture that clearly displayed a hand with five fingers—it looked like he was sucking his thumb! He was also a good, healthy size for his age in the womb. He is now a handsome, 6-foot tall Biology graduate venturing out into the world.

The sonogram of our second son was different. No matter where the transducer was placed, he didn't move. The technician said he was asleep and even used the transducer to "tap" on him to wake him, but he never moved. He was also considerably smaller than our first son at that age, but we shouldn't expect all our children to be six feet tall. The pictures that were taken were basically all the same, since he never moved. My maternal instincts were sending up warning bells, and only much later, when doing extensive thyroid research, did I learn that lack of adequate thyroid hormone during pregnancy can lead to cognitive and developmental problems for the child, including lower IQ and attention deficit and hyperactivity disorder.[20]

I did not have to deal with the stress of wondering if there was something wrong with my second son for six more months, because a week after the amniocentesis, I lost the baby.

Sulfa drugs

The following April when I was 38, I came down with a bad cold and was prescribed TMP/SMZ, a sulfa antibiotic. Within an hour of swallowing the first pill, my whole body puffed up and became red, hot, and itchy with hives. I called my HMO (Health Maintenance Organization) nurse's hotline, and she asked if my lips were swelling up. They were actually turning blue, so she suggested we go to the ER. I was getting worse by the minute so my husband drove like a race car driver to the ER. I think we ran a red light, after looking both ways (it was late and there was no traffic). I could barely make it to the front desk, because I was having difficulty walking in a straight line (like I was drunk), and there was a strong tremor in my hands (like I had Parkinson's). "I th-th-think I'm ha-ha-having an aller-ler-gic reac-ac-tion." I stood there, rocking and shaking. Eventually a nurse came and took my vitals, said my BP was low, and then took me to a patient area. I was given some Atarax, which is apparently used to control allergic skin reactions, and also serves as a sedative and antihistamine. I remember feeling incredibly cold, and at one point had four blankets on me. That reminded me of when I'd get the flu and have a fever . . . we actually feel coldest when we're most feverish. I don't know how high my temperature got that night. I was eventually released after my symptoms calmed down, but the next day I felt like I'd been run over by a truck—my entire body hurt. Patients with thyroid dysfunction often have hypersensitive reactions to drugs.[21] One study noted that fever is characteristic of *idiosyncratic sulfonamide hypersensitivity*, which would be the medical term for my reaction. It also noted that some patients became hypothyroid months after their reaction.[22]

Struggling adrenal glands

Some manual blood pressure checks from health fairs and blood donations at work over the next two years show my BP starting to drop (a sign of low cortisol): 104/72, 100/60, 100/60 mmHg. Sodium and potassium levels are starting to go in opposite directions (a sign of struggling adrenal glands), and the difference is only obvious when the numbers are looked at as a percentage in range. Sodium is 27% and potassium 67%. Levels normally rise and fall together. Sodium below the reference range and potassium above the reference range is a clear sign of adrenal insufficiency, and a marker for Addison's disease, where the adrenals produce little to no cortisol.[23]

Low thyroid and high altitude don't mix

In 1997, when I was 39, I went snow skiing for the first time in my life. My son was now eight, had seen skiing on TV, and asked if we could do that. We'd taken him on annual vacations so he'd already seen snow (leftover in the mountains in summer), but the thought of skiing had never ever crossed my mind, since we lived in Florida. After some research, I chose Winter Park, Colorado, because it was considered a good beginner's mountain, there were direct flights to Denver, and lift tickets and lodging were reasonable if you went late in the season, which coincided perfectly with his spring break. I knew nothing about skiing, rented the cheapest skis possible (you really *do* get what you pay for!), and took my first lesson two days after going from sea level in Florida to a base elevation of 9,000 feet. Needless to say, I had a horrible time, and by the end of the lesson, was nearly in tears. I couldn't breathe or think straight, my heart pounded, and with knock knees, I couldn't turn well on the cheap skis I'd rented and fell more than once.

Why am I telling you a ski story in a thyroid book? Because being low in thyroid hormone makes it especially difficult to function in high altitudes, because there's less oxygen. I was back down to a 75 mcg dose of levothyroxine and probably had less than optimal amounts of both T3 and T4, the two major thyroid hormones. In a normal person, the body somehow senses the higher altitude and increases thyroid output, resulting in more T4.[24] But since I have no thyroid function due to RAI, I was stuck with my sea level dose of 75 mcg. Since my body didn't have any more thyroid energy, it compensated for the lack of oxygen by raising both my heart rate and breathing, which is why I felt so out-of-breath with a fast, pounding heart rate. Of course, as soon as we returned home to sea level, my breathing and heart rate returned to normal.

Prednisone suppresses adrenal function

At 40, I injured my back at work by moving some heavy boxes and ended up with sciatica. Someone had placed a stack of heavy boxes right in front of the large printer-plotter that I used to print 3' x 4' maps. I remember bending over, lifting the box, and then swinging it over to the right. I felt something snap in my back, but didn't think anything of it. There was no immediate pain. However, with each passing day, the sciatica became more apparent. For those who are unfamiliar with sciatica, something "popped" in my lower back around my spinal cord, which is where multiple nerves are bundled; the area was now inflamed due to the injury, and touching the sciatic nerve that goes 45 degrees out from the back to the buttocks, and then straight down the leg to the ankles. At first, there was a sharp pain when I stood up from a seated position, going from the middle of my back to my buttocks. "What was that?" I thought, because I'd never heard of sciatica. I assumed it had to be related to that popping sensation I felt when moving the box. With each day, the pain became worse, until it was finally unbearable. When I would stand up from a seated position, it was like a hot poker would fire from my back, and then shoot all the way to my ankle before letting up. It was like a nerve had fired, and had to travel its whole length before it subsided. When I stood up, I would grab onto the desk with a white knuckle grip and exhale (like I was taught in Lamaze class!) until the nerve had finished firing. Only then was it ok to walk; the pain was only agonizing when rising from a seated position, because sitting would bend/stress my back right at the point of injury.

The Workmen's Compensation doctor immediately diagnosed me with sciatica, and told me to take eight ibuprofen a day to reduce the inflammation. It was obvious I hadn't broken my back, and he didn't think I'd popped a disc either, because my foot was not limp. Thinking eight ibuprofen a day was an overdose, I compromised and took four per day, or one every six hours. I was also fearful of taking so much because I'm allergic to aspirin; this allergy is related to the yellow 5 food color intolerance I mentioned earlier, and the sensitivity to both aspirin and yellow 5 has been noted in other individuals.[25] In any case, ibuprofen was too weak and I was still in excruciating pain. I was never given any days off, which meant I had to sit in my car for the one hour commute each way, and then sit at my desk job for the entire workday. In hindsight, I'm wondering if just lying flat on my back and not bending for three days would have allowed the inflammation to subside.

After three weeks had passed, my pain was worse than ever, and on a return visit, the doctor finally prescribed a prednisone pack to relieve the inflammation. This is a pack of prednisone pills in decreasing doses used to reduce serious inflammation. Prednisone can have some serious side effects, but my quality of life was now zero, and I honestly don't know how people live with chronic pain. They have my utmost compassion. I could not even put on or take shoes off, because that required bending. I couldn't lean over the sink to brush my teeth. Getting up from a chair was torturous. The only time I didn't hurt was when my body was straight—either lying down in bed or standing up. So I took the prednisone. And in two days, the pain was gone!

But this miracle drug had a hefty price. Suppression of the hypothalamic-pituitary-adrenal (HPA) axis is a documented side effect, and this adrenal suppression can persist for up to twelve months after corticosteroid therapy.[26,27] A "pred pack," by definition, is only taken for a few days, but I'm fairly certain it suppressed my natural cortisol production, which may already have been subpar, since I was on a suboptimal dose of thyroid hormone. Cortisol is a hormone produced by the adrenal glands, and works in conjunction with thyroid hormone. The adrenal glands of rats atrophied when they were made hypothyroid with anti-thyroid drugs,[28] and this downregulation of cortisol levels is confirmed, anecdotally, by many hypothyroid members on thyroid internet forums.

The prednisone gave me my life back, because I regained full function of my body, without pain, and life went on. But shortly after this incident, I noticed that my hair and eyebrows were noticeably thinning out, I felt brain-fogged, and I was gaining weight. I knew that these were low thyroid symptoms so asked my doctor to test my thyroid levels, and was told my TSH was just fine, right about mid-range, like 3.0 mIU/L. I didn't know anything back then, so just accepted his word that I was fine. My weight continued to creep up, until I weighed about 25 pounds more than usual. The only other time I'd weighed this much was when I was about six months pregnant! And I had to buy new clothes to fit, just like when I *was* pregnant!

Flu shots

My company offered free flu shots every fall, and some years I would get the shot, and others not. In any case, I'd had flu shots before, without incident. This time though, shortly after returning to my desk, I started to feel warm and itchy. The itching was on my inner thighs and I could feel that the skin was warmer there, and starting to get bumpy, meaning I was breaking out in hives. The hives started progressing upwards over my stomach, and my skin was getting more inflamed. I called my doctor's office and all they could think of was to take an antihistamine, which I'd already done. I was terrified, because this was not something I'd eaten which could just be upchucked. It was in me and there was no way to get it out. I just had to hope I didn't die of an allergic reaction. I called the department that administered the shots to determine what was in the flu shot. The shot is contraindicated for anyone who's allergic to eggs. But I love omelets, so that can't be what I was reacting to. What else is in the flu shot? Thimerosal, a mercury compound, is used as a preservative. I knew that word! That was the preservative in my soft contact lens solution that made my eyes bloodshot back in 1980, nearly 20 years earlier.[29] I am obviously sensitive to mercury! Apparently, so are a lot of other people, because most contact lens solutions today don't contain thimerosal. Well obviously I didn't die, but I haven't had a flu shot since. Mercury induces autoimmunity in susceptible individuals.[30]

Die by dye

Remember that sweet tooth I mentioned earlier? That hadn't changed, even though I was now 42. I was still pretty ignorant about healthy eating, and consumed the Standard American Diet (SAD). Bright yellow macaroni and cheese, lime gelatin, orange sherbet, pickles, and chocolate mint cookies with a green filling were some of the things I ate. Yellow 5, a food color, is in all these foods, but I wasn't aware that some people have severe reactions to a food color that is in so many packaged food products. While I had suffered from eczema since childhood, I was now suffering from something new—whole body hives! The hives were at a low level, but they were there all the time. Because of my past history of severe responses to something I'd ingested (beer, sulfa antibiotics, dried apricots with sulfur dioxide), I was sure I was consuming something I was allergic to, but just could not figure it out. The foods I named above are hardly in the same food group. Yes, macaroni and cheese and mint cookies would certainly contain gluten, a known allergen for some, but I'm pretty sure lime jello, orange sherbet, and pickles don't contain gluten! I could *not* figure this out and the itching was driving me crazy.

So I lived with the chronic itching for months. When it was bad, I would take an antihistamine every night. Even that wasn't really enough and I was not getting restful sleep because I was rolling around, scratching all night. The hives would flare and subside for no reason, as far as I could tell, because I had no idea what was setting it off. I had a varied diet and did not eat the same thing every single day. Then Halloween came around, and I bought the usual assortment of treats for the trick-or-treaters, and oops, got into the candy myself. I love peanut butter and chocolate, so I bought not only Reese's Pieces, but Reese's Cups, along with other candy. Like most people, I tended to snack at night in front of the TV. I'd been eating Reese's cups all week while watching TV at night, until eventually that bag ran out. So the next night, I opened up the bag of Reese's Pieces. Not five minutes had passed when the whole body hives started. The medical term for what I had is *dermatographic urticaria*, and is also known as *skin writing*, because wherever I scratched would become raised. I could actually write my name on my arm during these outbreaks.

I had always done well in science classes and knew I had just performed the diagnostic experiment that would tell me what I was allergic to. The empty bag from the Reese's Cups I had finished the night before was still in the trash can, and I had the new bag from the Reese's Pieces. I know I am not allergic to chocolate or peanut butter, because I've eaten those individually many times. So what ingredient is in Reese's Pieces that's not in Reese's Cups? Yellow 5 food color (also known as tartrazine or E102). OMG. I started to connect the dots of everything I ate, and how many things contained Yellow 5. I remembered I used to take a daily multi-vitamin that was bright orange, which meant I was probably ingesting Yellow 5 daily. The eczema I had from eating Starburst candy when I was a kid finally made sense. I loved lime gelatin (with pineapple), orange sherbet, and chocolate cookies with a mint filling. Turns out they all contain Yellow 5. I still had some eczema on my hand and had just been living with it for the past 30 years. Within two weeks of eliminating Yellow 5 from my diet, the eczema cleared, completely. But, I still had some very low grade itching. It was nowhere near the severity of the previous whole body hives outbreaks, but I was obviously still reacting to something. I had to think long and hard about everything I put into my mouth and it finally dawned on me. My Crest toothpaste, the toothpaste I'd used my entire life, since childhood, had Yellow 5. That's what gives it that light blue color. Once I switched brands, all the itching stopped. For 30 years, I had suffered from something that was legally in our food supply. I was stunned and appalled. I just hope this story may help someone else who may also have a Yellow 5 sensitivity.

I'd eaten the candy around Halloween, and now, in early 2001, completely free of hives and eczema, wanted to do something to get Yellow 5 out of our food supply. The internet was still fairly new, but I did find one site online for people who had reacted to Yellow 5. Eczema, asthma, and hives were the most common reactions, and it nearly killed a toddler when it triggered a severe asthma attack. I read that asthma cases are on the rise, and often wonder if these people unknowingly consume a lot of Yellow 5. I also wonder if asthma cases peak in October. Yellow 5 is not just in Reese's Pieces, but Butterfinger, M&Ms, Sweet Tarts, Skittles, Starburst, candy corn, and anything bright yellow-orange or light green. Can you guess what gives Halloween cupcakes that bright orange color? I noticed that several members on the internet Yellow 5 group were also taking Synthroid (a T4 thyroid medication). Looking back now, I'm guessing all of us were deficient in T3 (triiodothyronine), the most active thyroid hormone, and consequently, we were low in cortisol, which is a natural anti-inflammatory. As mentioned earlier in the prednisone section, cortisol is produced by the adrenal glands, which need adequate thyroid levels to function. Metabolism is also slower without sufficient T3, and toxins (Yellow 5) remain in the body for a longer time before being processed out.

The mother of that toddler who almost died submitted a petition to the Food and Drug Administration (FDA) in August 2001, requesting that Yellow 5 be taken off the market. Her son, at 20 months, had ingested eggnog that was colored with Yellow 5 and had a life threatening asthma attack. Doctors had to use a COPD drug (Chronic Obstructive Pulmonary Disease, usually seen in long-term smokers) to save his life. Her petition was assigned a number (Docket 01P-0345), but Yellow 5 was not removed from the food supply. I helped her publicize the petition and we did get the support of the Feingold Association. They're a non-profit organization dedicated to publicizing the side effects of synthetic food additives. They've designed a diet that is very helpful for anyone who reacts to food colors.

In June 2008, the Center for Science in the Public Interest (CSPI) submitted a more substantial, 30-page petition requesting that eight synthetic food dyes, including Yellow 5, be banned. Numerous studies detailing the adverse effects of food colors on behavior, learning, and health were cited, and the petition was signed by over a dozen Ph.D.s and M.D.s. It was assigned a new number (Docket No. FDA-2008-P-0349), but ultimately, resulted in the same response as the first petition—no changes.

Apparently Yellow 5 is not going away anytime soon and will remain in our food supply. I have found it in the most unlikely places, such as chocolate ice cream and facial lotions. Now I read every label of every product I come into physical contact with. Even so, I know that I have unwittingly ingested Yellow 5 since discovering my sensitivity, but I have never again reacted with whole body hives. I believe my higher, more optimal thyroid dose has something to do with that, and my metabolism is now more normal. Because of my sensitivity to food colors, I only use the 50 mcg doses of levothyroxine, which are the only strength made without any food colors. Tirosint is another brand of levothyroxine that has no food color in any strength.

A 77-year-old hypothyroid man in Korea apparently has the same problem I have. He was prescribed *Synthyroid*, a brand of levothyroxine made in Korea colored with tartrazine. (This is not the same *Synthroid* produced by Abbott Labs in the U.S.) He developed a rash within a day, which continued to worsen over five days. The doctors stopped the antibiotics he was on (since he'd displayed allergic drug rashes in the past), and started him on four types of antihistamines, with no improvement. Eventually, the *Synthyroid* was suspected and stopped. After 10 days on 30 mg prednisolone (a steroid), the rash finally subsided. Oral provocation tests confirmed he was reacting to something in the *Synthyroid*, and a switch to another brand of levothyroxine without any food colors was successful.[31]

Desiccated thyroid

I must've changed HMOs sometime around 2001, because my medical records show a different ob-gyn and GP (General Practitioner). My new GP was very talkative and open-minded, unlike many doctors I have encountered. When I went in for my first visit to get a refill on my levothyroxine (generic Synthroid), I asked him about my thinning hair (he's bald) and he began to tell me a story about the female pattern baldness in his family! I let him go on and on, but finally asked if maybe we could just raise my Synthroid dose, since hair loss is a known hypothyroid symptom. He agreed, and I raised from 75 to 88 to 100 to 112 mcg of levothyroxine at six week intervals. That is a significant increase in my dose, but there was little change in my hair.

Early in 2002, I saw an article in my local newspaper about Armour Thyroid, and how some hypothyroid patients were finding better symptom relief with it instead of Synthroid. I had never heard of this medication and didn't even know there were other options besides Synthroid. Since my hair was still thin, I had planned to ask for another levothyroxine increase on my next visit, to 125 mcg, but instead, showed the newspaper article to my GP, and started on 1.5 grains of Armour Thyroid. A *grain* is an older measurement of weight; most prescriptions today are dispensed in milligrams (mg) or micrograms (mcg).

I cut the pills in half, and took it twice a day: 3/4 grain on waking, and 3/4 grain before dinner. One thing I noticed, only three days after starting the Armour, was that the whites of my eyes became white again. They had been yellowish, even though I was then only 44-years-old. Yellow eyes are a form of jaundice, or suboptimal liver function, which my normal liver labs never indicated. I guess something in Armour improved my liver function.

What does Armour have that Synthroid doesn't? Desiccated thyroid contains both T4 (thyroxine) and T3 (triiodothyronine), the two thyroid hormones a normal thyroid gland produces. One grain has 38 mcg T4 and 9 mcg T3. Armour is made from dried (desiccated) pig thyroids, so it has all the components of a real thyroid, which would include not only T4 and T3, but all the other ingredients found in a normal thyroid gland: thyroglobulin, reverse T3 (rT3), diiodotyrosine (DIT), monoiodotyrosine (MIT), thyroperoxidase enzyme (TPO), hydrogen peroxide (H_2O_2), iodide, tyrosyl residues, and calcitonin (a hormone involved in calcium and bone metabolism). Contrary to what you may have read on the internet, desiccated thyroid does not really contain much T2 or T1, and if there is any present, it would only be in trace amounts. Synthroid is a manufactured product so only contains T4.

Figure 1-1 illustrates my T3 and T4 levels on 112 mcg levothyroxine, and then six weeks later, on 1.5 grains Armour Thyroid. On 1.5 grains Armour Thyroid, my total T3 was flagged as high for being considerably over the top of the reference range at 278 ng/dL (85-205), my glucose flagged as low at 62 mg/dL (65-109), and my ALT (alanine aminotransferase), a liver enzyme, was flagged as high at 64 IU/L (0-40). TSH was 4.66 uIU/mL (0.35-5.5), actually on the high side for me, which suggests a hypothyroid state in spite of the high T3 levels. High T3 levels can cause hyperthyroid symptoms, like a rapid heartbeat, while low T3 levels can cause hypothyroid symptoms, like a slow heartbeat. Low glucose or low blood sugar can often result from low cortisol, because that is the hormone that maintains blood sugar levels. In fact, high cortisol will tend to result in high blood sugar. And as I mentioned earlier, low cortisol can result from low thyroid function, which often happens to those taking T4-only medications. The high ALT value may be from the sudden energy the liver received from the T3 found in Armour. These labs are not typical for that small a dose of Armour, and reflect my body's shock from switching from 112 mcg T4 one day to 1.5 grains Armour the next. In hindsight, the switch should've been more gradual—lower the T4 dose some, while adding in ¼ grain of Armour, then lower it again to add another ¼ grain, pausing for 6 weeks between dose changes so the body can adjust.

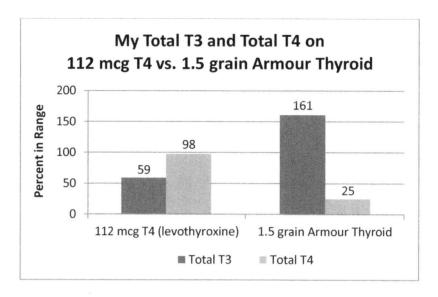

Figure 1-1. Comparison of my Total T3 and Total T4 on two different medications: 112 mcg levothyroxine and 1.5 grains Armour Thyroid. Note the inequality of the T3 and T4 expressed as a percent in range in the two different medications.   On only 1.5 grains Armour Thyroid, Total T3 exceeds the reference range, while Total T4 is only 25% in the reference range.

There's an obvious disparity in the graph illustrating my lab results on the two different medications. On levothyroxine, which is made of 100% T4, my T4 tests results are high (98% in range), while T3 is just above mid-range (59%). On Armour, which is about 80% T4 and 20% T3, the values are reversed, with T3 significantly over range (161%), while T4 is alarmingly low in range (25%). While the huge disparity is because my body had not yet adjusted to the Armour Thyroid, the graphs do bring up an important point. That is, that desiccated thyroid contains a much higher proportion of T3 to T4 because it is made from pig thyroids, not human thyroids. In fact, the T4:T3 ratio is 4:1 in pig thyroid, but 15:1 in the human thyroid gland.[32] The relative proportions are illustrated in Figure 1-2. In someone with fairly normal metabolism of thyroid hormones, this may cause much higher T3 than T4 levels, as illustrated by my lab results.

My GP had allowed me to try Armour Thyroid, but was alarmed by these lab results and immediately referred me to an endocrinologist. I was pleasantly surprised by this endocrinologist, who was not opposed to Armour and was familiar with it. This man is the Medical Director of a Diabetes Institute at a hospital in a major city. He took one look at my 4.66 mIU/L TSH and concluded that I was hypothyroid and needed an increase in my Armour Thyroid dose, in spite of the over range T3 levels. I guess he didn't even look at my T3 lab results, because (as so many patients say) endos typically only look at TSH. In all fairness, he did examine me quite thoroughly and did a test I've never seen before. He took a tuning fork, tapped it so it vibrated, then placed it on one of my bare feet. He told me to let him know when I couldn't feel the vibration anymore. I am slightly hard of hearing and could not hear the tone long before I lost the vibrating sensation, and in fact, never lost the feeling. But I sensed that I had already passed the test from the length of time that had elapsed. He told me that was the longest he'd ever seen anyone feel the vibration, but it's very likely that most of his patients were diabetic, and they often have diminished sensation in their extremities. Thyroid and diabetes symptoms overlap; in fact, low or high thyroid levels may cause problems with blood sugar.[33] In any case, he increased my dose from 1.5 grains to 1.75 grains for about two weeks, before it was again increased to 2 grains, taken as 1 grain upon waking, and another grain before dinner.

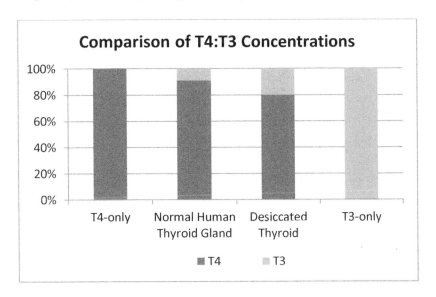

Figure 1-2. Comparison of the T4 and T3 content in different medications vs. what a normal human thyroid gland secretes. Note that no single medication, by itself, replicates the human thyroid gland.

As I mentioned earlier, those first labs were a bit of an anomaly, because my body hadn't had time to adjust—my T3 shouldn't have been so high on only 1.5 grains of Armour, and TSH tends to be suppressed (below the reference range) in those taking desiccated thyroid. Well sure enough, when I got my next set of labs while taking the prescribed two grains, my TSH had become suppressed, which, from my doctor's point of view, meant I was hyperthyroid. So my dose was cut to 1.75 grains. I managed to have a normal TSH for about another year and a half, before my TSH again fell below the reference range. I did ask what my Free T3 (unbound, usable form of T3) and Free T4 (unbound, usable form of T4) were at 1.75 grains, and they were both within the reference ranges—it was only the TSH that was too low. But the TSH ruled—I would not be *allowed* to stay on a dose with a TSH that was below the reference range, so my dose was cut, in spite of my protests. "You realize this will put me right back at the dose that I was on when I first came to see you, right?" Finally, back on 1.5 grains, my TSH was "normal." But I was cold and had to wear a jacket in the office all the time, my hair was still thin, and if I only knew then what I know now, I would've fought for a combination dose of both T4 and desiccated. All I had done was trade being slightly low in T3 on 100% Synthroid, to being low in T4 on 1.5 grains Armour. Contrary to what you might read on the internet, T4 does have some valuable properties,[34] especially on mood, brain function,[35] and hair. Even when I was on 2 grains, my hair was missing something—it was still thin. Hair loss is common in both hyper and hypothyroidism. Figure 1-3 clarifies the T4:T3 content found in different doses.

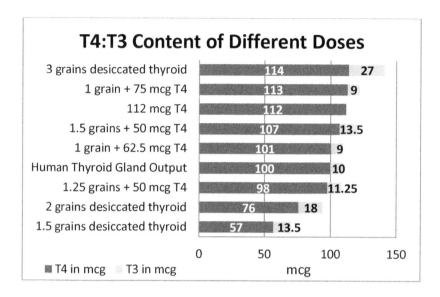

Figure 1-3. Comparison of the T4 and T3 content of different medication doses compared to a normal human thyroid gland's output. Note that 1.5 grains is relatively deficient in T4.

The higher amount of T3 in desiccated thyroid (compared to a human thyroid gland) has a suppressive effect on TSH.[36] The only way to get the TSH back up into the normal range is to take a smaller dose of T3, which in my particular case, was 1.5 grains. But, as Figure 1-3 illustrates, that leaves me seriously deficient in T4, compared to a normal thyroid gland's output. In fact, to truly replicate a human thyroid gland's output, some amount of T4 needs to be added to a small dose of desiccated thyroid.

Surgeries

In December 2004, I had a partial hysterectomy to remove uterine fibroids. They were first discovered on my annual visit in 2001, when I was still on levothyroxine, and did not diminish in size with the switch to Armour Thyroid in 2002. In fact, they continued to grow. I put the surgery off as long as I could, but they were becoming uncomfortable (I was constantly going to the bathroom and could no longer fit my jeans), and my periods bordered on hemorrhaging, so I finally consented to surgery. I was lucky there were no complications, and I recovered quickly. I was taking 1.75 grains at the time of surgery. Interestingly, hysterectomies were the most common surgery among hypothyroid women in an informal survey on a thyroid forum. Googling *hypothyroid* and *hysterectomy* also brings up several case studies where patients had both conditions. One study found a higher hysterectomy rate among patients with Hashimoto's (a hypothyroid autoimmune condition).[37]

Over Labor Day weekend in 2005, we laid tile down in our master bedroom, and I was on my knees for hours. Shortly after, my left knee became warm and swollen, and would not straighten. I had previously injured my knee in 1994 playing volleyball, when something in my knee popped when I attempted to save a low ball. After that, my knee would occasionally fall out from under me while walking, and there was occasional pain inside the knee for about a year after that, but with time, both of those problems went away. I guess the hours of kneeling flared something up, and in October 2005, I had arthroscopic knee surgery. The surgeon said he could find no meniscus shards (knee cartilage), which is what he had expected to find. I was still on 1.75 grains when I laid the tile, but my dose was dropped to 1.5 grains after surgery because of a suppressed TSH. Apparently, being low in thyroid hormone causes tendons to be too lax and knee and other joints can become problematic. Swollen knees can be a hypothyroid symptom.[38] Carpal tunnel is also a hypothyroid symptom, and I had a mild case at one point.[39]

Early retirement

Shortly after Thanksgiving in 2005, I was laid off and began early retirement at age 47. I managed to stay busy because it was December and I had Christmas chores to complete, and because I still had to drive into town for outplacement training. I was a database map analyst at a major newspaper—I analyzed large volumes of data looking for patterns, and then conveyed the data visually via large, plotter-sized maps. Which ZIP code had the highest concentration of newspaper readers? That would be a map the Circulation department would request. How many people lived within a 10 mile radius of a major grocery store? That's what a major grocery store advertiser would want to know. Where are the citrus canker cases, i.e., how widespread is the problem? That's a map Editorial would use in one of their stories. That job allowed me to use both my analytical and artistic skills, which is considered a rare combination.

During outplacement training, I learned that I had a very specific skill set, because very few business offices have mapping software and use large plotters. That meant I had to radically change gears if I wanted to be employed again. But the other thing I realized was that I was quite tired of my daily one-hour commute, and would gladly take a local job for lower pay. But there was nothing locally that used a similar skill set. My severance package gave me access to the online company training programs for several more months, and since I enjoyed creative computer projects, I used my days to finish online tutorials in website design and HTML (HyperText Markup Language). Little did I know they would come in handy, when TiredThyroid.com was born six years later.

If my TSH is normal, why don't I feel well?

In January of 2006, about three months after my dose had been reduced back to 1.5 grains, I noticed I was coughing a lot in the morning, like I had phlegm in my lungs, and that I was a little wheezy every night after dinner. I am not a smoker. I was also cold (it *was* January), and started wearing thermal underwear under my sweatshirt and sweatpants around the house. It made more sense for me to wear more clothes than to crank up the heat, which was kept at 68 degrees. Now that I read what I just wrote, it seems ridiculous. I was wearing thermal underwear when it was 68 degrees?! I was obviously undermedicated! It also turns out that asthma is another low thyroid symptom, and mine went away completely when I later raised my dose. One study found a correlation of anti-

TPO (thyroid peroxidase) antibodies with asthma, and even went so far as recommending that all asthmatic patients be checked for thyroid disease.[40]

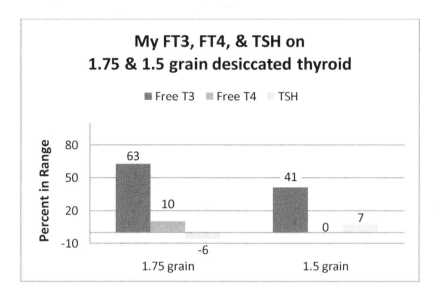

Figure 1-4. Comparison of my FT3, FT4 and TSH on two different doses of desiccated thyroid. My dose was lowered from 1.75 grains to 1.5 grains to bring my TSH back up. TSH did rise into the normal range, but my FT4 was now 0% within the reference range and I developed asthma.

Figure 1-4 clearly shows why some someone cannot be dosed by TSH while taking desiccated thyroid, or really, any thyroid medication. The bars on the left side of the chart show the percentage in the reference range of my lab values on 1.75 grains desiccated thyroid. Free T3 (FT3) is over six times higher in the range than Free T4 (FT4), which is only 10% above the bottom of the range at 0.9 ng/dL (.8-1.8). TSH is flagged as low on the lab report, because it's below the range at 0.09 mIU/L (.4-5.5). If the goal is to normalize the TSH value, then the most logical thing to do would be to lower my dose, because of the inverse relationship of TSH to thyroid levels. Someone who is hyperthyroid will tend to have a TSH below the reference range. Now look at the bars on the right that show my lab values on my reduced dose of 1.5 grains. Sure enough, my TSH has risen so that it is now within the reference range, but both my Free T3 and Free T4 have dropped, which would be expected on a lower dose. FT4 is now at 0% in the range at 0.8 ng/dL (.8-1.8) and FT3 also decreased. So my TSH is now normal, but my hair is falling out, I'm cold, and I've developed asthma. There are some obvious mathematical concepts here that the medical profession is not grasping. If my FT4 measures 0.8 ng/dL, and the normal range goes up to 1.8 ng/dL, I could literally double my FT4 to 1.6 ng/dL, and still be within the reference range. Double? And not be hyperthyroid? How could that be possible? Well it is possible if 1.6 ng/dL is actually a more normal level and .8 ng/dL is actually a hypothyroid FT4 level.

Let's look at this another way. A person's weight would be a good analogy. Let's multiply the .8-1.8 range by 100 and apply it to an average woman's weight. That would mean it would be *normal* to weigh anywhere from 80-180 lbs. I know very few healthy, normal-sized women that are either 80 or 180 lbs. Most cluster more towards the middle of that range, and I would guess that weights over 100 pounds are more normal than weights around 80 pounds. Logically, the bottom of the range needs to move up, so that 80 pounds would be flagged as unusually low. With a range of 100-180, the lowest number in the range could not be doubled, and still be considered *normal*. It would be a more valid reference range. When this concept is applied to the FT4 reference range, a lower range of 1.0 ng/dL might be more valid. I was certainly hypothyroid when my FT4 was 0.8 ng/dL. But according to the laboratory references ranges, I was "normal."

I just want a refill!

My Armour thyroid prescription was about to expire, which meant I had to make a doctor appointment with someone for a refill. It made no sense to see my old doctor, who was an hour away near my former place of employment. I also got a letter around that time saying he was no longer with the medical group I went to, which was certainly a sign I should look for someone closer to home. So I looked in my PPO (Preferred Provider Organization) list for a general practitioner in my area and picked one.

The doctor's receptionist was pleasant, and I filled out the standard paperwork upon arrival. When I finally met with the doctor, I showed him my current prescription bottle, which was for three ½ grains of Armour Thyroid (1.5 grains total daily), and said I just needed a refill. He picked up the bottle, looked at it, and said, "how come . . ."

I interrupted, "you mean, why aren't I taking Synthroid instead?" I then explained that some people don't convert their T4 to T3 as well as others, and Armour had pre-formed T3 in it, so worked better for someone like me.

He corrected me, "no, T3 converts to T4."

"I'm pretty sure T4 is what converts to T3," I said. We actually continued back and forth like this for a while, and I refused to budge, and so did he, until he eventually became angry, flung the door open, stormed out of the room to get his medical encyclopedia, brought it back into the exam room, and then found the page that said . . . T4 converts to T3. He read the page in silence and didn't share what he was reading! Did I get an apology? No, but I got my prescription refill and never went back.

Eventually that prescription ran out and I had to find another doctor. Since this is a fairly small town, I looked up the available GPs in my new PPO (the medical insurance had been through my employment, and was now through hubby's), then made a list (there were less than 10) and called them. My question to whomever answered the phone was simple: "will the doctor prescribe Armour Thyroid?" Most times I was put on hold, and the person would come back and say, "no, he doesn't." One woman even said, "what's that?" But another said, without even checking with the doctor, "if it's a prescription medication, he can write you a prescription." Wow, that was a refreshingly different point of view! I would guess that for every ailment, there are multiple prescription choices, just like there are multiple types of antibiotics. Why should the doctor care which one I took, as long as it does the job, and isn't killing me? So I made an appointment and have been with this doctor since February 2007. I am ever so grateful for finding this doctor, who lets me participate in my own health decisions.

Lack of thyroid hormone affects the entire body

I never did find another job and just found other projects to fill my day. For the first time, I got to be a stay-at-home-Mom! Too bad my son was already heading into his senior year of high school. But I did get to help him with his senior science fair project and participate in his school's Project Graduation.

I was still having asthma-like symptoms, and since I was home all day, started researching on the internet. I had an inkling it was connected to my thyroid dose being too low, because I'd never heard of an adult coming down with asthma; it usually presented in children. The asthma also only appeared when my dose was lowered back to 1.5 grains, which I knew from previous experience was too low a dose for me. And the only reason I was stuck on that dose was because of something called a TSH. I did find some studies that corroborated what I thought—that low thyroid levels can cause asthma.[41] Armed with this information, I asked my new GP if I could raise back to 1.75 grains again. He wrote me the prescription, but when I tried adding in this ¼ grain, I got hyperthyroid symptoms—both my heart rate and blood pressure increased and I felt nervous and anxious. In spite of the life history I've written here, I consider my life up to this point to have been fairly normal. Everyone has some sort of health issue today, it seems, and I don't consider anything in my health history to be catastrophic—I'd gone to college, married a great guy, raised a great kid, held a job, enjoyed family vacations, could swim, bike, ski, etc. and considered myself lucky to have such a good life. But I was soon to learn how important good thyroid levels are to a person's quality of life.

Because my heart rate was elevated, I thought I had become hyperthyroid again and lowered my dose back to 1.5 grains. I had taken 1.75 grains a few years earlier and had felt great—I had no idea what was wrong this time. I felt okay for a few days on the lower dose, but soon felt hyper with a fast heart rate again. I continued to lower my dose, each time feeling a little better initially, followed by feeling worse. In hindsight, the dose of desiccated thyroid I was on (1.5 grains) had left me seriously deficient in T4 for too long (my T4 was 0% in the reference range), and I may have developed a combination of low cortisol and iron deficiency anemia. Both conditions are associated with low thyroid levels and intolerance to supplemental thyroid hormone. Thyroid and cortisol levels usually rise and fall in tandem, and this has been demonstrated in animal studies. Rats displayed adrenal gland atrophy when given anti-thyroid drugs that lowered their thyroid function.[42] Likewise, a cat without an adrenal gland will die if given thyroid hormone.[43] Thyroid hormone speeds up cortisol clearance, and without adequate cortisol, supplemental thyroid hormone can induce an adrenal crisis: blood pressure and glucose can become dangerously low and the patient may become unconscious.[44]

Iron deficiency anemia will also cause an intolerance to supplemental thyroid hormone, and discontinuation of the thyroid medication until supplemental iron brings the iron levels up will usually correct the condition. Lab measurements show that norepinephrine is extremely elevated in some iron deficient hypothyroid patients,[45] and this would explain the elevated heart rate, blood pressure, and anxiousness I felt when trying to raise my dose by only ¼ grain. I wasn't hyperthyroid, I was hypothyroid! How did I become iron deficient? Well, the blood mobile showed up at my workplace on a regular basis, so I donated occasionally. Apparently, women donating as infrequently as twice within two years have a 14-fold increased risk for iron deficiency, as compared to first time blood donors.[46] This risk increases if they are still menstruating, which I still was at the time. In addition, my uterine fibroids were contributing to excessively heavy periods, so I was losing a lot of blood every month. I'd also read that eating a healthier, vegetarian type of diet might help reduce the fibroids, so I was eating less meat, which meant I was consuming less iron. Vegetarians have lower ferritin levels than non-vegetarians.[47] The hypothyroid state also causes prolonged heavy periods, known as menorrhagia,[48] and I was quite deficient in T4. And finally, the hypothyroid state itself causes low serum iron and ferritin levels.[49] I did take a daily multivitamin with iron, but apparently it was not enough.

Eventually, I was only taking ½ grain, which meant I was now seriously deficient in both T3 and T4. I had my first panic attack, which for me, was a hypoglycemic seizure. A couple of hours after a high carbohydrate leftover pasta breakfast (while I was surfing on the internet), my heart raced so fast I thought I would pass out, I broke out in a sweat, lost control of my body, shook like I was having a seizure, and lost my grip on the computer mouse. It was over in a few seconds. Did I just have a heart attack? Is this what people experience when they say they have panic attacks? It was frightening, because I had no control over my own body. Luckily I was home and just at my computer, but had I been driving . . . I shudder to think. I had three more panic attacks before I made the connection—I was having them about 2.5 hours after a high carb meal. Once I realized that, I ate low carb and ate frequently, so I was never more than two hours from my last meal. That helped tremendously, but really, the actual problem was that my thyroid levels were too low, which in turn caused my cortisol to be too low, and I was having hypoglycemic seizures.[50] Once I got back to a more optimal level, I could safely eat carbs again. All I can say is that you really can't understand how terrifying a panic attack is until you have one.

I went back to my doctor because my blood pressure was now 170/100 mmHg, pulse was 100 bpm, I felt anxious all the time, and I knew I was not well. Up till this point, I had always had rather low blood pressure, a low pulse, and was considered very laid back. I didn't understand how I could be hyperthyroid again when I'd already had RAI. But my doctor told me that he knew of patients who had had RAI three times, because their thyroid kept growing back. We even discussed my stopping the ½ grain I was on, but intuitively, it didn't make sense, so I stayed on it while waiting for my lab work. In hindsight, the high blood pressure and pulse were from the noradrenaline my body was secreting to compensate for the lack of thyroid hormone.[51]

One morning after waking, I headed to the bathroom, as I normally do. What was odd was that I couldn't walk in a straight line. Or rather, that while I could see the toilet and thought I was headed that way, my body was veering about 45 degrees to the right! I was completely off balance, and had to hold my head about 45 degrees to the right too, or I'd fall. The only way I made it to the toilet was to tell myself to veer 90 degrees left. That compensated for the imbalance and I made it. I had to lean my head against the wall at a 45 degree angle though, so the room wouldn't be off-kilter. The room was spinning, and cockeyed! Vertigo, or the sensation of movement when you are standing still, is another low thyroid symptom,[52] and went away once my dose was raised.

I developed benign paroxysmal positional vertigo (BPPV) from being so hypothyroid. I told my husband that even after all these years, kissing him still made my head spin.

The scientific explanation was that tiny particles had formed in my ear canals, and their movement whenever I tilted or turned my head (when we kissed) was causing the dizziness. A canalith repositioning procedure (CRP), where my head was quickly turned from one side to the other, moved the crystals into a benign position, and the dizziness has not returned.[53]

I've had occasional spells where I've thrown up, for seemingly no reason. It's not the flu, nor is it food poisoning, because no other family members are affected. It must be another low thyroid symptom, because others have reported this too.[54] Three times it was in the middle of the night, one time it was just a couple of hours after dinner. That time, my stomach felt empty and I felt hungry after throwing up, so I ate again and felt fine. These episodes were sporadic, happening months apart, and I think they're a low cortisol symptom, especially because they happened in the middle of the night, when cortisol is lowest. Nausea and vomiting are symptoms of Addison's, which is when someone has no cortisol.[55] Or perhaps I wasn't secreting enough acid to digest my meals, so my body hit the purge button. In any case, it's been almost two years since my last episode, thank goodness!

Another odd symptom was a whole body vibration. I laid down for a nap one afternoon and thought I'd lain on a vibrating bed, until I realized it was me that was vibrating. Other times, it was just a buzzing in my foot I would notice. These symptoms also went away when I was able to take more thyroid hormone. Peripheral neuropathy, or a tingling/ numbness of the extremities, is another hypothyroid symptom.[56]

One day, I noticed a white spot on my face, then another, then another one on my chest. Oh geez, another new symptom. What was this? It's vitiligo, an autoimmune disease of the skin, where skin loses its pigment, leaving lighter-colored patches. Some vitiligo patients displayed either high or low levels of T3 and T4, according to one study.[57] In any case, these spots only appeared on my face when my thyroid dose was too low, and some (not all) of them went away when my dose was raised again.

Another morning, I experienced what seemed like diabetes insipidus, which is not the blood sugar problem, but a water retention problem. Vasopressin, or ADH (antidiuretic hormone), is the hormone produced by the hypothalamus that helps retain fluid in the body. Without this hormone, the kidneys don't conserve any water when they filter the blood. I had an absolutely unquenchable thirst and probably drank a gallon of water in only 10 minutes, only to have it pass right through me. This was new, I thought. Since the only thing different in my biochemistry was a lower level of thyroid hormone, I concluded that I had gone too low and immediately took 1/8 grain of desiccated thyroid; I knew that thyroid hormone should be raised slowly. The unquenchable thirst stopped! I had now learned, firsthand, that low thyroid levels can cause hypoglycemia,[58] panic attacks,[59] high blood pressure,[60] vertigo, BPPV, vomiting, vitiligo, and diabetes insipidus.[61] It's also correlated with tonsillectomies and hysterectomies. OMG, I wonder how many people suffer from these symptoms and have no idea they're hypothyroid?

The lab results from my last doctor's visit finally appeared and my Free T3 was below the reference range, FT4 was shown as normal at 0% in range, and TSH was high, but within the range, so also "normal." A doctor who follows the TSH rule would say my normal TSH and FT4 meant I was just "fine." I knew I was not. So ever so slowly, I raised my desiccated thyroid by 1/8 grain increments. Eventually, I got back to 1.5 grains, which was where I was before I'd started to raise my dose. My hair was still thin, and now

I was thin too—rather gaunt looking, in fact. Hypoglycemia and low body weight are signs of Addison's disease, where the body is severely deficient in cortisol. Another sign is dark tanning on various parts of the body, and the area under my arms had darkened considerably. They had actually darkened several years before, when I first started taking desiccated thyroid. I did not have this tanning while I was on Synthroid.

Looking for health in all the wrong places

In August 2007, my son left home for college. Because he's an only child, we are very close, and I always enjoyed following his school activities and achievements throughout the years. All of a sudden that came to an end. And only two years after being laid off from my paid job, this felt like another layoff, with all activities (parenting) from this job abruptly ceasing too. That was very stressful.

While I had already raised my dose back to 1.5 grains (the highest dose of desiccated I could take and still have a normal TSH), I knew I still wasn't quite right but didn't know what exactly to fix. I'd already read quite a few books, but none of them really talked about the specifics of dosing. So I went online in 2007 and found a popular thyroid website that basically said: most thyroid patients need 3-5 grains of desiccated thyroid, T4 meds are crap, the TSH is useless, my Free T3 should be at the top of the reference range or higher, and most of us are simply undermedicated. Given those guidelines, I was grossly undermedicated on 1.5 grains! So with my doctor's permission, I slowly raised my dose to 2 grains.

Some of the books I'd read mentioned the importance of adequate cortisol levels when taking thyroid hormone. The thyroid internet group I'd joined also recommended saliva cortisol labs, so I had those tested by Diagnos-Techs in spring 2008, when I was taking 2 grains. I was surprised to find my rhythm and levels were normal—cortisol was highest in the morning and lowest at night, as it should be. Only the noon value was slightly elevated. Serum cortisol labs also looked good, close to the top of the range.

I'd also read that supplementing tyrosine would give me some energy, because it's one of the components of thyroid hormone, along with iodine. So I added tyrosine to my supplements. Bad idea. Adrenaline is made from tyrosine, and boy did I feel anxious and wired! Luckily it stopped as soon as I stopped the tyrosine.

The B vitamins were also mentioned as beneficial to thyroid metabolism, so I took some B6 (pyridoxine). Another bad idea. Some people don't process B6 properly, and it causes a tingling/neuropathy in their hands.[62] I'm one of those people. Fortunately, I didn't suffer any permanent damage.

Magnesium is another supplement that is frequently recommended. I was already taking magnesium, but it's easy to be led into thinking that more is always beneficial (it isn't). My bowel movements became very loose, like diarrhea, when I added another daily magnesium pill, even though I hadn't changed my thyroid dose. Eventually, I went back to one magnesium pill per day and my bowel movements returned to normal.

I started having typical menopausal symptoms in 2008, when I turned 50, and had to decide whether or not to try bioidentical hormone replacement therapy. I did extensive research, as usual, and determined that the benefits outweighed the risks. I could age naturally, but that meant I would slowly lose my bones,[63] brains,[64] and body.[65] Besides, I found the vaginal itching from vaginal dryness, the dribbles when I laughed or sneezed, and the inability to fall asleep rather annoying. So I started on topical, compounded tri-est and progesterone gels. With only a small dose, all those annoying symptoms went away!

My search continued. What was I searching for? Hair and eyebrows. Did I find them on 2 grains? No. My hair and eyebrows remained thin, so I thought I was still under-medicated, because I certainly wasn't taking the 3-5 grains "most" people take, according to some internet groups. I tried raising to 2.5 grains, and noticed sharp pains in my hip, and my back ached. My heart rate was also over 80 bpm (beats per minute), which I find uncomfortable. Since hip pain could be the first sign of osteoporosis, I dropped back to 2 grains. I had labs done while on 2 grains, and four tests were flagged as out of range. Fasting blood glucose was slightly high at 100 mg/dL (65-99), ALT (a liver enzyme) was high at 47 U/L (6-40), RBC (red blood cells), hemoglobin, and hematocrit (RBC density) were also over range, and of course, TSH was near zero. It was obvious that 2 grains of desiccated thyroid was too much for me. High blood sugar correlates with the hyper-thyroid state,[66] and so do high liver enzymes.[67] Surprisingly, my FT3 and FT4 are both within the reference range, though FT3 is almost four times higher in the range than FT4, as shown in Figure 1-5. Note that these results are about 8 hours after my last dose of ½ grain at bedtime, so it's entirely possible that my Free T3 peaked above the range in the middle of the night.

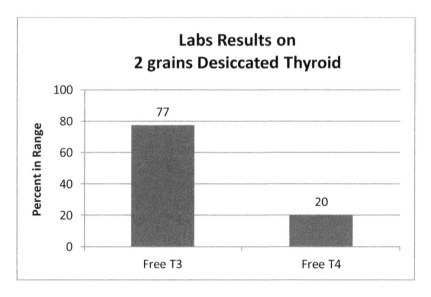

Figure 1-5. My Free T3 and Free T4 levels on 2 grains of desiccated thyroid. Note that FT3 is almost 4 times FT4 levels, as a percent in range.

I was alarmed by my lab results and didn't realize all my errant lab values were simply from too much thyroid hormone. After all, I was "only" taking 2 grains! So I went to a hematologist (doctor who specializes in blood disorders) to find out why my RBC, hemo-globin, and hematocrit tested so high. They were actually just barely over the range and only tested high whenever I took more than 1.5 grains of desiccated thyroid. It should have been obvious to me that it was just too much thyroid, because it had tested high in the past, but I was new to all of this, and was just following the guidelines on these internet forums to raise my dose up to 3 grains.

The hematologist was the most arrogant doctor I have ever met in my life. He was a know-it-all and talked to me in a very condescending manner. Hematologists deal with a lot of cancer patients, and I thought, how sad if my last days on earth were spent dealing with this jerk! His diagnosis was that I had polycythemia vera or erythrocytosis. Polycythemia vera is a condition that older men get; they appear very red in the face (from the excess red blood cells) and have increased platelets. I had none of those characteristics. The doctor did run more diagnostic tests though.

Elevated RBC, hemoglobin, and hematocrit are also known as erythrocytosis, and are a known side effect of testosterone replacement therapy in men.[68] But I wasn't a man nor was I taking any testosterone! It turns out erythrocytosis is also a side effect of too much thyroid hormone.[69] Erythropoietin is a hormone produced in the kidney that stimulates red blood cell production. Apparently, the hyperthyroid state raises erythropoietin levels, which causes the higher levels of red blood cells. Likewise, hypothyroid patients have lower levels of red blood cells for their weight, and are often anemic.

While waiting for the labwork and my follow-up visit, I did my own research, as usual. I had copies of my labwork from 2005, and there was a clear trend. In September 2005, while taking 1.75 grains desiccated thyroid, my labs showed erythrocytosis. My dose was reduced because of the TSH, and the next three sets of labs from November 2005-February 2007 at 1.5 grains show nothing out of range. I stayed at that dose through 2007, and all labs were normal. In November 2007, after I raised back to 1.75 grains, my labs showed erythrocytosis, but they were barely over range, so we dismissed it. But a year later (November 2008), while on 2 grains, my labs again showed erythrocytosis, along with other abnormalities.

When I went for my follow-up visit with Dr. Arrogant, he told me that I didn't have the genetic mutation that could cause polycythemia vera, nor did I have elevated erythropoietin, so he didn't know what was wrong with me, and suggested I could go to Shands Hospital (which is four hours away) if I wanted to pursue it. I told him I'd done some of my own research and concluded I was just taking too much thyroid hormone and had already reduced my dose and was feeling better. "Where did you find that?" he asked. "Online," I said. So he pulled up PubMed on the computer in the exam room and looked it up, and sure enough, there were some studies verifying what I'd just said. Of course, he didn't say anything. And it didn't stop this "brilliant" man from sending me a bill for his "consult," even though I was the one who figured out why I had erythrocytosis.

I had asked Dr. Arrogant to test my iron levels, because thyroid patients often have low or high iron levels contributing to their problems, but he'd refused, so I went back to my primary care doctor for more tests, since my whole body ached. My iron panel and ferritin were fine, but I did test positive for Antinuclear Antibodies (ANA). They were also positive when tested many years ago. Good grief, what are those? ANA tend to be positive when someone has an autoimmune disease, though the test doesn't specifically say which one. It is often used to diagnose lupus, but I've never had the distinctive butterfly rash on my face, nor am I in any way anemic. Some of the other symptoms for lupus, like fatigue and hair loss, are identical to hypothyroid symptoms. I still have some Graves' antibodies, so that may be why the ANA test was positive.

When I asked other members on the thyroid internet groups about my ferritin of 137 ng/mL, I was told that it was high, and that I should donate blood. It had been four years since I'd had a period, and I'd never donated blood in that time period, so it seemed like a good idea. I donated twice within five months: in February and July. When I tested my ferritin two months later in September 2009, it had dropped to 31 ng/mL, which is considered low (but normal) by most standards. I now wonder how low it was right after my second donation. A normal person who does not load iron, like me, cannot donate blood more than once a year without depleting their iron stores.[70] Adequate iron and ferritin levels are essential to thyroid metabolism. Before donating blood, the blood bank tests your hemoglobin (which is produced with iron), but that is not the same as checking your levels of iron and ferritin, which are the raw materials for some essential enzymes; producing hemoglobin is only one of iron's many functions.

Sex hormone testing: serum vs. saliva

On the day I went in for another round of bloodwork (serum), I also did a saliva test with ZRT Labs for my sex hormones, just to see how the two results would compare. I followed their instructions precisely and was meticulous about not getting any of my topical tri-est or progesterone gel on my fingers for several days preceding the saliva labs.

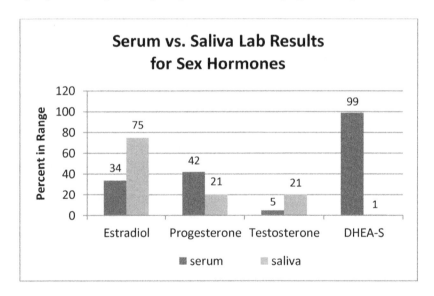

Figure 1-6. Comparison of sex steroid hormones by serum and saliva testing. Note the disparity between the two types of testing.

The results in Figure 1-6 show why there are so many arguments over which test is best. Sometimes the serum result is higher, other times the saliva, so it's impossible to say which one is more accurate. The most divergent result was the DHEA-S (Dehydroepi-androsterone Sulfate), a steroid hormone produced primarily by the adrenal glands. Yes, that really is a 99% in range result by serum, and a 1% in range result by saliva. According to Salimetrics, a saliva testing company, DHEA-S does not readily pass into saliva because of the attached sulfate group.[71] The larger molecule size might explain why only 0.1% of plasma DHEA-S levels are found in saliva. Therefore, according to Salimetrics, my serum value from my blood draw is more valid.

Combining T4 with desiccated thyroid

People on desiccated thyroid with a rather low FT4 and rather high FT3 (like mine) are told they have low cortisol by some thyroid internet groups. My saliva cortisol test was not low. This was when I started to realize that a lot of what I was being told was simply not true. I clearly could not take 2 grains—I didn't feel good *and* my labwork confirmed it. I was clearly underdosed on 1.5 grains, with completely "normal" labs but thin hair and asthma. Then the eureka moment hit me. I could take a lower dose of desiccated thyroid combined with levothyroxine (T4), which would help even out my T3 and T4 levels. I started taking 1.25 grains of desiccated thyroid combined with 50 mcg of T4 and ran new labs in April 2009. For the first time in my life, both my Free T3 and Free T4 levels were close to each other, in terms of where they fell in the reference range; my labs weren't so lopsided (see Figure 1-7). But I still didn't feel 100%.

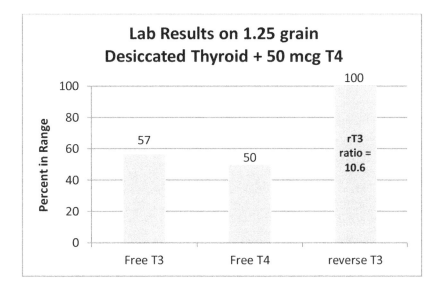

Figure 1-7. My Free T3, Free T4, and reverse T3 on 1.25 grains desiccated thyroid combined with 50 mcg levothyroxine. FT3 and FT4 are closer to each other, as a percent in range, but rT3 is at 100%.

The reverse T3 hoax

I had just learned about reverse T3 (rT3), so had that tested too, and sure enough, my levels were high and at the top of the reference range. What exactly is rT3? It's a by-product of T4, formed when one iodine atom is removed from T4 by an enzyme. Molecules are three-dimensional, so which particular iodine atom you remove makes a difference; T3 and rT3 are stereoisomers—they have the same number of atoms but they're arranged differently. Your left and right hands are examples of stereoisomers. They both have a palm, with five fingers attached. But although identical in number of attached fingers, one thumb faces left, while the other faces right. They are mirror images—similar but not the same. You cannot put a left hand into a right glove or vice versa. T3 and rT3 are not mirror images, but the concept is the same; they are different molecules and rT3 does not fit into a cell's T3 receptor, but is bounced out of the cell and returned to the bloodstream.[72] It does not block T3 from the cell receptor. If it were stuck in the cell receptors, it wouldn't be measurable in serum.

My rT3 ratio was 10.6. The FT3/rT3 ratio should be greater than 20, say the proponents of the T3-only protocol. They say my low ratio means my cellular thyroid hormone receptors are all "blocked" with rT3, because rT3 fits into the T3 receptor, keeping T3, the active hormone, from reaching the receptors. They also say I was taking too much T4, which is a "useless" hormone, and that's why my rT3 was so high. Again, I didn't know any better back then, and there was no research disproving anything these people were spouting, so I bought into it. Surely they must know what they're talking about, right?

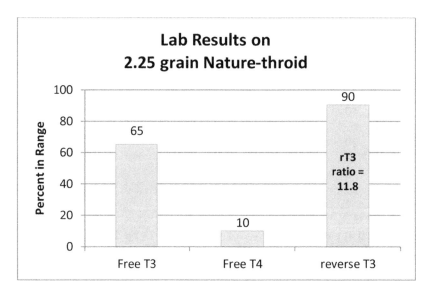

Figure 1-8. My Free T3, Free T4, and reverse T3 on 2.25 grains Nature-throid. Note that FT3 is more than 6 times higher than FT4 as a percent in range, but rT3 is still very high.

Because I still had my doubts about rT3 and the T3-only protocol, I did not switch over to 100% T3, but raised my desiccated thyroid dose instead and took 2.25 grains Nature-throid. This was an increase from my previous dose of 2 grains, because I still had hypothyroid symptoms. My next labs show everything is "normal," except my TSH is less than 0.01 mIU/L. And of course, my labs are lopsided again, as shown in Figure 1-8. My rT3 ratio had only increased to 11.8, a little over one point, even though my FT3 was now over six times higher in the range than my FT4. This was when I started to question the validity of the rT3 ratio rule. I would occasionally google *reverse T3 receptors*, but never once found any *legitimate* research study to corroborate the statement that "rT3 blocks the T3 receptors."

Armour Thyroid was reformulated late in 2009, and according to patients on the thyroid internet forums, it was ineffective and making people sick. Then it just disappeared and was unavailable. Patients were told both Armour and Nature-throid (another desiccated thyroid brand) were on backorder and could not get refills from their pharmacies, so I switched to Canadian Erfa Thyroid. I had no problems with the Canadian brand and used it for three years.

My thyroid lab results on Erfa Thyroid were lopsided as well (see Figure 1-9), as they are on any desiccated thyroid, but my FT3/rT3 ratio was increasing, which I thought was a step in the right direction. My hair and eyebrows were still thin, so I finally decided I needed to "clear" my rT3, as several thyroid internet groups recommend, by taking a higher than normal dose of T3, to push out the rT3 that was "blocking" my T3 receptors.

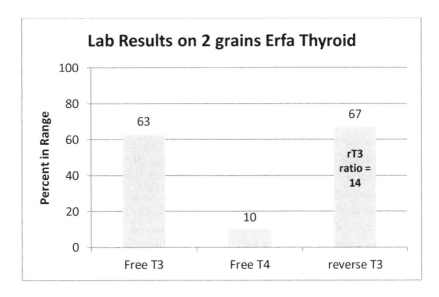

Figure 1-9. My Free T3, Free T4, and reverse T3 on 2 grains. Note that Free T3 is over 6 times higher, as a percent in range, than FT4. Reverse T3 is improving (decreasing).

My plan was to make the switch to 100% T3 gradually, so I slowly reduced my Erfa Thyroid down to 1 grain, while adding T3 in 5 mcg increments, until I was taking 25 mcg T3 per day in addition to the 1 grain of desiccated thyroid. I was then taking a total of 36 mcg T4 + 33 mcg T3. Figure 1-10 shows what that looks like graphically in comparison to a normal thyroid gland's output of 100 mcg T4 and 10 mcg T3.

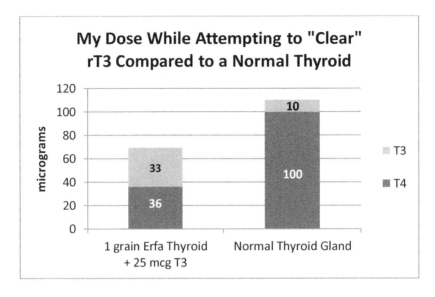

Figure 1-10. My T4:T3 dose compared to a normal thyroid gland's output. Note that my T3 dose is over 3 times normal, while T4 dose is about 1/3 normal.

At 33 mcg T3, I was actually taking more than three times a normal thyroid gland's output of T3. My heart rate became slightly elevated, but that was tolerable, because it was only 80+ bpm. What was absolutely frightening was that I lost my brain/memory. When I was about ten years old, I was taught by my engineer father how to calculate tax and percentage discounts, and make change in my head when shopping. Back then, cash registers showed you a total, but did not calculate change. That was counted out manually; registers weren't computerized yet. So whenever I bought anything, I was able to calculate my cost and change before I got to the register. And I could certainly calculate change from a dollar in my head. I'd been doing it since I was ten! Well, on this T3-only protocol, I lost all my mathematical ability. I was at a produce store and could not, absolutely could not figure out that if I gave the clerk $5, and my produce cost $4.87, that I was owed 13 cents. I remember running the numbers through my head while driving home. The change from $4.87 is? is? is? I felt like an old record that was scratched and stuck on the same note, unable to move forward without a nudge. I also stopped at the drug store on the way home, and also couldn't make the right amount of change; the clerk said something about an extra dollar I gave her.

Later that afternoon, I checked in on the thyroid internet forums, and posted a reply to someone's question. It popped up a couple minutes later and I read the reply, agreed with it (imagine that!), and then noticed that I was the author. Really? I did not remember writing it, even though the time stamp was only a couple of minutes ago. Now that was scary. Alarmed, I remembered my inability to add earlier in the day and thought I must be losing my mind. As usual, I started researching, and sure enough, there's something called *hyperthyroid dementia*. Too much T3 causes cognitive dysfunction.[73] No more T3-only protocol for me! In a normal person, when T3 becomes too high, any available T4 will convert to rT3 to protect the body (and brain) from an excessive level of thyroid hormone. As you can see from the chart above, my T3 levels were excessive and were likely overloading my brain circuits, causing the inability to compute, or remember.

There was also very little T4 to convert to rT3 anyway, only about a third of a normal person's level.

The human brain was designed to run primarily on T4, not T3. Alzheimer's patients have lower levels of T4 in their cerebrospinal fluid (the fluid that bathes the brain) compared to controls, though the serum T4 levels don't show this difference.[74] Their T3 and TSH levels in the cerebrospinal fluid did not differ significantly from the controls. I did not know all of these facts back then, so went back to 100% desiccated thyroid. After all, that's the best thyroid medication out there, according to some popular thyroid websites. I was not thinking clearly because of all the T3 I'd been taking, so still believed (or wanted to believe) what I was being told: that desiccated thyroid was the superior thyroid replacement, that wellness was found at 3-5 grains, and that I needed to have my FT3 at the top of the reference range, or even above it. So I pushed my dose even higher and worked up to 2.5 grains Erfa Thyroid. My labs show I was clearly overmedicated (see Figure 1-11), with my FT3 over the reference range at 492 pg/dL (230-420). FT4 is again low in range relative to FT3; in other words, my labs are lopsided again. This is a consistent finding for me on desiccated thyroid. But look, my rT3 ratio is finally around 20! This must mean I'm completely well, and rT3 is no longer blocking my receptors. NOT!

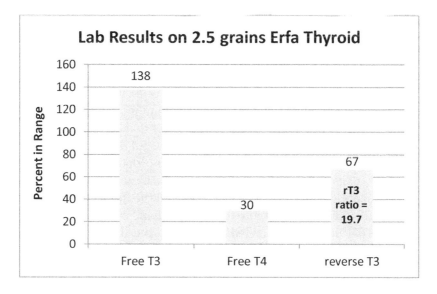

Figure 1-11. My FT3, FT4, and rT3 on 2.5 grains Erfa Thyroid. FT3 is clearly over range, and more than 4x the FT4 level, as a percent in range. Reverse T3 ratio rounds up to 20, which is considered ideal by the rT3 proponents. But I didn't feel well.

Reverse T3 does not block the T3 receptors. There are deiodinase enzymes at the cell membrane that either accept or reject incoming T4, depending on the cell's needs.[75] T4 is either converted to T3, which makes its way to the nuclear receptor, or T4 is converted to rT3, and then expelled out of the cell. There is nothing to clear because nothing was being blocked!

People should realize that anyone can make up anything and publish it on the internet. That doesn't make it true. It is easy to draw erroneous conclusions if the underlying physiology isn't understood. Political sites are an excellent example of questionable conclusions drawn from blurred "facts," but unfortunately, many medical sites fall into this category too.

Hello? Does anyone understand thyroid physiology?

My mother told me I always did well in science classes and expected I would end up doing something in that field. I always enjoyed the intrigue of performing science experiments in school, never quite knowing what results we were supposed to get, but always fascinated with what results we did get. Then we had to correlate our results with known scientific facts/theories and draw some conclusions. That's basically what I was doing with all these different thyroid medications and protocols, except this time I was the experimental subject. I had now tried all three types of thyroid medications (T4, T3, and desiccated thyroid), and it was time to draw some conclusions about thyroid advice given by some websites and forums on the internet.

1. Can I take the recommended 3-5 grains? No.
2. Is it because I have low cortisol? According to saliva labs from two different companies, no.
3. Should I keep my Free T3 at the top of range or higher? I could, but it clearly induces erythrocytosis in me, and well before I'm at the top of range. Fasting blood sugar and liver enzymes also become elevated. So no.
4. Is T4 "crap"? According to all the research I've done, a normal thyroid secretes mostly T4 and only a little T3, so no, I don't think it's crap.
5. Is taking a lot of T3 ok? Not for me; it blew out my brain.
6. Does getting my rT3 ratio about 20 or higher make me feel better? No. Figure 1-11 shows my rT3 ratio was finally about 20, but only because my FT3 was way over range and FT4 low in the range. This "optimal" ratio did not result in normal hair and eyebrows again, which was my whole reason for experimenting with different medications in the first place. Reverse T3 cannot fit into a T3 receptor any more than my left hand can fit into a right glove.
7. Is the TSH useless? No. TSH stimulates the deiodinase enzyme (D2) that converts T4 to T3,[76] and rT3 to T2 at the cellular level.[77] So ideally, *some* TSH would be desirable.[78] Many who take desiccated thyroid end up with high rT3 levels and then are told they need to take T3-only to correct it—another myth. Desiccated thyroid's high T3 levels suppress TSH, which then suppresses the D2 enzyme which degrades rT3 to T2. So it's not that more rT3 is made, rather that less is degraded, and the lack of TSH causes this imbalance. Likewise, hyperthyroid patients have the highest levels of rT3,[79] and they also have a TSH close to zero. The high rT3 is actually from too much T3 (which suppressed the TSH), not too much T4! My rT3 levels have actually gone down (and my ratio improved), as I lowered my T3 and raised my T4. Others have reported the same thing. However, I don't think anyone should be dosed by their TSH levels, which is actually a different issue. TSH is useless in determining one's optimal dosage because it's so variable. A high TSH indicates that someone does not have enough thyroid hormone. But a low TSH (below the reference range) is not that clear cut. For a variety of different reasons, someone can

have a low TSH, but they could be anywhere from severely hyperthyroid (Graves' disease) to severely hypothyroid (pituitary problems or non-thyroidal illness), or actually feel fine (taking desiccated thyroid or any T3 supplementation).

8. Is desiccated thyroid a superior medication because it contains T2, T1, and calcitonin, in addition to T4 and T3? No, this is actually misleading information. Desiccated thyroid is composed of whatever is in a pig's thyroid gland. Thyroid glands manufacture T4 and T3 by joining two molecular building blocks together: MIT (monoiodotyrosine) or DIT (diiodotyrosine). It is impossible to produce T1 when either of these two building blocks are joined, because 1+1 cannot = 1 (T1). T2's presence in the body is primarily from deiodination or conversion (by removal of one iodine atom) from T3 and rT3; in other words, the thyroid gland is not the primary source of T2.[80] Calcitonin does not have an effect when taken orally; in fact, prescription calcitonin is administered nasally, rectally, or by injections, because it degrades and does not absorb well through the gastrointestinal tract.[81] Does anyone take their desiccated thyroid nasally (up their nose) or rectally (up their butt)? I didn't think so! And finally, the ratio of T3:T4 in desiccated thyroid is much greater than that found in a human thyroid gland, which explains the consistent imbalance in my T3:T4 levels on desiccated thyroid.

Like many other thyroid patients looking to improve their health, I eagerly followed all the advice listed above only to find out none of it was true! I'm sure there are other thyroid patients out there who found some of the above statements to be helpful, so these guidelines were beneficial to them. Obviously, they were not beneficial to me, and I wasted several years of my life searching for my optimal dose, which was nowhere to be found in the advice I was given from these thyroid internet groups.

Was the advice from doctors any better?
1. When my TSH was within the normal reference range, did I feel fine? No, unless you consider having brain fog, dry skin, weight gain, and thin hair and eyebrows "fine." A statistical analysis showed that TSH in T4-treated patients did not correlate to the same levels of FT3 and FT4 in untreated patients, making TSH in T4-treated patients a questionable diagnostic.[82]
2. Does a TSH below the reference range cause osteoporosis? No, TSH is not a thyroid hormone, it's a pituitary hormone, so it doesn't have any thyroid effects. True hyperthyroidism, or T3 and T4 levels significantly above the reference range will cause bone loss, but so will low T3 and T4 levels.[83] Unfortunately, the TSH often doesn't correlate with T3 and T4 levels.
3. When my FT4 was in the normal reference range, did I feel fine? No, I had hypoglycemic seizures/panic attacks, high blood pressure, vomiting, vertigo, and diabetes insipidus when my FT4 *and* TSH were both *normal*. The lower end of the FT4 reference range is probably too low, and the upper end of the TSH reference range is probably too high.
4. Are the reference ranges logical? No, not when the top value is more than twice the bottom value. Mathematically, that doesn't make sense.

5. Does taking 100% T4 work for me? No, I still had hypothyroid symptoms. It turns out a normal thyroid gland manufactures some T3, so both T3 and T4 should be components of a thyroid hormone replacement program, which is essential for someone like me, who had RAI and produces no thyroid hormone. T3 stimulates the dciodinase enzyme (D1) that converts T4 to T3 and degrades rT3 to T2.[84] Likewise, T4 is the most potent inactivator of the D2 enzyme (which also converts T4 to T3), which explains why higher and higher doses of T4 don't increase T3 very much.[85] The small amount of T3 that a normal thyroid releases, about 10 mcg, provides a synergy which is essential for normal cellular conversion. This may explain why patients on T4-only do not have physiological T4/T3 ratios. There is always too much T4 in proportion to T3, when compared to an untreated patient.[86]

6. Do doctors normally prescribe T3? No. In fact, medical guidelines clearly state that T4 (levothyroxine or Synthroid equivalent) is what should be prescribed. The following is from the 2012 *Clinical Practice Guidelines for Hypothyroidism in Adults: Cosponsored by the American Association of Clinical Endocrinologists and the American Thyroid Association.*[87]

A serum thyrotropin [TSH] is the single best screening test for primary thyroid dysfunction for the vast majority of outpatient clinical situations. The standard treatment is replacement with L-thyroxine. The decision to treat subclinical hypothyroidism when the serum thyrotropin [TSH] is less than 10 mIU/L should be tailored to the individual patient.

Just the facts, ma'am

I knew I would get nowhere with doctors, because of their reliance on the TSH. So I had turned to the internet and joined some thyroid support groups. Ironically, while they rail against doctors, they have their own erroneous dogma that in my case, made my condition worse. I had now rejected almost everything I'd been told. So what was left? Only what I could figure out myself, from research. Real research from medical journals; I would have to learn thyroid physiology myself and learn the real facts. Not "made up facts," which is all I'd been told.

After my analysis, it became clear to me that the only way I could get both FT3 and FT4 about mid-range or higher was to take both T4 (gasp!) *and* desiccated thyroid. Most doctors are dead set against desiccated thyroid, and many patient groups are dead set against T4. I felt like I was undertaking another experiment when I started combining the two in 2010, with positive results. How did I know I needed to be mid-range or higher in the reference range? Well, one day, I left a question about the reference ranges on the website for the laboratory where all my testing was done. I could not believe it when the phone rang and I was able to talk to the Director of Quality Assurance, a clinical pathologist. He explained to me that the distribution curves for the thyroid lab ranges were not normal (equal, symmetrical distributions), but were negatively skewed. In other words, most of the values were in the upper half! When I asked why they didn't just move the bottom of the range up, he replied that it wasn't that simple, and that he alone could not set ranges. Multiple doctors from different fields (endocrinology, gynecology, etc.) had a say, and the ranges are a compromise of multiple opinions.

I'm confident my optimal dose will always consist of both T3 and T4, though I'm not sure of the exact proportions of each yet, because too many variables keep changing. I'd been on Canadian Erfa Thyroid for three years, but the second year, the price doubled. This year, it is three times what it cost when I first ordered it, so I decided to go back to a U.S. source. I'd been on generic Mylan levothyroxine but switched pharmacies this year, and the new pharmacy gave me generic Lannett brand, which was either weaker or stronger, so that changed things too. Different brands of thyroid medications have different fillers, and that can sometimes result in the same dose of medication having a stronger or weaker effect. Adding new supplements also affects conversion rates; like many of you reading, I am a work in progress.

Figure 1-3 earlier in this chapter shows all the combinations I've tried, except for 3 grains. That's in the graph just to illustrate the T3:T4 content of that "recommended" dose. I recently started taking 1 grain + 62.5 mcg T4, but only time will tell if that becomes my optimal dose. I am sleeping better since lowering the desiccated thyroid and raising the T4. I tried taking 1.5 grain + 50 mcg T4 in the past, but my FT3 was too high on that dose, and my lab results showed erythrocytosis, which means it's too high a dose for me. I've also tried 1.5 grain + 37.5 mcg T4 (still had erythrocytosis) and 1.25 grain + 50 mcg T4, but neither of those doses felt quite right either. I have added and changed supplements along the way too, and those may affect conversion, which would then change how much T3 I need. Since lowering my dose of desiccated thyroid and raising my T4 levels, both my hair and eyebrows have improved. I also feel the T4+T3 combo has helped tremendously with my brain function, and I don't believe I could've built a website or written a book without my T4 being higher in the reference range. I remember reading research articles when I was taking 1.5 - 2 grains of desiccated thyroid just a few years ago, and not understanding what I'd read. I can now read and understand the same articles, and the only difference is that I've added some T4 to my dose. My FT4 was at 0% in the reference range on 1.5 grains.

After doing a *lot* of research, I concluded that this T4+T3 combo best replicated what a normal thyroid produces. I joined the groups in 2007, and when I wasn't reading forum posts from other members and the advice given by moderators, I was reading thyroid books from the library, or doing my own research with PubMed and Google Scholar. After a while, it became quite clear to me that a lot of what I was told, by both doctors and patients, was just flat out wrong. Patients complained that their doctors didn't understand how to properly test and treat thyroid disease, but my observation was that patients sometimes didn't understand what they were talking about either. Both sides were making up their own nonsensical rules, and this nonsense has propagated across the internet. Even doctors have their own websites, some spouting the same misinformation found on patient websites. Very few doctors or patients truly understand endocrine physiology because it is ridiculously complex and all the hormones are intertwined. I have now studied it *ad nauseam* for over six years and I still don't know everything there is to know, and probably never will. Many doctors think that as long as our TSH is in range, we're fine. Many patients think that if they just stop their T4 medications and take 3-5 grains of desiccated thyroid that they'll be fine. I can say that neither approach worked for me, and just caused more health problems. In fact, combining those two ideas was one of the worst things to do! Doctors let me take desiccated thyroid but kept my dose low to keep my TSH in range. That resulted in a T4 deficiency and I developed asthma to go along with my already dry skin, thin hair, and eyebrows.

When I would post differing viewpoints on patient forums, I would be "corrected" with the prevailing dogma, and eventually be put on moderation (my posts would need approval before they'd be posted). New ideas were not welcome. Some of these forums are similar to cults, with all-knowing leaders and loyal, obedient subjects who don't question anything. Sadly, this is quite similar to some doctor-patient relationships. I watched from the sidelines as new members joined the groups, then became worse following the group's protocols. I could not believe people really believed what they were reading. Whatever happened to common sense? The flaws of the protocols could not be explained in a simple post. It would take a book to do that! But I did have a platform to express my opinion and eventually wrote the following post on my blog:

Beware of Dogmatic Thyroid Internet Groups and Cognitive Dissonance

Posted on July 29, 2011 by barb

Someone looking for thyroid advice can go through the following stages when they land on internet forums dispensing advice:

1. The Journey Begins – don't feel well
2. Seek Help – most likely from a medical doctor
3. Disappointment/Disillusionment – not getting any better, and may have spent a fortune on doctors
4. Seek Alternatives – find thyroid internet support/chat groups
5. Hope – maybe their protocol will work
6. Caution – some will be wary and questioning, but others go straight to
7. Enchantment – buy-in, assimilation, commitment to protocol
8. Love – they experience some improvement after starting and want to share the process with everyone and give advice, just like they were given; some become the "new" moderators
9. Plateau/Decline – as time passes, improvement stops and some get worse as they take their dosages higher and higher, thinking more is better
10. Crash and Burn – now worse than before any treatment
11. Angry/Disgusted/Frustrated – what am I doing wrong?
12. Blame The Patient – groups/moderators blame the patient for not getting better; it is not that their protocol is faulty, but that some other electrolyte or hormone is too high or too low and preventing thyroid optimization
13. Realization – I am so messed up, and I've been had
14. Hit Bottom – Now what?
15. Questions and No Answers – some who complain or question the protocols are actually "booted" out of the group and left to fend for themselves; some migrate to other groups still in search of answers. Sadly, many actually blame themselves for not "correctly" following the protocol. Very few consider that the protocol itself could be flawed and might not work for everyone, or that it is so complicated, that few can make it work.

What is my point in writing all of this? It is to caution people that there are sources of terrible thyroid misinformation out there, and I have watched in horror as more sick, innocent people continue to fall prey to these groups. Just because someone says it's so doesn't make it so. Where did this advice come from? Did someone make it up years ago and it's just been passed on like some old wives' tale? Is there any research to back up these protocols? Do the people posting sound like they're getting better or worse?

Every now and then a new member will ask where the success stories are. The answer given is that people regain their lives, get better, and then no longer post. Little do they know that some leave in disgust, worse than ever, or that others have been banned from the group because they questioned the protocol when it didn't work for them. This is where cognitive dissonance, or rationalization and denial, comes into play. I see people floundering, who are in such a vulnerable, sick position, that they are willing to try anything to regain their health, and they completely discount and ignore all the obvious red flag warnings and their own intuition. One red flag warning is a group that moderates every single post. What don't they want you to see? People believe what they want to believe, because they need hope that some protocol somewhere will restore their health. Mainstream medicine didn't work, but maybe, just maybe, this will! Especially if they have already started on the protocol, they may gloss over any negative side effects they may be experiencing, and continue on, hoping things will improve. To acknowledge that what they are doing could be wrong, would also mean acknowledging that they did something foolish. The brain cannot handle belief in polar opposite arguments, so rational arguments and research will be discounted and dismissed.

My advice? Question everything! Listen to your body and your intuition and never go against your better judgment. Be warned that both too much and too little thyroid hormone can greatly affect your brain and ability to think and reason. Once you embark on these protocols, you may not be able to think clearly. Are you prepared for that? Is there someone who can help you monitor your progress? Who can pick you up in case you stumble? There *are* some groups giving good, knowledgeable advice based on sound principles, but they are not as popular as those that are sources of terrible thyroid misinformation. Do your homework and listen to your body, not some person on the internet with a "god" complex as a moderator. Your health is at stake. A moderator or group that has only one protocol, theirs and only theirs, cannot possibly give good advice. Be wary of rigid, dogmatic, authoritarian, "because I said so" answers. Only trust groups whose moderators are open-minded and willing to engage in discussions. We are all so different that no one protocol, nor one medication, should be expected to fit all of us.

There is also much sincere, but misguided advice given by patients to other patients. Be warned that some of the sickest patients give the most advice. Here are some of the most memorable, misinformed posts (paraphrased) I can remember reading:

Is your hair falling out? Then don't wash it so often or brush it too much.

Your body will only absorb as much thyroid meds as it needs.

I am on 162.5 mcg T3 and my heart is racing. What am I doing wrong?

I am on 12.5 mcg T4. Why do I feel like crap?

Again, my point is that some patients, while well-meaning and wanting to share, may know nothing about thyroid physiology and how thyroid hormone affects the entire body. Or worse, in their brain fog, they have all the concepts mixed up! A little knowledge is a dangerous thing. Doctors may know some thyroid physiology, but are often overly reliant on misleading TSH and lab ranges. Unfortunately, you will have to educate yourself and be your own patient advocate. That is the current state of thyroid treatment today. I sincerely hope that everyone reading this finds the answers they seek. We all deserve better health!

Iodine

Iodine was the one thing I hadn't tried on my journey. I already knew, from reading thousands of thyroid internet posts, that iodine is a very polarizing supplement for thyroid patients. Some people rave about its health benefits, and say it even cured their cancer. Other patients are furious, because they say it induced hypo or hyperthyroidism in them. As usual, I did some research, and it appeared that while some benefit from supplementing iodine, others end up either hypo or hyperthyroid after taking high doses of iodine. And yes, that is in spite of taking the required additional supplements of selenium, Vitamin C, magnesium, and sea salt. I was already hypo from RAI, so that was not an issue, and if I went hyper, I could always just reduce my current thyroid dose, so that was also not an issue, so I bought a bottle of 2% Lugol's iodine to try.

Initially, I did feel better, but when I increased the Lugol's to three drops (7.5 mg) daily, I developed a few spots of what looked like bad acne on my face, neck, and chest; they were raised, pustular, larger than a regular pimple, but did not really have a "head." The medical term for this is *iododerma*. The high-dose iodine proponents will tell you that you are detoxing bromide. But I wasn't taking any bromide, I was taking iodine! Bromide does cause a very similar condition called *bromoderma*,[88] but is slightly different in appearance. Bromoderma tends to cover a larger area on the lower extremities, like the legs, with a border of pustules; iododerma tends to be on the face,[89] and consists of individual pustules. My nasal passages also seemed inflamed, my eyelids were puffy, and my problem knee swelled up again. I also developed a chronic cough, as if my asthma was returning. I had no idea this was from the Lugol's, till I read about iodine toxicity.[90] The high-dose iodine proponents insist that any symptoms are due to bromide detoxing, and that I just needed to take more sea salt. Once I dropped back to two drops daily, the symptoms went away, and when I later raised back to three drops daily, they returned, but it was less severe. Once again, I started to question the science behind a protocol and my research findings are summarized in Chapter 18 on Iodine. Anyone who is considering the Iodine Protocol should take the time to read it. Some of it is eye-opening.

Research studies confirm that iodine is indeed helpful in battling cancer, and since there's a history of cancer in my family, I probably stayed on the iodine longer than I should have, thinking it would be beneficial for me. I thought the chronic runny nose, coughing, chest congestion, and wheezing I was experiencing were from the spring pollen season; I didn't even realize how much I was coughing until my husband pointed out that I was "gacking" a lot. I was reacting to the iodine. How is that possible? Iodine is an essential element, isn't it? Well yes, it is, but Lugol's and Iodoral are manufactured products. And they are manufactured in a process using sulfur dioxide and sulfites,[91] which I'm highly sensitive to. By consuming a low concentration of sulfites daily (which my body considers a toxin), I brought my asthma back. I cannot begin to tell you how thrilled I was when I realized what had happened. As usual, I started to research the topic, and my findings on Asthma are in Chapter 7. The other possibility is that my symptoms were simply those of iodine poisoning, or iodism. Even dairy cattle display symptoms of coryza (cold symptoms such as nasal congestion) and coughing when fed a high iodide diet.[92]

Iodine can be toxic to humans. Businesses that handle potassium iodide (chemical manufacturers and distributors, etc.) are required to have a Material Safety Data Sheet (MSDS) on file, which lists potential hazards of working with the material in an occupational setting. The U.S. Centers for Disease Control (CDC) and Prevention lists iodine as a chemical hazard.[93] Of course, they are talking about exposure at high levels, but for some individuals, like me, the high-dose iodine protocol recommended by iodine proponents *is* a toxic exposure. The following is from the CDC website:

> *Exposure Routes: inhalation, ingestion, skin and/or eye contact*
>
> *Symptoms: irritation eyes, skin, nose; lacrimation (discharge of tears); headache; chest tightness; skin burns, rash; cutaneous hypersensitivity*
>
> *Target Organs: Eyes, skin, respiratory system, central nervous system, cardiovascular system*

I feel that iodine damaged my respiratory system, and I can only hope that I didn't do any permanent damage to my lungs. It's been over eight months, and the asthma is finally receding (though I still "gack" occasionally). My GP, at a routine checkup last year, first made me aware that something was wrong. After listening to my chest and looking up my nose, he said, "Do you have asthma? I can hear a rattle and your nostrils are really inflamed." Since I've been his patient for over five years, and he'd never mentioned it before, I knew it had to be an iodine side effect. When I got home, I used a flashlight to see what the inside of my nose looked like, and it was bright red! That is inflammation that I could see myself—I shudder to think what my lungs looked like. Fast forward a year and I just had my annual check-up; my GP said my lungs sounded clear, so hopefully they're finally healing.

How I determine if my thyroid dose is too high or low

Are there any signs from the body that say a thyroid dose is too high or low? For me, bleeding gums are a sign I'm too low, along with hard stools, rough, dry heels, dry skin, acid burps, or a lot of gas. I tend to mix up the first consonants in pairs of words when I'm too low—I'll say "dig bog" instead of "big dog," for example. My heart tends to "pause" while I'm sleeping too, which wakes me up. Raising by only ¼ grain or 12.5 mcg T4 has always stopped it. I also get "attack" types of dreams when I'm too low. A dog lunging at me, a person about to run into me, that sort of thing. I always wake with my heart racing when that happens, and it also goes away with a small dose increase. Feeling too hot when sleeping and throwing off the covers in the middle of the night is another sign that I'm too low. On the other hand, I don't sleep well when my dose is too high either, and I'll tend to wake multiple times throughout the night.

Another interesting test is the knee reflex; take a wooden spoon and lightly tap below your knee to see the speed of the reflex. A rapid kick up might mean you're on too much thyroid hormone. Too little response might mean you need more thyroid hormone. The Bristol Stool Chart (Google it) categorizes stools from hard to liquid. Since I've been both hyper and hypothyroid, I can say that the chart is a pretty accurate representation of how thyroid hormone levels affect the stool. Stools that are too loose and approaching diarrhea (Type 7) are a sign you could be on too much thyroid hormone; dry pellets that only come out with a lot of pushing are a sign of too little thyroid hormone (Type 1). Lactose intolerance and celiac disease may also impact stool consistency, as can supplements like magnesium and Vitamin C; stool would then not be a good indicator. My eyes feel gritty and a little too wide open if my dose is high; kind of a deer in the headlights look. My fingernails also start to detach from the nail bed at the far (white) end if my dose is too high; it's like the fingernail is lifting up. This is called onycholysis.[94] I also get heart palpitations, where the heartbeat is irregular, when my dose is too high. This is different from the "heart pause" I feel when my dose is too low. That literally feels like a momentary pause, after which the heart starts beating in a normal rhythm. The palpitations, when my dose is too high, feels highly irregular. It's not a momentary pause, but more like flip flops, in different rhythms. I also feel short of breath when exercising when my dose is too high. These are all important indicators for me, because lab results only reflect serum levels of thyroid hormones, and do not reflect what's going on at the cellular level. But everything I've just described reflects thyroid hormone's effect at the cellular level: it affects my heart, eyes, fingernails, sleep, stool, speech, etc.

Magical mushrooms

Finally, I wanted to talk about taking a mushroom complex. Research shows that mushrooms have beneficial effects on the immune system, from lowering allergic responses to improving survival in cancer patients.[95] I've read conflicting theories on autoimmunity—that it's from an overactive immune system, so the immune system should *not* be stimulated; to the opposite theory that the immune system is compromised, and that it *should* be stimulated. Mushrooms are considered immunomodulatory, so they would work either way. I've noticed that my white blood cell count tends to be near the bottom of the reference range, which indicates, to me, that I have lowered immunity. So I went with the theory that my immune system could use all the help it could. There are reports on thyroid forums of patients who have greatly lowered their antibodies by taking LDN (low dose naltrexone), and LDN works on the immune system. Mushrooms are supposed to work in a similar fashion, and because I could buy a mushroom complex over-the-counter (LDN must be compounded and requires a prescription), I decided to give that a try first.

I had RAI in 1993, but 17 years later, in 2010, I still had measurable TSI (Thyroid Stimulating Immunoglobulin), which are a measure of the potency of Graves' antibodies. After taking the mushroom complex, my TSI dropped from 107% stimulation down to 26%, and my TPO (thyroid peroxidase) and Thyroglobulin antibodies also decreased. Also worth mentioning is that my seasonal allergies were minimal while I was taking the mushrooms. According to the local newspaper, last spring was *the* worst for oak pollen, and allergists' offices were completely booked. I normally get pretty congested, my eyes water, and I sneeze a lot during oak season, but while on the mushrooms, I didn't have to deal with that, for the first time in my life! I'm not sure if I should take the mushrooms daily, or just use them when I need more immunity, during allergy and flu season, for example. I will, as usual, continue to research and experiment.

TiredThyroid's beginnings

TiredThyroid.com went live in February 2011 from the support of a fellow Graves' patient I'd met on a forum. Since I had been unemployed since 2005, it was a low budget endeavor, researched, written, and designed by me. My goal was to educate people about thyroid physiology—how a thyroid gland *really* works. Every assertion has a reference supporting it.

That picture on the website of the skier lying flat on the bench? That's me. After crashing healthwise in 2007, I thought I'd recovered after three years and planned a ski trip in 2010 for my 25th wedding anniversary. I was still taking way too much T3 and as a result did not have much stamina, nor could I handle the altitude. My heart was pounding so hard and fast after a simple run that I laid down on an outdoor bench. Of course, hubby saw a great photo op! Little did he know he was taking the perfect picture for my new website!

In June 2012, I attended my niece's high school graduation party and met a journalist. She asked what I did, and after I described my website, she asked if it made any money. I said "no, not really, unless you count $10 a month from Google ads." She said I just needed to write a book. Since I'd just put everything I knew into a public, free-access website, I didn't see what material there'd be for a book!

In August 2012, a retired dermatologist found my site (his wife is hypothyroid) and contacted me. He said my site was a Ph.D. thyroid thesis and that I must write a book. Here we go again, I thought. "Everything I know is already on the website, what would I put in a book?"

"You tell your story, and how you figured everything out."

"But I'm nobody, and I'm not a doctor. Why would anyone read a book I wrote?"

"That's precisely *why* they would read your book. They'd identify with you."

Well that put an entirely different spin on things. But it still wasn't an outline for a book I'd buy myself. I spent the next month mulling ideas around and investigating what would be involved in publishing a book. Did I need an agent? Not in this day and age. Everything's digital and books can be printed on demand, as they are ordered. So I don't even have to keep an inventory in my house. And I won't have to lay out thousands of dollars for printing costs either. I might be able to do it on a shoestring, just like the website. I just had to write the book.

In September 2012, the eureka moment came. There are already thyroid books written by doctors and patients. But what there isn't, is something along the lines of a textbook—a thyroid training manual that both doctors and patients could refer to, with references. Something that patients could relate to, with case studies of people with similar thyroid health issues. And it would explain, with charts and graphs, why some of the current thinking on both sides is erroneous—and more importantly, what *is* true and works (at least for me). It would be the book I wished I'd had when I started this journey, one that presented the *real* facts. There are two sides to every issue, not two sides to every fact. At one point, I considered calling this book *I Call Bull Sh*t!*, but figured it might not go over too well. To say that I had been misled, by both doctors and patients, is a *gross* understatement, and this book is my attempt to share what I've learned, so others won't have to suffer too. And guess what? My eyebrows are growing back in!

Key points

- Topical cortisone creams may help with eczema, but may inhibit natural cortisol production.
- Hearing loss can be a low thyroid symptom; it may be correctable if the thyroid deficiency is corrected early enough.
- Quite a few hypothyroid patients have had tonsillectomies.
- Menstrual cycles more than 28 days apart may be a symptom of hypothyroidism; cycles less than 28 days apart may be a symptom of hyperthyroidism.
- Autoimmune diseases are associated with celiac disease or gluten intolerance
- Stress can be a trigger for Graves' disease.
- Radioactive iodine treatment makes you radioactive for a while; this may damage the thyroid of others (even animals) that you come in contact with.
- Hypothyroid women who become pregnant while on thyroid medication should have their doses increased by approximately 50%, and their thyroid levels monitored throughout the pregnancy.
- Insufficient thyroid hormone during pregnancy can lead to cognitive and developmental problems for the child, including lower IQ and attention deficit and hyperactivity disorders.
- Hypothyroid patients often have hypersensitive reactions to drugs like sulfa antibiotics.
- Low blood pressure and lab results that show sodium low in range and potassium high in range are early indicators of adrenal dysfunction.
- High altitudes are difficult to tolerate when hypothyroid.
- Prednisone can suppress adrenal function for up to a year.
- Low thyroid levels lead to adrenal gland atrophy and low cortisol.
- Mercury induces autoimmunity in susceptible individuals.
- Yellow 5 food coloring can cause eczema, asthma, and hives in susceptible individuals.
- Desiccated thyroid has all the components of a thyroid gland, including T4, T3 and reverse T3. T2 and T1 are not manufactured in the thyroid gland so would only be present in trace amounts.
- Thyroid dosage changes should be made gradually, so the body can adjust.
- Desiccated thyroid has a much higher proportion of T3 to T4 than a normal human thyroid gland. The T3 in it will cause TSH suppression, even though the T4 levels may be suboptimal.

- Hysterectomies appear to correlate with Hashimoto's or hypothyroidism.
- Lax tendons that cause carpal tunnel syndrome and knee problems can be a symptom of hypothyroidism.
- Asthma can be a hypothyroid symptom.
- TSH is a poor guideline for determining the right dose of thyroid hormone.
- Low cortisol and/or low iron will cause an intolerance to thyroid hormone.
- A pre-menopausal hypothyroid woman can easily become iron deficient by donating blood more than once per year, having heavy menstrual periods, and eating a vegetarian diet.
- Low thyroid levels can cause hypoglycemic seizures, which may be similar to panic attacks.
- A fast pulse and high blood pressure may actually be symptoms of low thyroid levels; noradrenaline, not excessive T3, is the problem.
- Vertigo and BPPV (benign paroxysmal positional vertigo), or the sensation that the room is spinning, especially when the head is moved or tilted, is another low thyroid symptom.
- Nausea and vomiting can be signs of low thyroid, probably related to low cortisol.
- Vitiligo, an autoimmune skin disorder where the skin loses its pigment, can be triggered by low thyroid levels.
- Peripheral neuropathy, or a tingling/numbness/buzzing of the extremities, is another hypothyroid symptom; some report a whole body vibration.
- Hypothyroidism can cause diabetes insipidus, or a problem with water retention.
- Weight loss (a gaunt look), hypoglycemia, and darkened skin areas are signs of very low cortisol.
- Tyrosine is a component of adrenaline, so it's not wise to supplement.
- B6 can cause peripheral neuropathy (tingling in the hands) in susceptible people.
- Bioidentical hormone replacement therapy can help preserve a woman's bones, brains, and body; it also eliminates vaginal dryness, incontinence, and insomnia.
- Erythrocytosis, or high RBC, hemoglobin, and hematocrit can be caused by high thyroid levels.
- Iron and ferritin are measures of iron in the body; hemoglobin is created from iron, but measures a different blood component. A person's hemoglobin may be normal while iron/ferritin levels may be quite low.
- DHEA-S is best measured in serum, not saliva.
- Too much T3 may cause hyperthyroid dementia or memory loss and an inability to think logically.
- The rT3 target ratio of 20 or more is not based on any real science.
- Reverse T3 does not block T3 from reaching the nuclear receptor; rT3 is shaped differently from T3 and does not fit the receptor any more than a right hand fits into a left glove.
- 3 grains of desiccated thyroid is an overdose for some people.
- Both doctors and patients have misconceptions about thyroid physiology.
- Patients should question everything they're told and not blindly follow protocols just because it worked for someone else.
- T4 is not crap, and is what the brain was designed to run on.

- T3 is important too; heart failure patients exhibit the *low T3 syndrome.*
- TSH is not useless; it triggers T4 to T3 conversion at the cellular level.
- Without TSH, rT3 levels build up, because TSH stimulates rT3 to T2 conversion.
- High levels of T3 (desiccated thyroid has high levels of T3) will induce high levels of rT3; it's a protective mechanism.
- Hair loss can be from both too much *or* too little thyroid hormone.
- Mushrooms can help with immunity and lower antibodies; they may also help with allergies.
- Iodine is helpful to some, harmful to others, and can be toxic in high doses; the toxic threshold differs for each individual.
- Those with a sulfite sensitivity should be cautious with iodine.
- Bleeding gums, hard stools, rough, dry heels, acid burps, attack type dreams and slow reflexes suggest a thyroid dose may be too low.
- Diarrhea, gritty eyes with a wide-eyed look, and fingernails that are detaching from the nailbed suggest a thyroid dose may be too high.

---

[1] Gulec, Mustafa, et al. "Chronotype effects on general well-being and psychopathology levels in healthy young adults." Biological Rhythm Research_ (2012).

[2] Fort, P., et al. "Breast and soy-formula feedings in early infancy and the prevalence of autoimmune thyroid disease in children." *Journal of the American College of Nutrition* 9.2 (1990): 164-167.

[3] Tarlo, S. M., and G. L. Sussman. "Asthma and anaphylactoid reactions to food additives." *Canadian Family Physician* 39 (1993): 1119.

[4] Queille, Catherine, Renée Pommarede, and Jean-Hilaire Saurat. "Efficacy versus systemic effects of six topical steroids in the treatment of atopic dermatitis of childhood." *Pediatric dermatology* 1.3 (2008): 246-253.

[5] Hickson, V. M. "Improvement in neonatal hearing loss following treatment with thyroxin." *Archives of Disease in Childhood* 96.Suppl 1 (2011): A31-A32.

[6] Śpiewak, Radoslaw, and Jacek Dutkiewicz. "Occupational airborne and hand dermatitis to hop (*Humuluslupulus*) with non-occupational relapses." *Ann Agric Environ Med* 9 (2002): 249-252.

[7] Nissimov, J., and U. Elchalal. "Scalp hair diameter increases during pregnancy." *Clinical and experimental dermatology* 28.5 (2003): 525-530.

[8] Alexander, Erik K., et al. "Timing and magnitude of increases in levothyroxine requirements during pregnancy in women with hypothyroidism." *New England Journal of Medicine* 351.3 (2004): 241-249.

[9] O'Leary, Peter, et al. "Longitudinal assessment of changes in reproductive hormones during normal pregnancy." *Clinical chemistry* 37.5 (1991): 667-672.

[10] Thornton, M. J. "The biological actions of estrogens on skin." *Experimental dermatology* 11.6 (2002): 487-502.

[11] Dittrich, Ralf, et al. "Thyroid hormone receptors and reproduction." *Journal of reproductive immunology* 90.1 (2011): 58-66.

[12] Tektonidou, M. G., et al. "Presence of systemic autoimmune disorders in patients with autoimmune thyroid diseases." *Annals of the rheumatic diseases* 63.9 (2004): 1159-1161.

13 Low white blood cell count. mayoclinic.com. Accessed 1/14/14. http://www.mayoclinic.com/health/low-white-blood-cell-count/MY00162/ DSECTION=causes

14 Ch'ng, Chin Lye, M. Keston Jones, and Jeremy GC Kingham. "Celiac disease and autoimmune thyroid disease." *Clinical medicine & research* 5.3 (2007): 184-192.

15 Falgarone, Geraldine, et al. "Role of emotional stress in the pathophysiology of Graves' disease." *European Journal of Endocrinology* (2012).

16 Acharya, Shamasunder H., et al. "Radioiodine therapy (RAI) for Graves' disease (GD) and the effect on ophthalmopathy: a systematic review*." *Clinical endocrinology* 69.6 (2008): 943-950.

17 Valeria C, Benavides, and Rivkees Scott A. "Myopathy associated with acute hypothyroidism following radioiodine therapy for Graves' disease in an adolescent." *International journal of pediatric endocrinology* 2010 (2010).

18 De Groot, Leslie, et al. "Management of thyroid dysfunction during pregnancy and postpartum: an endocrine society clinical practice guideline." *Journal of Clinical Endocrinology & Metabolism* 97.8 (2012): 2543-2565.

19 Escobar-Morreale, Héctor F., et al. "Treatment of hypothyroidism with combinations of levothyroxine plus liothyronine." *Journal of Clinical Endocrinology & Metabolism* 90.8 (2005): 4946-4954.

20 Klubo-Gwiezdzinska, Joanna, et al. "Levothyroxine treatment in pregnancy: indications, efficacy, and therapeutic regimen." *Journal of Thyroid Research* 2011 (2011).

21 Gupta, Abhya, et al. "Drug-induced hypothyroidism: the thyroid as a target organ in hypersensitivity reactions to anticonvulsants and sulfonamides." *Clinical Pharmacology & Therapeutics* 51.1 (1992): 56-67.

22 Pickert, Curtis B., Craig W. Belsha, and Gregory L. Kearns. "Multi-organ disease secondary to sulfonamide toxicity." *Pediatrics* 94.2 (1994): 237-239.

23 Penrice, Juliet, and S. S. Nussey. "Recovery of adrenocortical function following treatment of tuberculous Addison's disease." *Postgraduate medical journal* 68.797 (1992): 204-205.

24 Richalet, Jean-Paul, Murielle Letournel, and Jean-Claude Souberbielle. "Effects of high-altitude hypoxia on the hormonal response to hypothalamic factors." *American Journal of Physiology-Regulatory, Integrative and Comparative Physiology* 299.6 (2010): R1685-R1692.

25 Grzelewska-Rzymowska, I., et al. "Sensitivity and tolerance to tartrazine in aspirin-sensitive asthmatics." *Allergol et Inmunopathol* 14 (1986): 31-36.

26 Schuetz, Philipp, et al. "Effect of a 14-day course of systemic corticosteroids on the hypothalamic-pituitary-adrenal-axis in patients with acute exacerbation of chronic obstructive pulmonary disease." *BMC pulmonary medicine* 8.1 (2008): 1.

27 Drugs.com. Prednisone, Prescribing Information For Professionals. Accessed 12/29/13. http://www.drugs.com/pro/prednisone.html

28 Sarwar, Ghulam, and Sughra Parveen. "Carbimazole-induced hypothyroidism causes the adrenal atrophy in 10 days' prenatally treated albino rats." *Journal-College Of Physicians And Surgeons Of Pakistan* 15.7 (2005): 383.

29 Patrizi, Annalisa, et al. "Sensitization to thimerosal in atopic children." *Contact Dermatitis* 40.2 (2007): 94-97.

30 Hybenova, Monika, et al. "The role of environmental factors in autoimmune thyroiditis." *Neuroendocrinol. Lett* 31 (2010): 283-289.

31 Young Hwan Choi, et al. "Drug rash induced by levothyroxine tablets." *Thyroid* 22.10 (2012): 1.

32 Kenneth Woeber. Treatment of Hypothyroidism. Werner And Ingbar's The Thyroid: A Fundamental And Clinical Text, Chapter 67. 9th edition, 2005. Lippincott Williams & Wilkins. P. 864.

49

[33] Kapadia, Kunal B., Parloop A. Bhatt, and Jigna S. Shah. "Association between altered thyroid state and insulin resistance." *Journal of Pharmacology & Pharmacotherapeutics* 3.2 (2012): 156.

[34] Davis, P. J., F. B. Davis, and H-Y. Lin. "L-Thyroxine acts as a hormone as well as a prohormone at the cell membrane." Immunology, Endocrine & Metabolic Agents in Medicinal Chemistry (Formerly Current Medicinal Chemistry-Immunology, Endocrine and Metabolic Agents) 6.3 (2006): 235-240.

[35] Caria, Marcello Alessandro, et al. "Thyroid hormone action: nongenomic modulation of neuronal excitability in the hippocampus." *Journal of neuroendocrinology* 21.2 (2009): 98-107.

[36] Appelhof, Bente C., et al. "Combined therapy with levothyroxine and liothyronine in two ratios, compared with levothyroxine monotherapy in primary hypothyroidism: a double-blind, randomized, controlled clinical trial." *Journal of Clinical Endocrinology & Metabolism* 90.5 (2005): 2666-2674.

[37] Phillips, D. I. W., J. H. Lazarus, and B. K. Butland. "The influence of pregnancy and reproductive span on the occurrence of autoimmune thyroiditis." *Clinical endocrinology* 32.3 (2008): 301-306.

[38] Gillan, M. M., R. H. Scofield, and J. B. Harley. "Hashimoto's thyroiditis presenting as bilateral knee arthropathy." *The Journal of the Oklahoma State Medical Association* 95.5 (2002): 323.

[39] Eslamian, Fariba, et al. "Electrophysiologic changes in patients with untreated primary hypothyroidism." *Journal of Clinical Neurophysiology* 28.3 (2011): 323-328.

[40] Samareh, Fekri M., et al. "Association between anti-thyroid peroxidase antibody and asthma in women." *Iranian journal of allergy, asthma, and immunology* 11.3 (2012): 241.

[41] Dr. David Derry Answers Reader Questions. Brought to you by Mary Shomon, Your Thyroid Guide. Topic: Asthma and Thyroid Hormone. http://thyroid.about.com/library/derry/bl10.htm

[42] Dehghani, Farzaneh, et al. "Protective effect of Brewer's yeast on methimazole-induced-adrenal atrophy (a stereological study)." *The Tokai journal of experimental and clinical medicine* 35.1 (2010): 34.

[43] Peterson, Ralph E. "The influence of the thyroid on adrenal cortical function." *Journal of Clinical Investigation* 37.5 (1958): 736.

[44] Choudhary, Nidhi, et al. "Thyroxine replacement precipitating adrenal crisis." *Endocrine Abstracts*. Vol. 19. 2009.

[45] Shakir, K. M., et al. "Anemia: a cause of intolerance to thyroxine sodium." *Mayo Clinic Proceedings*. Vol. 75. No. 2. Elsevier, 2000.

[46] Brittenham, Gary M. "Iron deficiency in whole blood donors." *Transfusion* 51.3 (2011): 458-461.

[47] Alexander, D., M. J. Ball, and J. Mann. "Nutrient intake and haematological status of vegetarians and age-sex matched omnivores." *European journal of clinical nutrition* 48.8 (1994): 538.

[48] Kaur, Tajinder, Veena Aseeja, and Sujata Sharma. "Thyroid Dysfunction In Dysfunctional Uterine Bleeding." (2011).

[49] Demir, Tiroid Fonksiyon Bozukluğu Olan Hastalarda. "Iron Metabolism In Patients With Impaired Thyroid Function." *J. Fac. Pharm* 32.4 (2003): 221-230.

[50] Bryce, Gillian M., and Fiona Poyner. "Myxoedema presenting with seizures." *Postgraduate medical journal* 68.795 (1992): 35-36.

[51] Fommei, Enza, and Giorgio Iervasi. "The role of thyroid hormone in blood pressure homeostasis: evidence from short-term hypothyroidism in humans." *Journal of Clinical Endocrinology & Metabolism* 87.5 (2002): 1996-2000.

[52] Bhatia, P. L., et al. "Audiological and vestibular function tests in hypothyroidism." *The Laryngoscope* 87.12 (1977): 2082-2089.

[53] Kim, Yoon Kyung, Jeong Eun Shin, and Jong Woo Chung. "The effect of canalith repositioning for anterior semicircular canal canalithiasis." *ORL* 67.1 (2005): 56-60.

[54] Sweet, Chris, Abhishek Sharma, and George Lipscomb. "Unusual presentation of more common disease/injury: Recurrent nausea, vomiting and abdominal pain due to hypothyroidism." *BMJ Case Reports* 2010 (2010).

[55] Locher, R., et al. "[Tiredness, hyperpigmentation, weight loss, nausea and vomiting. Polyglandular autoimmune syndrome (PAS) type 2]." *Praxis* 99.20 (2010): 1223.

[56] Magri, Flavia, et al. "Improvement of intra-epidermal nerve fiber density in hypothyroidism after L-thyroxine therapy." *Clinical Endocrinology* (2012).

[57] Subba, K., D. Karn, and R. Khatri. "Triiodothyronin, Thyroxine and Thyrotropin in Vitiligo." *Kathmandu University Medical Journal* 9.2 (2012): 7-10.

[58] Samaan, N. A. "Hypoglycemia secondary to endocrine deficiencies." *Endocrinology and metabolism clinics of North America* 18.1 (1989): 145.

[59] Kikuchi, Mitsuru, et al. "Relationship between anxiety and thyroid function in patients with panic disorder." *Progress in Neuro-Psychopharmacology and Biological Psychiatry* 29.1 (2005): 77-81.

[60] Mordi, Ify, and Nikolaos Tzemos. "Subclinical hypothyroidism as a cause of resistant hypertension." *Cardiovascular Endocrinology* 1.2 (2012): 31-32.

[61] Macaron, Chamel, and Olufunsho Famuyiwa. "Hyponatremia of hypothyroidism: Appropriate suppression of antidiuretic hormone levels." *Archives of Internal Medicine* 138.5 (1978): 820.

[62] Dalton, Katharina, and Michael John Thomson Dalton. "Characteristics of pyridoxine overdose neuropathy syndrome." *Acta neurologica scandinavica* 76.1 (2009): 8-11.

[63] Mikkola, Tuija M., et al. "Influence of long-term postmenopausal hormone-replacement therapy on estimated structural bone strength: A study in discordant monozygotic twins." *Journal of Bone and Mineral Research* 26.3 (2011): 546-552.

[64] Toran-Allerand, C. Dominique, et al. "17α-Estradiol: A Brain-Active Estrogen?." *Endocrinology* 146.9 (2005): 3843-3850.

[65] Ronkainen, Paula HA, et al. "Postmenopausal hormone replacement therapy modifies skeletal muscle composition and function: a study with monozygotic twin pairs." *Journal of Applied Physiology* 107.1 (2009): 25-33.

[66] Potenza, Matthew, Michael A. Via, and Robert T. Yanagisawa. "Excess thyroid hormone and carbohydrate metabolism." *Endocrine Practice* 15.3 (2009): 254-262.

[67] Khan, Tariq Mehmood, Saqib Malik, and Inayat Ullah Diju. "Correlation Between Plasma Thyroid Hormones and Liver Enzymes Level in Thyrotoxic Cases and Controls in Hazara Division." *J Ayub Med Coll Abbottabad* 22.2 (2010).

[68] Coviello, Andrea D., et al. "Effects of graded doses of testosterone on erythropoiesis in healthy young and older men." *Journal of Clinical Endocrinology & Metabolism* 93.3 (2008): 914-919.

[69] Das, K. C., et al. "Erythropoiesis and erythropoietin in hypo-and hyperthyroidism." *Journal of Clinical Endocrinology & Metabolism* 40.2 (1975): 211-220.

[70] Brittenham, Gary M. "Iron deficiency in whole blood donors." *Transfusion* 51.3 (2011): 458-461.

[71] "Salimetrics Publish DHEA and DHEA-S: An Introduction to their Function and Measurement." http://salimetricseurope.blogspot.com/2012/08/salimetrics-publish-dhea-and-dhea-s.html Monday, 20 August 2012. Accessed 1/14/14.

[72] Gereben, Balázs, et al. "Cellular and molecular basis of deiodinase-regulated thyroid hormone signaling." *Endocrine Reviews* 29.7 (2008): 898-938, Figure 7.

[73] Fukui, Toshiya, Yukihiro Hasegawa, and Hiroki Takenaka. "Hyperthyroid dementia: clinicoradiological findings and response to treatment." *Journal of the neurological sciences* 184.1 (2001): 81-88.

[74] Johansson, Per, et al. "Reduced cerebrospinal fluid level of thyroxine in patients with Alzheimer's disease." *Psychoneuroendocrinology* (2012).

[75] Gereben, Balázs, et al. "Cellular and molecular basis of deiodinase-regulated thyroid hormone signaling." *Endocrine Reviews* 29.7 (2008): 898-938.

[76] Ikeda, Tadasu, et al. "Effect of thyrotropin on conversion of T4 to T3 in perfused rat liver." *Life sciences* 38.20 (1986): 1801-1806.

[77] Wu, Sing-Yung, R. Reggio, and W. H. Florsheim. "Characterization of thyrotropin-induced increase in iodothyronine monodeiodinating activity in mice." *Endocrinology* 116.3 (1985): 901-908.

[78] Kabadi, Udaya M. "Role of thyrotropin in metabolism of thyroid hormones in nonthyroidal tissues." *Metabolism* 55.6 (2006): 748-750.

[79] Kaplan, Michael M., Martin Schimmel, and Robert D. Utiger. "Changes in serum 3, 3′, 5′-triiodothyronine (reverse T3) concentrations with altered thyroid hormone secretion and metabolism." *Journal of Clinical Endocrinology & Metabolism* 45.3 (1977): 447-456.

[80] Gavin, Laurence A., et al. "3, 3′-Diiodothyronine production, a major pathway of peripheral iodothyronine metabolism in man." *Journal of Clinical Investigation* 61.5 (1978): 1276.

[81] Buclin, Thierry, et al. "Bioavailability and biological efficacy of a new oral formulation of salmon calcitonin in healthy volunteers." *Journal of Bone and Mineral Research* 17.8 (2002): 1478-1485.

[82] Hoermann, Rudolf, et al. "Is Pituitary Thyrotropin an Adequate Measure Of Thyroid Hormone-Controlled Homeostasis During Thyroxine Treatment?." *European Journal of Endocrinology* (2012).

[83] Wojcicka, Anna, J. H. Bassett, and Graham R. Williams. "Mechanisms of action of thyroid hormones in the skeleton." *Biochimica et Biophysica Acta (BBA)-General Subjects* (2012).

[84] Debaveye, Yves, et al. "Regulation of tissue iodothyronine deiodinase activity in a model of prolonged critical illness." *Thyroid* 18.5 (2008): 551-560.

[85] Salvatore, Domenico. "Deiodinases: keeping the thyroid hormone supply in balance." *Journal of Endocrinology* 209.3 (2011): 259-260.

[86] Gullo, Damiano, et al. "Levothyroxine monotherapy cannot guarantee euthyroidism in all athyreotic patients." *PloS one* 6.8 (2011): e22552.

[87] Garber, Jeffrey R., et al. "Clinical Practice Guidelines for Hypothyroidism in Adults Co-sponsored by the American Association of Clinical Endocrinologists (AACE) and the American Thyroid Association, Inc.(ATA)." *Thyroid* ja (2012).

[88] Maffeis, Laura, Maria Carmela Musolino, and Stefano Cambiaghi. "Single-plaque vegetating bromoderma." *Journal of the American Academy of Dermatology* 58.4 (2008): 682-684.

[89] Ogretmen, Zerrin, Serhat Sari, and Murat Ermete. "Use of topical povidone-iodine resulting in a iododerma." *Indian Journal of Dermatology* 56.3 (2011): 346.

[90] Backer, Howard, and Joe Hollowell. "Use of iodine for water disinfection: iodine toxicity and maximum recommended dose." *Environmental Health Perspectives* 108.8 (2000): 679.

[91] Faust, John B. "The Production of Iodine in Chile." *Industrial & Engineering Chemistry* 18.8 (1926): 808-811.

[92] Hillman, Donald, and A. R. Curtis. "Chronic iodine toxicity in dairy cattle: Blood chemistry, leukocytes, and milk iodide." *Journal of dairy science* 63.1 (1980): 55-63.

[93] Centers for Disease Control and Prevention. NIOSH Pocket Guide to Chemical Hazards. Iodine. Accessed 1/15/14. http://www.cdc.gov/niosh/npg/npgd0342.html

[94] Puri, Neerja. "A study on cutaneous manifestations of thyroid disease." *Indian Journal of Dermatology* 57.3 (2012): 247.

[95] Ramberg, Jane E., Erika D. Nelson, and Robert A. Sinnott. "Immunomodulatory dietary polysaccharides: a systematic review of the literature." *Nutr J* 9.54 (2010): 1-22.

2

Peter's Perplexing Pituitary Problem

Your labs are normal and you're just fine.

—conclusion of four different doctors: an endocrinologist, neurologist, rheumatologist, and infectious disease expert

Peter, a 55-year-old Canadian, has not felt well for most of his life, but his health deteriorated significantly when he was 46. He suffered from physical exhaustion with weak, sore, and cramped muscles. He couldn't concentrate and his short-term memory had deteriorated. His eyebrows and cheeks would twitch, and he'd wake in the middle of the night, drenched with sweat, his heart racing, shaking in tremors, and feeling like bugs were crawling under his skin

Peter wasn't always this way. His endocrine problems started after a head injury when he was 9-years-old. He had just learned that carrots grow underground, and he and a group of friends were lying in the dirt, looking at a mound where the carrot tops were sticking out. Another boy arrived, and seeing them lying on the ground, picked up a nearby boulder and dropped it on the back of Peter's head. Of course he blacked out, there was blood everywhere, and he was rushed to the hospital, where he was sewn back together. X-rays showed a 2 x 2 cm bone spur in the back of his skull at the point of impact and multiple fractures. He had headaches for weeks, but obviously survived. What on earth would possess the other boy to do this? Well, it turns out he was hyperactive and a fan of Road Runner/Wile E. Coyote cartoons. Remember how the Coyote was always trying to drop something on the Road Runner, like anvils, boulders, etc? Apparently some kids shouldn't watch cartoons!

Miraculously, Peter's skull grew back together, but his pituitary gland, which is located at the base of the skull, was probably damaged from the trauma. The pituitary gland releases Thyroid Stimulating Hormone (TSH) for the thyroid, Luteinizing Hormone (LH) and Follicle Stimulating Hormone (FSH) for the testes and ovaries, Adrenocorticotropic Hormone (ACTH) for the adrenal cortex, and Growth Hormone (GH), to name just a few. The pituitary is only about the size of a pea, but without its signals, none of these other hormones would be produced. Someone with limited pituitary function is said to be hypopituitary. Any head injury can damage the pituitary. Car accidents or head trauma from sports activities are common causes. In women, severe blood loss during childbirth (known as Sheehan's Syndrome) can cause pituitary tissue to die.

When Peter's skull was fractured, he became hypopituitary, but the formal diagnosis wasn't made until he was in his 50s, when all his hormones were found to be low. Hormones are essential for growth, development, and maturation, so it's not surprising that Peter started to have symptoms shortly after the accident. For two years, he couldn't sleep between midnight and 6 a.m. (probably from a disturbed cortisol rhythm).[1] He started gaining weight (probably low thyroid),[2] and even his teeth are shorter than normal (probably low growth hormone).[3] Lack of growth hormone limits skull growth, and Peter has a small face. He buys children's ski goggles, because the adult sizes are too big for him. His jaw is small too, and his lower wisdom teeth never grew in. The upper wisdoms broke through the gums when he was 25, were impacted and had to be removed. Dentists have mentioned that his teeth are short, and his dental arches are small, like a child's. All his facial features remained childlike, with a much smaller nose, eyes, and ears than would be expected for an adult. At 5' 7", he is shorter than both his brother and father by three inches. He has struggled with his weight, going from 180 pounds at age 16, to 293 pounds by age 19. He didn't know he was hypopituitary and starved himself in an attempt to keep his weight down, but the pounds just kept piling on.

Lack of thyroid and growth hormone negatively affects bone and dental health[4] and Peter's teeth became full of cavities when he was 17-19 years old. He also began grinding his teeth at night, which is known as bruxism. Children with bruxism often have lower levels of morning cortisol.[5] He did not sleep well and woke exhausted most mornings.

In spite of his condition, Peter was quite active and exercised diligently. He ran marathon distances (27 miles) a few times fueled only by youth (age 19), willpower, and determination. But his doctors still blamed his weight problems on poor diet and insufficient exercise, so Peter basically starved himself, and lost 100 pounds in a six-month period. His fatigue never diminished his passion for the outdoors, and he skied, sailed, and was more physically active than most of his friends.

Peter found university work challenging because of his limited attention span. He noticed he had to reread things a lot, and in discussions with classmates, noticed he didn't remember sections of material right after the lecture! He retained written material far better than spoken material. Anecdotally, many who are hypothyroid report the same thing, and also have trouble speaking articulately, because word recall is a problem.[6] With unwavering perseverance (and a lot of coffee), Peter earned an MBA. He has had a successful career in a sports field his whole family enjoys, and married his childhood sweetheart when he was 27. They celebrated their 28th wedding anniversary this year.

When he was in his 40s, Peter started having bouts of prostatitis, or an inflamed prostate that causes painful urination. The pain and inability to void were sometimes intolerable, and he was occasionally given morphine, because doctors didn't know what was wrong. He was hospitalized and put on antibiotics more than once. The antibiotics always helped, but after a month or so, the same symptoms would return. Studies show that high estradiol (a form of estrogen) is implicated in prostatitis,[7] and Peter has gynecomastia[8] (male breasts from high estradiol) because of his head injury. When a hormone doctor (an MD/DO who specializes in hormones and anti-aging) tested his sex hormones, his testosterone was very low and his estradiol was high and significantly above the reference range. Now that Peter takes Arimidex (a prescription aromatase inhibitor that lowers estradiol), he says he hasn't had a single problem with his prostate and no longer has any pain.

Peter's hypopituitary condition started to take its toll in his late 40s, when his low hormone levels were compounded with the normal, age-related decline. He had chronic back pain, his whole body ached, his joints were stiff, his muscles cramped, and he couldn't think clearly. Peter had his hormones tested by an endocrinologist, but since his lab results were always within the reference range, he was told he was normal, and not to get so "stressed out." In spite of Peter's protests and a recital of all his symptoms, his endocrinologist insisted that he was fine, gave him the "you're crazy" look, and told him that his symptoms didn't matter.

He was referred to a neurologist who performed muscle biopsies and six electromyograms (EMG). An EMG measures the electrical activity of muscles at rest and during contraction. In addition, nerve conduction studies measure how well and how fast the nerves can send electrical signals. The neurologist felt something wasn't quite right and retested him in six months. Unfortunately, test results were always "normal," so he was offered prescription muscle relaxants and anti-psychotics, which he refused. A referral to a rheumatologist also resulted in a normal diagnosis. Next was a visit to the Head of Infectious Disease, because after some intensive research of his own, Peter suspected he might have Lyme disease. He remembers a bulls-eye rash behind his knee (a common marker for Lyme) which appeared after he walked some deer trails in Maine. It never itched or bothered him, and eventually disappeared. Lyme is a bacterial infection transmitted by tick bites and causes flu-like symptoms, such as muscle aches and pains, which Peter certainly had. In fact, many Lyme disease symptoms are identical to hypothyroid symptoms: fatigue, joint and muscle aches, hair loss, ringing in the ears, constipation, sleep difficulties, memory loss, etc.[9] The Canadian Head of Infectious Disease declared Peter normal.

Then one morning, Peter heard a discussion of Lyme disease on the radio. Apparently, in Canada they use a test that produces a false negative 95% of the time, which means most with Lyme disease are never correctly diagnosed or treated.[10] But Lyme Literate Doctors (LLMDs) are able to diagnose and treat this complicated disease successfully. Peter did extensive research on the internet after hearing about this, and presented the information to his endocrinologist, thinking he had found the source of his problem and that he would then get the appropriate tests. The endocrinologist's response? Peter didn't have Lyme, his labs were perfect, there was nothing wrong with him, it was all in his head, and he'd better suck it up and get on with life. Peter was shocked and never spoke with that doctor again.

Peter felt sure that he had Lyme, but questioned his own judgment because the endocrinologist had been so dismissive. His continued research only made him more certain that he had Lyme, and he eventually made an appointment with an LLMD just across the border in the U.S. Unlike the negative Canadian test, he was diagnosed as positive in three different ways: by the CDC (Centers for Disease Control) standard, Igenex standard, and by his clinical symptoms. He completed his Lyme treatment within a year. On his final appointment with the LLMD, she mentioned that his thyroid levels looked low, and that he should explore thyroid treatment.

The Lyme treatment brought many improvements: his sleep was better, the night sweats and racing heart stopped, and his skin was no longer so dry and itchy. However, his muscles were still stiff and weak, and he often had muscle cramps. While his thoughts were clearer, he still felt a little brain fogged. So he started researching thyroid treatment and realized there were two completely different schools of thought. Current mainstream medicine diagnoses and treats thyroid patients by the TSH (Thyroid Stimulating Hormone) lab value, while treatment before the mid-1970s was based upon elimination of symptoms. Peter joined several thyroid internet groups and noticed that many on these groups were not happy when their treatment was based on a "normal" TSH. Most felt better when their symptoms were relieved, which usually correlated with an "abnormal" (too low) TSH! Before starting on thyroid medication, Peter's TSH was 1.26 mIU/L (considered normal) and his Free T3 (FT3) was 3.4 pg/mL (also within the normal reference range of 2.8-7.1 pg/mL). FT3 is a measurement of the active, unbound thyroid hormone that is readily available to the cells. His previous primary care physician, who was also an endocrinologist, thought these results were fine, even though his FT3 was only 14% in the reference range.

Peter's blood sugar was at the top of the reference range and had been that way for years, so he was considered pre-diabetic. His lipids were also not ideal—total cholesterol, triglycerides, and LDL (low-density lipoprotein) were high, while HDL (high-density lipoprotein) was low. In spite of a good diet and exercise (tennis with his endocrinologist!), his lipids never changed. So this endocrinologist prescribed statins so that Peter could control his "genetic" problem, but they only caused additional muscle pain. When Peter realized that friends and family members were getting heart bypass operations even though they'd been on statins for years, he weaned himself off of these drugs. He figured that there was no point in suffering from additional muscle pain if he was going to end up having bypass surgery anyway. He had also read enough negative information on statins to question the entire pharmaceutical industry—he believes they are in business to generate profits, not to help patients. It's possible that those with high cholesterol are simply hypothyroid and need thyroid hormone and/or testosterone, not statins. High cholesterol and heart disease correlate with low thyroid levels and low testosterone, and cholesterol levels can actually be manipulated with thyroid hormone and testosterone. A hypothyroid patient's high cholesterol levels will drop after thyroid hormone is prescribed, and a hyperthyroid patient's low cholesterol levels will rise after anti-thyroid drugs or radioactive iodine (that destroys the thyroid) is prescribed.[11] Total and LDL cholesterol levels correlate inversely with Free T4 levels. In other words, lower Free T4 levels result in higher total and LDL levels and vice versa.

Peter's hormone doctor prescribed ½ grain (30 mg) of Canadian Erfa Thyroid, a natural desiccated thyroid product (similar to Armour Thyroid) which is made from dried pig thyroids. A grain is an older measurement of weight; most prescriptions today are dispensed in milligrams (mg) or micrograms (mcg). Desiccated thyroid contains both T4 and T3, the two thyroid hormones a normal thyroid produces. Peter raised his dose by ½ grain increments every 10 days until he was taking 3.5 grains. This is the equivalent of 133 mcg T4 and 31.5 mcg T3. After two months on Erfa Thyroid, his symptoms worsened—he was in more pain than ever. His doctor lowered his dosage from 3.5 grains to 2 grains, but it didn't really help. Peter had been following a thyroid internet group that claims high reverse T3 (rT3) is a problem for many people taking thyroid medications containing T4, so he decided to follow their protocol to "clear" the rT3 by stopping the desiccated thyroid and taking only T3.

What exactly is rT3? It's a byproduct of T4, formed when one iodine atom is removed from T4 by a deiodinase enzyme. Molecules are three-dimensional, so which particular iodine atom is removed makes a difference; T3 and rT3 are isomers—they have the same number of atoms but they're arranged differently. Left and right hands are an example of isomers; both have a palm with five fingers attached, but although identical in number of attached fingers, one thumb faces left, while the other faces right. They are mirror images—similar, but not the same. (T3 and rT3 are not mirror images, but the concept is the same.) A left hand will not fit into a right glove or vice versa. Likewise, rT3 does not fit into the T3 nuclear cell receptor, but is bounced out of the cell and returned to the bloodstream.[12] It does not "block" T3 at the cell receptor.

Labs in Canada do not perform the rT3 test, so Peter just began the protocol assuming high rT3 was his problem. Peter stopped the Erfa Thyroid and began taking Cytomel (synthetic T3) instead. He increased the T3 until he was taking 125 mcg of T3 daily and no T4. A normal thyroid produces about 6 mcg of T3 and 100 mcg of T4 daily.[13] Higher levels of T3 (around 30 mcg) are found in the body, but this is from conversion of the T4 to T3, primarily by the liver and kidneys. In any case, 125 mcg of T3 is a very high dose.

While Peter felt his brain was clearer on this new T3-only protocol, it gave him chronic diarrhea (a hyperthyroid symptom), and he was more irritable. He felt this was a small price to pay though, and stayed on this protocol for about five months because it relieved some of his pain. His thyroid labs reflected his new dose (see Figure 2-1), with a Free T3 significantly over the reference range, a Free T4 below the reference range, and a TSH of 0.01 mIU/L (considered hyperthyroid by traditional doctors).

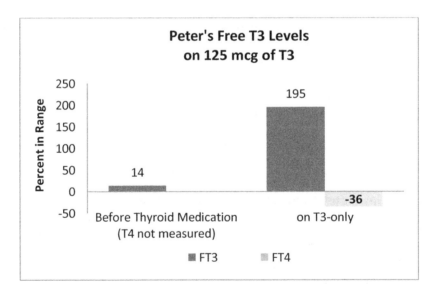

Figure 2-1. Peter's Free T3 measurement before starting on any thyroid hormone was very low, but still 14% within the reference range. Free T4 was not measured. When he took 125 mcg of T3 and no T4, his labs reflected the imbalance, with his FT3 levels testing at 195% of the reference range, and his FT4 levels testing 36% below the reference range.

Taking the advice of the thyroid internet groups, he tested his iron levels, because low iron levels can affect thyroid function. Many people with low thyroid levels are anemic,[14] and someone with low iron levels will not be able to tolerate supplemental thyroid hormone.[15] Peter's total iron, iron binding capacity, percent saturation, and ferritin were all at good levels, so Peter did not have an iron problem. Then he took a cortisol saliva test, which is considered by members of the thyroid internet groups to be the only reliable way to test cortisol. Low cortisol, like low iron, will also cause intolerance to supplemental thyroid hormone.[16] His cortisol was low at each of the four measured times. Two readings were at the bottom of the reference range, while the other two were actually below the reference range (Figure 2-2).

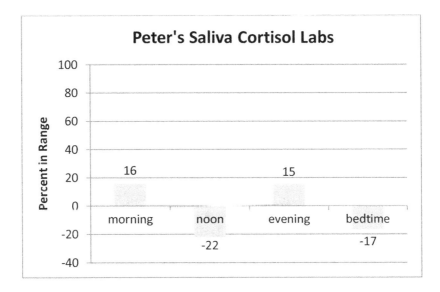

Figure 2-2. Peter's saliva cortisol labs from ZRT labs, December 2010. His rhythm is highly irregular, because a normal cortisol lab is highest in the morning, and then trends down towards the day, being lowest at bedtime. His labs are barely within the reference range in the morning and evening, and fall below the reference range at noon and bedtime.

Cortisol, a natural anti-inflammatory, is a hormone produced by the adrenal glands in response to an ACTH signal from the pituitary gland. But remember, Peter's pituitary was damaged when he was 9-years-old, so any ACTH signal was probably insufficient. Even though his cortisol labs were very low, his MD thought he was fine, although his hormone doctor thought that he might benefit from a supplement. Peter thought his levels were low enough to warrant treatment, so he started treating himself with hydrocortisone (HC) to raise his cortisol levels. Most of his back pain disappeared shortly after starting the HC, and back pain is a common symptom for people with low cortisol.[17]

After Peter had been taking T3-only and HC for 12 weeks, his hormone doctor noticed that his testosterone lab tests were also very low and suggested testosterone replacement therapy (TRT). Because he still didn't feel 100% better, Peter agreed and started with a compounded topical cream. Unfortunately, lab tests four months later showed his testosterone levels were actually lower than before he started! This is actually quite common, because many men who are low in testosterone are also hypothyroid. Hypothyroid skin is thicker than normal and doesn't absorb topical creams effectively. For others, topical creams seem to lose their effectiveness over time. Peter was then switched to injectable testosterone cypionate, which he injects subcutaneously every third day. Only then did he start to feel the benefits of more normal testosterone levels. He built up

15-20 pounds of muscle, some of his pain disappeared, his belly fat decreased, and his pants are now looser than ever. He knows he is much stronger today because he can easily lift items today that he could barely carry before. Unfortunately, one of the side effects of TRT is high levels of one of the estrogens, E2 (estradiol), which has its own set of undesirable side effects. Peter is now learning how to properly dose a prescription aromatase inhibitor, which prevents testosterone from converting to estradiol.[18]

Peter knew that low thyroid and low testosterone cause some of the same symptoms, and that there is a synergy between the two hormones in relieving symptoms. Now that he'd added testosterone, he knew he might be able to reduce his thyroid dose. He was also informed on a men's internet group that the T3-only protocol was raising his Sex Hormone Binding Globulin (SHBG), lowering his free testosterone, and raising his estradiol levels.[19] He also became aware of TiredThyroid's position that too much T3 can be detrimental, and that a normal thyroid produces primarily T4. So Peter started reducing his T3 dose and raising his T4 dose. He lowered his dose of 125 mcg T3 to 37.5 mcg and added 50 mcg Synthroid (T4), but didn't feel any differently. This brought his FT3 down into the normal range, and his FT4 came up slightly, but was still well below the reference range. He held his T3 dose at 37.5 mcg and continued to raise his T4 dose over the next six months until he was taking 175 mcg of T4. As his T4 levels increased, many symptoms began to disappear. His fingernails and toenails became harder (they used to be so soft he could bend them), the ridges on his nails disappeared, his constipation disappeared (he has suffered from hard stools for as long as he can remember), his thinking became clearer and he's less forgetful, his beard is now darker and he looks younger, his skin is softer and less dry so he's not as itchy as he used to be, and his hair is fuller and just looks healthier. These changes all happened after his T3 dose was reduced and his T4 dose was increased. Sadly, his hormone doctor doesn't think T4 has any beneficial properties and will accept a FT4 at the bottom of the reference range because he believes T3 is the only active hormone. This is simply not true; T4 has beneficial effects at the cell membrane before it converts to T3.[20] Other cells obtain most of their T3 by conversion from T4 at the cellular membrane.[21] Anecdotally, higher levels of T4 seem to have a positive effect on hair, and Peter's improved hair after adding T4 echoes the experience of many others.

Peter was able to fine-tune his dose from 37.5 mcg T3 + 175 mcg T4, to 33mcg T3 + 210 mcg T4, and stabilized on that dose for a while. If he lowered his T3 dose below that level, his myofascial pains (pain in the muscles or fascia throughout the body) returned. His pain is especially pronounced in the sides and back of his scalp.

Later in the year, Peter lowered his testosterone dose, and subsequently had to lower his thyroid dose to 25 mcg T3 + 200 mcg T4. His thinking became clearer and his memory improved noticeably on this lower dose. Overmedication, especially of T3, negatively affects the brain, and cases of hyperthyroid dementia have been reported by hyperthyroid Graves' patients. The brain has a very narrow range of T3 that it considers optimal, and cognitive problems (especially memory) appear when levels are too high.[22] On this lower dose, he also noticed his hair was thicker and growing faster. It had been quite thin, and seemed like it had stopped growing for a while.

Before Peter started on TRT, he was taking Metformin (an anti-diabetic drug) because his fasting blood sugar consistently tested at 120-140 mg/dL (less than 100 is ideal). However, once his testosterone reached more normal levels, his blood sugar became so low that he had dizzy spells and had to reduce the Metformin. He was taking the maximum dosage of 500 mg five times a day, but has now completely weaned off of Metformin. His blood sugar is now in the 80s, even after a meal. It is low and stable all the time now that his testosterone levels are higher in the reference range. TRT is beneficial to Type 2 diabetics—it lowers blood sugar and insulin resistance.[23]

His cholesterol and triglyceride levels have also come down into the normal range since starting TRT, and this time, without statins! A recent study corroborates Peter's experience—TRT reduced total cholesterol levels over and above the effect of statins, and triglyccrides were also significantly lowered.[24]

Peter's small facial features indicate he is obviously low in Growth Hormone (GH), but GH is expensive, difficult to dose, and comes with a multitude of side effects. The latest protocol to increase GH is to supplement the peptides that can stimulate natural GH release. Peter has only been taking Growth Hormone Releasing Hormone (GHRH) for a few months, but says he is sleeping better and his lower back pain is gone. His mood has improved and he feels positive, optimistic and upbeat now. He has been down so many roads trying to balance his hormones, and hopes this will be the final one that adds a synergy to all the other hormones he's taking.

Peter seems happier and more optimistic today, and others have noticed. While he never considered himself depressed before, he rarely wanted to do anything or go anywhere, and now he does! He and his wife recently went on vacation—the first time in five years!

Peter's health and quality of life have continued to improve as he has fine-tuned his hormone levels. Now that he can think clearly again, he questions a medical system that has failed him and so many others. He feels that mainstream medicine has too many policies and protocols to actually help a sick person. Medical guidelines say that a "normal" TSH test rules out hypothyroidism (the TSH Rule), and therefore no further investigation is necessary. Yet someone like Peter, who had minimal pituitary function, tested with a normal TSH of 1.26 mIU/L! He feels far too much emphasis is placed on lab results when doctors should be examining the patient in front of them. Lab reference ranges go so low that very few people have a chance of being diagnosed as deficient in any hormone, not just thyroid. Peter's testosterone levels were also "normal" when first tested. He feels current ranges don't help patients because they don't specify what the "optimal" values are and go so low as to include being almost dead.

At least Peter has a good working relationship with his hormone doctor. Over the last two years, the relationship between Peter and his doctor has changed, for the better. Peter spends considerable time educating himself and shares his findings with his doctor. Peter brings a list of items to discuss to each appointment, and the items are discussed together, as a team. If Peter opposes any of his doctor's suggestions he says so, and says why. If there are protocols that Peter wants to try, he brings it up. Peter is the one who pushed for higher doses of T4, not his doctor. Peter is also the one who educated his doctor about the different stages of adrenal insufficiency, and continues to use HC for effective pain relief. While it took a little time for his doctor to get adjusted to the concept of a patient-doctor partnership, he now considers Peter his most informed patient and treats him with respect. This is the kind of patient-doctor relationship we should all strive for.

Key points

- When multiple hormones are low (thyroid, cortisol, testosterone for men, estradiol and progesterone for women), the patient's pituitary function should be checked and hormone replacement discussed.
- Small facial features, short teeth, and child-size dental arches should have been a dead giveaway to a dentist that Peter suffered from a growth hormone deficiency.
- Lack of thyroid hormone can negatively affect teeth.
- Word recall and difficulty concentrating or remembering can be caused by low thyroid levels.
- Back pain may be a sign of low cortisol levels.
- Repeated bouts of prostatitis should be investigated with testosterone and estradiol testing; if estradiol levels are high, an anti-estrogen drug may relieve symptoms. Painful urination can also be caused by bladder cancer and should be investigated too.
- Symptoms of Lyme disease (a bulls-eye rash followed by muscle aches and fatigue) should not be ignored, and a Lyme Literate MD should be sought out for diagnosis and treatment.
- High cholesterol can be treated with thyroid hormone or TRT instead of statins.
- The T3-only protocol negatively affects men's hormones—it raises estradiol and SHBG, leaving less Free Testosterone available to the body.
- Too much T3 can negatively affect the brain, causing cognitive and memory issues.
- TRT may help build muscle and strength, but may also result in higher estradiol levels, which will then need to be controlled with other drugs or supplements.
- T4 is not useless and has positive effects on fingernails, hair, skin, and brain function.
- T3 may help relieve myofascial pains (muscle pain throughout the body).
- TRT lowers blood sugar and triglycerides.

---

[1] Balbo, Marcella, Rachel Leproult, and Eve Van Cauter. "Impact of sleep and its disturbances on hypothalamo-pituitary-adrenal axis activity." International journal of endocrinology 2010 (2010).

[2] Tran, Anh, et al. "The spectrum of presentations of hypothyroidism in primary care." Endocrine Abstracts. Vol. 28. 2012.

[3] Atreja, Gaurav, et al. "Oral manifestations in growth hormone disorders." Indian Journal of Endocrinology and Metabolism 16.3 (2012): 381.

[4] Nield, Linda S., James P. Stenger, and Deepak Kamat. "Common pediatric dental dilemmas." Clinical pediatrics 47.2 (2008): 99-105.

[5] Castelo, Paula Midori, et al. "Awakening salivary cortisol levels of children with sleep bruxism." Clinical biochemistry (2012).

[6] Correia, Neuman, et al. "Evidence for a specific defect in hippocampal memory in overt and subclinical hypothyroidism." Journal of Clinical Endocrinology & Metabolism 94.10 (2009): 3789-3797.

[7] Ellem, Stuart J., and Gail P. Risbridger. "Aromatase and regulating the estrogen: androgen ratio in the prostate gland." Journal of steroid biochemistry and molecular biology 118.4-5 (2010): 246-251.

[8] Johnson, Ruth E., and M. Hassan Murad. "Gynecomastia: pathophysiology, evaluation, and management." Mayo Clinic Proceedings. Vol. 84. No. 11. Mayo Foundation, 2009.

[9] Cameron, Daniel J. "Proof that chronic Lyme disease exists." Interdisciplinary Perspectives on Infectious Diseases 2010 (2010).

[10] Halperin, John J., Phillip Baker, and Gary P. Wormser. "Common Misconceptions About Lyme Disease." The American journal of medicine 126.3 (2013): 264-e1.

[11] Diekman, M. J. M., et al. "Changes in plasma low-density lipoprotein (LDL)-and high-density lipoprotein cholesterol in hypo-and hyperthyroid patients are related to changes in free thyroxine, not to polymorphisms in LDL receptor or cholesterol ester transfer protein genes." Journal of Clinical Endocrinology & Metabolism 85.5 (2000): 1857-1862.

[12] Gereben, Balázs, et al. "Cellular and molecular basis of deiodinase-regulated thyroid hormone signaling." Endocrine Reviews 29.7 (2008): 898-938, Figure 7.

[13] Escobar-Morreale, Héctor F., et al. "Treatment of hypothyroidism with combinations of levothyroxine plus liothyronine." Journal of Clinical Endocrinology & Metabolism 90.8 (2005): 4946-4954.

[14] Cincmre, Hakan, et al. "Hematologic effects of levothyroxine in iron-deficient subclinical hypothyroid patients: a randomized, double-blind, controlled study." Journal of Clinical Endocrinology & Metabolism 94.1 (2009): 151-156.

[15] Shakir, K. M., et al. "Anemia: a cause of intolerance to thyroxine sodium." Mayo Clinic Proceedings. Vol. 75. No. 2. Elsevier, 2000.

[16] Murray, Jonathan Stephen, Rubaraj Jayarajasingh, and Petros Perros. "Deterioration of symptoms after start of thyroid hormone replacement." BMJ 323.7308 (2001): 332-333.

[17] Muhtz, Christoph, et al. "Cortisol response to experimental pain in patients with chronic low back pain and patients with major depression." Pain Medicine (2012).

[18] Rhoden, E. L., and A. Morgentaler. "Treatment of testosterone-induced gynecomastia with the aromatase inhibitor, anastrozole." International journal of impotence research 16.1 (2004): 95-97.

[19] Pugeat, Michel, et al. "Sex hormone-binding globulin gene expression in the liver: drugs and the metabolic syndrome." Molecular and cellular endocrinology 316.1 (2010): 53-59.

[20] De Vito, Paolo, et al. "Nongenomic effects of thyroid hormones on the immune system cells: New targets, old players." Steroids (2012).

[21] Maia, Ana Luiza, et al. "Type 2 iodothyronine deiodinase is the major source of plasma T-3 in euthyroid humans." Journal of Clinical Investigation 115.9 (2005): 2524.

[22] Miao, Q., et al. "Reversible changes in brain glucose metabolism following thyroid function normalization in hyperthyroidism." American Journal of Neuroradiology 32.6 (2011): 1034-1042.

[23] Brooke, J., et al. "Testosterone replacement therapy: a safety audit of clinical practice including men with Type 2 diabetes and cardiovascular disease." Endocrine Abstracts. Vol. 29. 2012.

[24] Brooke, Jonathan, et al. "Testosterone replacement therapy has beneficial effects on cardiovascular risk factors and liver function in hypogonadal men." Endocrine Abstracts. Vol. 28. 2012.

3

The Woe of Vertigo

The thyroid doesn't affect your brain at all.

—Jane's primary care physician, unaware that hypothyroidism is associated with dementia, memory impairment, psychosis, depression, and disorientation.[1]

Jane is 86-years-old and has been taking Synthroid for 30 years, since she was diagnosed with Hashimoto's disease (an autoimmune hypothyroid condition) in her fifties. I have known her for a long time, and because we live in different time zones, we often communicate by email. She contacted me because she knew I had done a lot of thyroid research and might be able to help her. For whatever reason, she kept very detailed medical records over the years and was kind enough to share them with me for this extremely educational case study. Her dose has been increased and decreased as her Thyroid Stimulating Hormone (TSH) levels have risen and fallen throughout the years. She was initially started on 100 mcg of Synthroid 30 years ago, which she took for nearly twenty years, but she has also been prescribed 88 or 75 mcg in the last ten years, depending on her TSH. She has seen six endocrinologists in her lifetime and has also been prescribed Levothroid (another brand, like Synthroid) and generic levothyroxine at different times. In 2011 she started having debilitating bouts of vertigo and vomiting.

She remembers fainting twice in her lifetime--once as a child and once as an adult in her forties. She may already have been borderline hypothyroid then; low thyroid levels may cause heart abnormalities and a slow heart rate which can lead to fainting from an atrioventricular (AV) block. Levothyroxine treatment has corrected this problem in some patients.[2]

There were other symptoms before her hypothyroid diagnosis at age 55. She ate rock salt straight from the bag as a child and did not care for sweets. A craving for salt (hyponatremia) may be caused by hypothyroidism.[3] As a teenager she noticed she would gain a lot of weight if she ate normal-sized meals, so simply ate less. She could go all day without getting hungry or thirsty. In her late forties, she felt extreme tiredness and noticed she had a puffy face. She would sometimes mix her words up. She was also irritable and temperamental, often arguing with her colleagues. At work, she sometimes had trouble climbing the stairs to the second floor. All of these are common hypothyroid symptoms.

When Jane was 55 in 1982, she was diagnosed with breast cancer and had a modified radical mastectomy. Her mother had also had breast cancer, as did many other female relatives on her mother's side of the family. There is a history of rheumatoid arthritis, autoimmune thyroid disease (both Graves' and Hashi's), Parkinson's, diabetes, and knee problems in the extended family. Research has shown there is a strong genetic influence to autoimmune diseases,[4] and it can be clearly seen in Jane's family. In spite of this, Jane has led a fairly active life as a working, single mother, and managed a family business in her retirement. She still walks three blocks each way (some of it uphill!) to buy fresh eggs and visit her bank, and recently renewed her driver's license. She is also an avid gardener.

A month after her mastectomy, she was diagnosed with Hashimoto's disease. Her surgeon noticed that her thyroid gland was enlarged (2.5 times normal size) and she was started on 100 mcg of Synthroid. Researchers have long noted an association of thyroid disease and breast cancer.[5] Dr. David Derry considers hypothyroidism the second stage that causes cancer to metastasize; iodine deficiency is the first stage.[6]

Fast forward 17 years to 1999, when Jane is 72. She felt more tired and couldn't think as well as she used to, and wondered if her thyroid dosage needed adjusting. Her thyroid lab tests were declared "normal," so her dose was not changed.

Osteoporosis drugs

Jane had a bone scan in 1997 and was diagnosed with osteopenia (low bone mineral density), but she declined to take any medication for it. However, four years later, at the age of 74, she was prescribed 35 mg of Actonel for the osteopenia by her ob-gyn, and took the drug for nearly eight years. It was shortly after starting that drug that she began to lose her memory and couldn't remember where she parked her car, forgot to pay her bills on time, couldn't balance her checkbook, lost her checkbook, perspired profusely, had blurred vision occasionally (a documented Actonel side effect[7]), constantly fell asleep while reading at the kitchen table, couldn't remember what drawer or cabinet her dishes belonged in, and had her first panic attack while at a restaurant buffet, when she couldn't find her way back to her table. She remembers being disoriented and confused, and people's faces blurring. She became passive and apathetic in her daily life and was unable to think clearly or make decisions. She simply vegetated—didn't want to do anything, and didn't care to socialize either. These are all hypothyroid symptoms, and even in her state, she knew something was wrong. She had her thyroid levels tested again, but her endocrinologist did not change her dose. Her labs show a disconnect, because her TSH is flagged as low at <0.1 mIU/L, but her thyroid hormones, Total triiodothyronine (T3) and Free thyroxine (T4), are within the normal reference range, although her Total T3 is on the low end of the range. A very low TSH could be a sign of hyperthyroidism, or high thyroid levels, but hers are not high at all. Her TSH is not accurately reflecting her thyroid levels. Her Total T3 is less than half the level of Free T4, as a percent in range, as shown in Figure 3-1. This is expected with her near zero TSH, since TSH stimulates T4 to T3 conversion.[8]

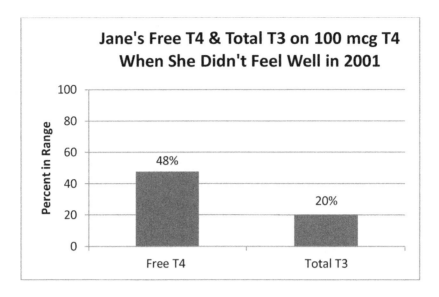

Figure 3-1. Jane's Free T4 and Total T3 on 100 mcg T4 when she didn't feel well. Her TSH was near zero, and as expected, her Total T3 is very low in the reference range; TSH stimulates T4 to T3 conversion and most people do not feel well at Jane's low levels.

Jane feels the Actonel prescribed in 2001 somehow interfered with her thyroid medications and started her health decline. She is diagnosed today with Barrett's esophagus, a precursor to esophageal cancer, which has been associated with oral bisphosphonate use (Actonel is a bisphosphonate).[9]

Because Jane felt sure that her thyroid dose was too high and causing her physical problems, she saw another endocrinologist in 2002, at the age of 75, hoping that the new endocrinologist might reduce her dose. He did lower her dose to 88 mcg from her previous 100 mcg. However, looking at her lab work now, it would be my guess that she was actually too low in thyroid hormone (particularly T3), rather than too high. To compensate for the lack of thyroid hormone, the body secretes norepinephrine[10] which can result in hyperthyroid symptoms. Too much norepinephrine feels almost the same as too much T3: a rapid heart rate, high blood pressure, and feeling revved up and anxious are typical. Norepinephrine triggers more T4 to T3 conversion during cold spells to keep the body warm.[11] A hypothyroid person in this state may sweat when it's not even hot, as Jane did. The biggest clue that she was undermedicated and not overmedicated was her apathetic and vegetative state; a hyperthyroid person tends to bounce off the walls, at least in the early stages. When she informed her endocrinologist that she was still experiencing periods of confusion, she was referred to a geriatric physician who diagnosed her with mild dementia and prescribed Aricept, which is used to treat Alzheimer's and other memory impairments. She did not feel she had a definitive diagnosis for Alzheimer's so refused to take the medication. Jane thought she had just been overmedicated on thyroid hormone and wanted to see if the new lower dose would help with her symptoms. It did! Her short-term memory improved, she was able to balance her checkbook again, and she could remember where she parked her car (but these improvements only lasted a year). Both low and high thyroid levels will cause cognitive dysfunction.[12]

Cholesterol drugs

At the end of that year, tests showed she had high cholesterol (over the reference range), which she'd never had before. She was prescribed the first of many types of cholesterol-lowering drugs by her primary care physician, starting with Lipitor, a statin. Two months after starting Lipitor, she had a nose bleed at 3 a.m. and thought she just had a runny nose because she has a chronic post-nasal drip. It was only after she woke the next morning that she was able to see a wastebasket full of bloody tissues. She also coughed up a blood clot the size of a quarter the next morning. She had never had a nose bleed before. She was told that hers was a posterior nosebleed, which generally doesn't stop on its own and usually requires a trip to the ER. She stopped the Lipitor but it still took a full week for the bleeding from her nose to taper off and finally stop. Her doctor then had her try various other brands of cholesterol-lowering drugs between 2002-2007: Lescol, then Niaspan, Zetia, Welcol, and Omocor. Because she had side effects on every single brand, she eventually stopped taking any cholesterol-lowering drugs and just lived with her high cholesterol. High cholesterol is often a symptom of low thyroid levels and was used a century ago to diagnose the severity of the hypothyroid condition; the higher the cholesterol, the lower the thyroid levels.[13]

Jane also had problems standing up in the morning shortly after starting Lipitor—her legs would collapse under her weight (she weighs less than 100 pounds), and she had to brace herself against the walls to walk out of her bedroom. Her neck muscles seemed to "freeze," and she could only look straight ahead without pain; it was excruciating to turn her head either to the right or left. The pain got progressively worse until she stopped the Lipitor, but there was still slight pain for a year afterwards. Her neck made knuckle-cracking sounds all day, even when she was perfectly still. Her knees also became stiff and occasionally made cracking sounds, her muscles tightened, and she was unable to bend her knees at times. There was pain in her knee, and it caused difficulty walking. Looking back now, 10 years later, many of the aches and pains brought on by Lipitor have now resolved, but Jane is now also on a better dose of thyroid hormone, including some much needed T3. Many others have reported similar muscle and joint pains after starting statins.[14]

She had problems with her eyes too. She had trouble focusing, and images would alternate between sharp and blurred. This was especially notable while watching TV, when words would be clear one minute and blurred the next. Her vision problems had started after taking Actonel for her osteopenia, but the Lipitor may have compounded the problem. At her annual eye exam, she was told she'd lost 50% of the vision in her left eye, and that she would need cataract surgery within a couple of years. The cataracts had been present for over 20 years, but had been very slow growing up till this point. She had difficulty sleeping and she noticed she was constantly opening the wrong kitchen drawers and cabinets when putting things away, as if her brain couldn't get the message to her hand quickly enough. When she told this to her endocrinologist, he told her that her mind/hand coordination problem might be a neurological one. Others have reported cognitive problems that started when they were prescribed statins; their diagnosis of dementia or Alzheimer's reversed when they stopped their statins.[15]

It appears that the hypothyroid state amplifies the problems caused by statins,[16] but the irony is that, as noted earlier, high cholesterol may simply be a symptom of hypothyroidism, so correcting the hypothyroid condition would negate the need for statins in the first place.

Blood pressure drugs

In 2003 she had a colonoscopy where a rectal tumor was found. Because her blood pressure was high (her systolic was 175 mmHg and desirable is less than 130), her surgeon requested that she be placed on a blood pressure medication before the surgery. Her primary care physician chose and prescribed Verapamil (a calcium channel blocker type of blood pressure medication). When someone is hypothyroid, noradrenaline, adrenaline, and cortisol levels may increase, and all are known to elevate blood pressure.[17] If she had just been prescribed more thyroid medication and some much needed T3, her blood pressure may have normalized. Instead, the Verapamil just compounded her problems. Verapamil inhibits ACTH (Adrenocorticotropic Hormone), the pituitary hormone that stimulates cortisol production, because ACTH synthesis requires calcium and Verapamil is a calcium channel blocker.[18] With suboptimal ACTH stimulation, cortisol levels will drop, and cortisol is essential to thyroid metabolism. Not surprisingly, lack of cortisol is associated with fatigue.[19] While she does not have a Total T3 to compare with previous thyroid labs that year, she does have a Free T4, and that is lower, so it could be assumed that the Total T3 is also lower, especially since she is now on a lower dose of Synthroid (88 mcg from previous 100 mcg). Jane may not have enough thyroid hormone in her body for normal metabolism in all tissues.

The addition of the blood pressure medication, Verapamil, created new symptoms. Jane could not stay awake as a passenger in any moving vehicle. She also falls asleep during TV programs and at the kitchen table while reading the newspaper. While she never sweated in the past, she now perspires to the point where her hair is wet and sweat is dripping down her face simply from raking the yard; on rare occasions, she would be comfortable one minute, and then suddenly hot the next. As stated earlier, she was having a problem simply putting dishes away, for example, opening the cabinet for cups when she was putting away a plate.

She assumed, from her overheating, that her dosage was too high, so cut her dosage on her own by taking her Synthroid right before eating, instead of over an hour before eating. The food in her stomach effectively reduced her dose. The result? Her mind/hand coordination improved somewhat, but was still off half the time. She was less sleepy, but still catnapped throughout the day. She was still sweating, and had minor periods of confusion and disorientation, but did not experience another panic attack. Her primary care physician then prescribed Reminyl, an Alzheimer's drug, which she refused to take. She was not happy with her gerontologist, so found another endocrinologist. Routine testing at age 77 in 2004 returned normal thyroid results, and her dose of 88 mcg of Levothroid was not changed. Jane felt her blood pressure medication was too high, and her own readings with a blood pressure machine confirmed that, so her new endocrinologist switched her over to 5 mg of Altace, an ACE (Angiotensin-Converting-Enzyme) inhibitor blood pressure medication. These drugs work by inhibiting an enzyme, which allows the blood vessels to dilate and results in lower blood pressure.

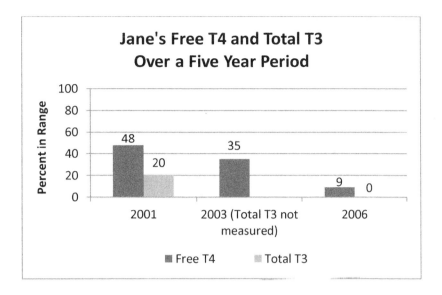

Figure 3-2. Jane's thyroid levels are declining over the years, which correlate with the increase in her health problems. While there was a decrease in her T4 dose from 2001 (100 mcg) to 2003 (88 mcg), the 2006 lab results reflect the effect of taking the same T4 dose (88 mcg) after breakfast, instead of one hour before, as she had done in the past. Her Total T3 in 2006 is actually 0% in the reference range or 77 ng/dL (77-178).

This new blood pressure medication gave her strong coughing spells 4-5 times a day that lasted until 2-3 a.m. She had so much phlegm that it would sometimes take 3-5 minutes of coughing to clear her throat. Because of these coughing attacks, she had paper cup spittoons all around the house. In public, people would withdraw, afraid of catching her "cold." Her mouth would get so dry while sleeping that she'd have to wake and moisten her mouth with water. She also lost some of her sense of taste. These are documented side effects of ACE inhibitors.[20]

Her health continued to deteriorate and she was having difficulty sleeping at night, balancing her checkbook, and recalling where her car was parked again. She again thought she was overmedicated so moved her thyroid dose to after breakfast, instead of before breakfast on an empty stomach. This further lowered her effective dose (see Figure 3-2) because Synthroid should be taken on an empty stomach for best absorption.[21] Her limited improvements each time she lowered her Synthroid dose may be due to the interaction of thyroid hormone on cortisol levels. Increased thyroid levels will increase the clearance of any cortisol,[22] and since her cortisol levels are suppressed by the blood pressure medication she was taking, her body can only handle a limited amount of thyroid hormone. Reducing her thyroid dose would effectively raise her cortisol levels, making her feel better. Cortisol is an essential hormone, and if the body can't produce the amount of cortisol needed, it can result in a fatal adrenal crisis.[23]

Surgeries

In 2005, at age 79, Jane had cataract surgery on her right eye, and was told she would need to have her left eye done later. Bisphosphonates such as Actonel have documented side effects that may threaten vision. These include scleritis (inflammation of the sclera, or the whites of the eye), uveitis (inflammation of the middle layer of the eye), blurred vision, and general irritation of the eye.[24] Jane stopped taking Actonel in 2008 and in 2010, she was informed that cataract surgery for her left eye was no longer necessary.

Colonoscopies were repeated in 2004, 2007, and 2008, after her rectal tumor was removed in 2003. Her 2008 colonoscopy was declared normal, so she will not be checked again until 2013. Surgery has been shown to cause cognitive dysfunction by inducing the low T3 syndrome, where both T3 and T4 become much lower than they normally are, and TSH does not rise in compensation to stimulate more thyroid hormone production. The liver, which does a large part of the conversion of T4 to T3, may be busy processing anesthetic drugs, resulting in reduced T4 to T3 conversion, which results in cognitive impairment.[25] An adjustment in thyroid medication may help this condition, but no changes were made to her dose.

A normal TSH while severely hypothyroid

Thyroid testing in 2006 showed her Total T3 had now fallen to 0% of the reference range, Free T4 was 9% in the reference range, TSH was 2.1 uIU/mL, and total cholesterol was high at 225 mg/dL (less than 200 is desirable). Because her TSH is within the broad reference range, no changes were made to her thyroid dose of 88 mcg. As stated earlier, high cholesterol can be a symptom of low thyroid levels. If Jane's symptoms or her actual lab result numbers were examined in terms of where they fell within the reference range, it would be obvious that an increase in her thyroid medication was warranted, and perhaps, even the addition of some much needed T3. But all her thyroid numbers were within the reference range, so no thyroid lab values were flagged, and her thyroid levels were considered "normal" from a statistical point of view.

In 2007, her TSH was a very normal 2.71 uU/mL (.28-4.02), yet several items on her routine lab work are flagged as outside the normal reference ranges:

- glomerular filtration rate (GFR) is flagged low at 57 mL/min
  (normal is greater than 60)

- CO_2 (carbon dioxide) is flagged high at 31 mEq/L
  (normal is 23-29)

- total cholesterol is flagged high at 273 mg/dL
  (< 200 is desirable)

- LDL (low-density lipoprotein) is also flagged as high at 182 mg/dL
  (< 100 optimal)

A reduced GFR from the kidneys is associated with hypothyroidism,[26] high carbon dioxide (CO_2) levels may be a result of impaired breathing that is correctable with thyroid hormone,[27] and high cholesterol levels are associated with hypothyroidism.[28] Even though her TSH at 2.71 would not be considered high or low, many other lab values are screaming that she is dangerously hypothyroid. High levels of carbon dioxide in the blood are known as *hypercapnia*. Hypercapnia is associated with myxedema, or the severest form of hypothyroidism that precedes coma and subsequently, death. It is caused by respiratory failure from low intracellular T3.[29]

A suppressed TSH while severely hypothyroid

In 2008, Jane's TSH disappeared (Figure 3-3). Even though Total T3, Free T3, and Free T4 were basically in the bottom third of the reference range, her TSH came back as 0.02 uIU/mL. A number that low may indicate that someone is hyperthyroid, or that they are taking too much thyroid hormone. Jane obviously was not, so her TSH would be expected to be much higher. Her endocrinologist then tested her FSH (Follicle Stimulating Hormone), another pituitary hormone, to see if her pituitary was working. Her FSH was high, as it should be, since she is well past menopause, which ruled out the hypopituitary theory.

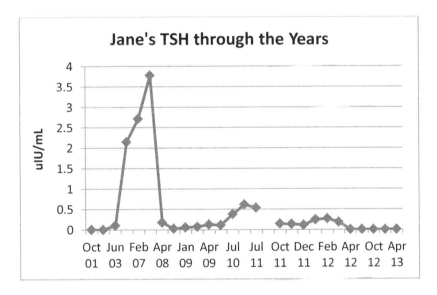

Figure 3-3. For over a decade, Jane has had very little TSH, except for three times between 2006-07. Her TSH has been below the reference range nearly the entire rest of the time. Jane was only taking Synthroid until March 2012, when 5 mcg of T3 was added to her dose. There is no datapoint for September 2011 because a TSH test was not run.

Why else would someone's TSH be so low? There is something called non-thyroidal illness, or the low T3 syndrome, which often presents in people who are ill. The thyroid may be completely operational, but the illness takes control of the thyroid and down-regulates TSH and thyroid hormone output. Surgery was already given as an example of a condition that would induce this syndrome, and Jane had four colonoscopies and cataract surgery previous to this point in time. Jane's TSH was 3.78 in October 2007. In January 2008 she had a normal colonoscopy. In April 2008, her TSH was 0.17, or below normal. As stated earlier, TSH stimulates T4 to T3 conversion, so is essential in someone who is not taking any T3 medication, which Jane was not.

The medical term for a low or suppressed TSH with normal free or total T4 and T3 levels is *subclinical hyperthyroidism*. It was thought that this was a precursor to actual hyperthyroidism, but in one study, only 6% of patients progressed to true hyperthyroidism after one year. In other words, 94% of the people who tested with a low or suppressed TSH at one time were not truly hyperthyroid.[30] When tested again later, some had a normal TSH, while others continued to have a suppressed TSH. TSH fluctuates and changes throughout the day[31] and there is even a seasonal variation.[32] It really should not be used as rigidly as it is to determine thyroid doses.

In a study of people older than 60 years of age, TSH only had a 12% positive predictive value for hyperthyroidism. When TSH was used in conjunction with T4, the predictive value increased fivefold to 67%. A low or suppressed TSH is far more common in older persons than actual hyperthyroidism.[33] In other words, a TSH test alone cannot be used to diagnose or manage an older person's thyroid dose.

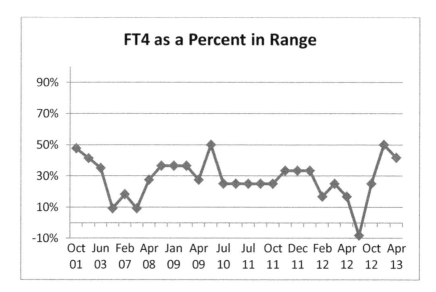

Figure 3-4. Jane's Free T4 has never exceeded 50% in the reference range, meaning it has always been in the bottom half or even below the reference range (July 2012). I see no correlation to her TSH. When a patient's TSH is suppressed, they'd be expected to have a high (above the reference range) FT4, FT3 or both. Jane has neither.

Pharmaceutical drugs, such as the Verapamil Jane was taking for her high blood pressure, can also interfere with thyroid hormones, or in this case, TSH. Verapamil inhibits the TRH (Thyrotropin-Releasing Hormone) signal from the hypothalamus that stimulates pituitary TSH production.[34] The release of TSH is calcium dependent, and Verapamil is a calcium channel blocker.[35] As stated earlier, TSH stimulates T4 to T3 conversion, which is absolutely essential for someone who does not take any T3, like Jane.

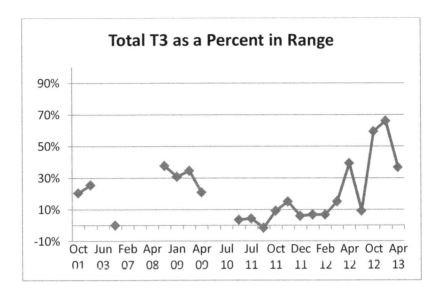

Figure 3-5. Jane's Total T3 has only recently surpassed the 50% in range mark, when 5 mcg of T3 was added to her dose in March 2012. While FT4 was always tested, Total T3 was only occasionally tested, hence the missing datapoints. Visually, this graph shows no correlation with the TSH graph, but does appear to somewhat follow the FT4 graph.

Jane's dose of Synthroid was raised back to 100 mcg in January 2009, then her dose was cut to 88 mcg in June 2009, then 75 mcg in February 2010, then back up to 88 mcg in August 2010. I'm not sure what the rationale was for the changes, other than that by lowering a dose, TSH *usually* comes up (the TSH rule). Her cholesterol was still consistently over the reference range at all doses, which indicates that Jane was still hypothyroid at any of these doses.

The vertigo begins

Jane's initial dose of Verapamil was 240 mg in 2003; it was lowered to 180 mg in 2005 at her request because she felt overmedicated, raised back to 240 mg in 2007, before this last raise to 360 mg in January 2011. Keep in mind that Jane barely weighs 100 pounds. Six months after the last increase in Verapamil, in June 2011, Jane had her first case of vertigo, where the world appeared to be spinning, causing her to feel very unbalanced and unable to walk. She was walking home from some errands and had to hang on to a tree branch to keep from falling. Luckily, a passing neighbor was able to help her walk home. Throughout the year, Jane had intermittent vertigo spells, noticed that her sense of taste was gone, and that two of her fingernails were flat. The last year had been very emotionally stressful for her for several reasons. Jane had lived in her home by herself for over a decade, but that was about to change, and the preparations were stressful. Her backyard garden, one of her passions, had also changed when a large tree was taken down, and the backyard tilled. The bad economy had also taken its toll and the family business was struggling. So there was a culmination of financial, emotional, and physical stress. As stated earlier, her blood pressure medication, Verapamil, was lowering her TSH and cortisol, both of which are essential for thyroid metabolism in someone taking only T4. Adequate thyroid hormones (especially some T3) supply the adrenal glands with the energy they need to secrete cortisol, and Jane has very little. To recap, because of Verapamil, Jane now has minimal TSH and as a result, minimal T3; she also has minimal ACTH and as a result, minimal cortisol. Hormonally, she is out of gas.

In September 2011, Jane's vertigo progressed to vomiting and diarrhea and she was taken to the ER, where she was prescribed anti-nausea pills. The vertigo prevented her from walking normally and she staggered around like a drunk. Ataxia, or unbalanced, uncoordinated walking, has been documented in severe hypothyroidism.[36] Because Jane was not having a vertigo episode when she saw her primary care physician (PCP) 10 days later, he declared her fine and scheduled her for another routine visit in three months. He dismissed her thyroid as a cause of any of her symptoms, but did ask if she wanted a flu shot, noted her blood pressure was fine, and thought her vertigo probably wasn't anything serious. When Jane asked if maybe her low thyroid levels were causing her dementia and inability to remember things, she was told that the thyroid had nothing to do with brain function, that her last thyroid tests were normal, and that everyone eventually becomes demented. After all, we lose 100,000 brain cells every day. That adds up over time, and he pointed out that she was 85 years old. Her Total T3 in January was 84 (80-200), or 3% in the reference range. Both hyper and hypothyroidism are known causes of reversible dementia.[37]

Jane left with no change in her thyroid dosage, but another order for more lab work. As expected, her thyroid hormone levels were low, and her Free T3 could be considered dangerously low, since it's 22% below the reference range, as shown in Figure 3-6. Her iron panel, ferritin, and Vitamin B12 are all at good levels. Cortisol, however, is also at the very bottom of the reference range at 7.7 ug/dL (6.0-25.0). Surprisingly, her sodium and potassium are fairly balanced; adrenal insufficiency (which could cause nausea and vomiting) would show as low sodium and high potassium. Her primary care physician does not prescribe thyroid hormone and prefers that an endocrinologist manage that part of her healthcare, so Jane decided to look for another endocrinologist.

Jane has her first appointment with a new endocrinologist in October 2011. Dr. Beta asks Jane a few questions, and then runs the typical thyroid labs. Her TSH is below the reference range at 0.14 uIU/mL (0.27-4.2), so the doctor considers her hyperthyroid, or overmedicated. This is in spite of the fact that her Free T3 tested at 0% of the reference range. She makes no change to Jane's prescription and schedules more lab work in a few weeks, even though Jane now has two sets of lab work, a month apart, that confirm she is dangerously low (below the reference range) in T3.

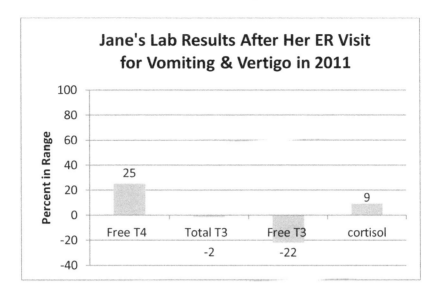

Figure 3-6. Jane's lab results after her ER visit for vomiting and vertigo show that she is dangerously low on hormones. Both her Free and Total T3 are below the reference range, which qualifies her as having the low T3 syndrome, which is a very unhealthy state. Cortisol is also at a low, unhealthy level.

Because Dr. Beta did not give Jane any more T4 or T3, she started taking Vitamin C,[38] Vitamin D,[39] and selenium,[40] since those are known to help with cortisol, autoimmunity, and thyroid hormone conversion from T4 to T3. With no change in dose, it looks like the supplements did have some positive effect on the T4 to T3 conversion (see Figure 3-7), because the next lab tests show her Total T3 and Free T3 have improved slightly, but are still too low to be considered healthy for most people.

When Dr. Beta heard that Jane was taking Vitamin C, Vitamin D, and selenium, she said it was causing her labs to be inaccurate, and that she should stop the supplements so she could be retested. Jane didn't want to be disagreeable, so she stopped the supplements. As expected, her thyroid levels dropped again, as shown in Figure 3-7. Keep in mind that throughout this entire time, Jane is having periodic episodes of vertigo, dizziness, and vomiting. She is a prisoner in her own home, because she's afraid to go out, lest she have another episode. People who have never experienced vertigo don't understand how debilitating it is.

On Jane's third visit with Dr. Beta, she is no longer taking any supplements, but her TSH is still suppressed. When Jane asks to try some form of T3, be it desiccated thyroid or Cytomel, Dr. Beta tells her that her TSH is too low, and that she would only consider giving her T3 if her TSH was in the normal range. In fact, because of Jane's low TSH, which can be a hyperthyroid indicator, Dr. Beta deduces that Jane is on too much medication and lowers Jane's T4 dose from 88 mcg to 75 mcg! From her point of view, the TSH is the only value that matters, even though TSH is a *pituitary* hormone, and does not in any way give the body the energy that *thyroid* hormone supplies. T3 and T4 are the actual thyroid hormones, and those are the only levels that should count when determining a patient's dose. As Jane's case illustrates, one can have very little TSH and be dangerously hypothyroid, the complete opposite of what would be expected.

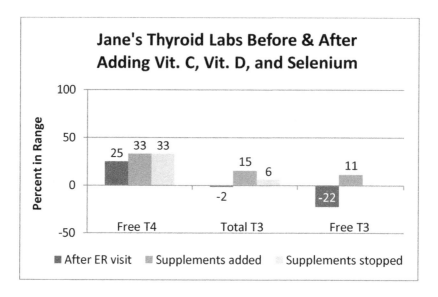

Figure 3-7. The addition of Vitamin C, Vitamin D, and selenium have a positive effect on Jane's Total and Free T3 levels with no change in actual thyroid medication dose.

Miraculously, Jane manages to survive on barely any thyroid hormone, and continues to have periodic episodes of nausea, dizziness, vertigo, and vomiting. These symptoms have been documented in others who were severely hypothyroid.[41] None of her doctors believe that low thyroid levels could be causing her symptoms and order tests to check for other possible causes of her vertigo. Dr. Beta orders an MRI of her brain and internal auditory canals (normal), and her primary physician orders an abdominal ultrasound (normal gallbladder, liver, pancreas, kidney, spleen) and an upper gastrointestinal series (normal esophagus, stomach, and duodenum, no reflux). There is even a referral to a cardiologist for a stress test, but Jane felt she was too dizzy and nauseous to complete the test, so it was never performed. Instead, her heart was monitored for 24 hours. Jane does not return to Dr. Beta, and instead, finds a new doctor in January 2012, a gerontologist, to see if her symptoms are due to her old age. Two of her fingernails have no curvature and are flattened out. Scoop fingernails (koilonychia) can be a hypothyroid indicator.[42] Her hands and heels are so dry the skin cracks. And she bounced another check. Her doctors refuse to see the enormous elephant in the room!

In February 2012 she had another bad episode of vomiting and a test of her cortisol levels came back high and over the reference range. When her cortisol levels were tested just a few months ago, after the ER visit, her cortisol was near the bottom of the reference range. That would imply adrenal insufficiency, but this current lab result refutes that diagnosis. ACTH was also tested and came back at the bottom of the reference range at 7 (6-58). Remember that Jane's blood pressure medication, Verapamil, is known to inhibit ACTH, but no one has put that particular piece of the puzzle together yet.

Between February and March, Jane had regular dizzy/vomiting episodes, sometimes as many as three in a week; the episodes were increasing in frequency and becoming debilitating. I had suggested to Jane that she badly needed some T3, but she didn't know how to get any doctor to prescribe it for her. Her cardiologist mentioned that Jane's last endocrinologist (before Dr. Beta) was actually a nice, decent man, and may be more open to trying alternatives. Had she tried asking Dr. Alpha to prescribe T3? She had, but he had dismissed the idea. Because he had been dosing her by TSH all these years, which probably contributed to her decline in health, she had looked for another endocrinologist but only ended up wasting time with Dr. Beta. Jane decided she might as well give Dr. Alpha, her last endocrinologist, another try.

In March 2012, Jane returned to Dr. Alpha and told him she was desperate, and wanted to try an alternative like pig (desiccated) thyroid because she obviously needed something more than the Synthroid she was on—the vertigo and vomiting had become chronic and she couldn't function anymore. Dr. Alpha felt that her problems were due to old age and that dizziness was not considered dangerous. Seriously? Jane was extremely fortunate she never had an attack while driving and didn't injure herself or anyone else. She was also lucky she didn't injure herself at home, because during an attack, it is difficult to walk without bumping into walls. He also told her that Armour Thyroid is not always consistent, so he doesn't prescribe it. When Jane visited Dr. Alpha, her TSH was .18 uIU/mL; this is below the reference range and could indicate that she is on too much medication. But since she was desperate, he prescribed her 5 mcg of Cytomel (synthetic T3) in addition to her 75 mcg Synthroid, in spite of her low TSH.

Only five days later, Jane wrote in an email:

> *I was able to accomplish a lot today after being useless for almost 10 months. Now I can get my papers and house in order. It's like a pig sty here. I had never heard of Cytomel. I think he prescribed it because I asked if he would prescribe Armour and I was desperate to try any alternative med. He told me he wouldn't prescribe Armour because it was not reliable and told me to try Cytomel maybe as a supplement to the Synthroid which he reduced to 75 mcg from 88 mcg. I asked him if he knew about Erfa and he said he didn't. I know the supplements made changes in the lab tests but toward the end it didn't help because I got dizzy and vomited on a regular basis every week. This is what I don't understand. Maybe he prescribed it as a supplement to Synthroid and because it is a thyroid medication. Did he test me for T3? Perhaps he was willing to try any other thyroid medication since I told him I was desperate to try something and told him after all the tests, they couldn't find anything wrong with me. He mentioned that the only test I didn't get was from a neurologist.*

Jane felt better and went in for routine lab work in April to see the effects of the new dosage. Her T3 was coming up nicely, but unfortunately, her TSH was now even lower at < 0.07, which concerned her endocrinologist.

Jane wrote:

> *I have a choice of staying as is or go back to 88 mcg Synthroid and drop*
> *Cytomel because I am now overdosed. My good days on Cytomel were*
> *much more "normal" than those that preceded Cytomel and since the pills*
> *are so expensive and I still have lots left, I might as well give it a longer*
> *trial period. He told me I could go for a third opinion but that's a waste of*
> *time. The quality of life in the good days on Cytomel is much better because*
> *I regain my sense of taste and can work to get things done.*

Even though Jane's T4 and T3 levels were in the bottom half of the reference range, her endocrinologist is declaring her overmedicated and recommending that she drop the Cytomel because of her low TSH. He is following the TSH rule that he was taught. Jane chose to stay with the 75 mcg T4 + 5 mcg T3, and yet her next set of labs in July are dismal. I'm not sure if her body adapted to and used up the 5 mcg Cytomel, or if it was from the additional stress of visiting out-of-town family members and activities during that time period. It's even possible that those particular labs were drawn *before* she took her daily medication, while the other results were taken shortly *after* her morning dose. Jane doesn't remember. In any case, even with her very low thyroid levels in July, her TSH was still < 0.07 uIU/mL. I knew her endocrinologist would want to lower her dose based on that TSH, so I pointed out that Jane hasn't had any TSH for the last five years and really shouldn't be dosed by TSH. When Dr. Alpha looked at her actual T4 and T3 levels, he agreed to raise her dose to 88 mcg T4 + 10 mcg T3.

Jane was grateful that she would finally be getting more medication and that she might feel better soon. But when she tried to raise her T4 dose from 75 mcg to 88 mcg, the vertigo episodes increased. She hadn't even raised the additional 5 mcg of Cytomel yet, because that was raised by a third of a pill at a time. She was clearly not overmedicated: her blood pressure was 110/60 and her pulse 64. So she returned to her dose of 75 mcg, and raised slowly, by adding in an 88 mcg pill every 7 days, then every 6 days, etc., until she had switched completely over to 88 mcg every day. She also slowly raised the Cytomel, by cutting the 5 mcg pill into thirds and then only adding 1/3 pill at a time for a few days, before adding another 1/3 pill.

Jane still had intermittent dizzy, vertigo, and vomiting spells in July while she was ramping up her thyroid dose. In August, after she reached the new dosage of 88 mcg T4 and 10 mcg T3 daily (two 5 mcg Cytomels), she reported that her muscle tone had improved and she no longer felt so dehydrated. She noted that she has had a sweet tooth for the past year, and wondered if that meant anything. Hypoglycemia, or low blood sugar, can be caused by low cortisol levels.[43] Cortisol is the hormone that keeps blood sugar stable; if cortisol is low, someone will feel the need to eat all the time, especially sweets. ACTH is the pituitary hormone that stimulates cortisol production, and Verapamil, her blood pressure medication, is known to inhibit ACTH.

She had vertigo twice in August 2012 and another vomiting episode in September, so something was still not right. Low thyroid is a documented cause of some of her symptoms, like vomiting, vertigo, and dizziness (I've had all of them too), but now that she is taking some T3 and more T4, it seemed like we were still missing something. I looked up Verapamil and found it inhibits ACTH and cortisol secretion. Everything finally made sense. The Verapamil had been suppressing her natural cortisol function, which is why she had such a hard time raising from 75 to 88 mcg T4. Verapamil was inducing a form of secondary borderline adrenal insufficiency (insufficient ACTH stimulation from the pituitary resulting in insufficient cortisol), which was compounded by a form of primary borderline adrenal insufficiency (insufficient cortisol output from the adrenal gland) caused by a natural downregulation of adrenal function because she was so hypothyroid. The adrenal cortex (where cortisol is made in the adrenal gland) shrinks in animals that are made hypothyroid by thyroidectomy or anti-thyroid drugs.[44]

- Her morning ACTH result on 2/17/12 was 7 pg/mL (6-58) or 2% in range

- Her morning cortisol result on 9/27/11 was 7.7 ug/dL (6-25) or 9% in range

Cortisol must be adequate when adding or raising levothyroxine because thyroid hormone raises cortisol clearance rates, and if cortisol goes too low, it can trigger an adrenal crisis, where the patient would lose consciousness.[45] In serious cases, it could be fatal.[46]

In September 2012, Jane convinced her gerontologist to lower her Verapamil dose from 360 mg to 240 mg and the dizziness stopped. She wrote:

> Started 240 mg last night and didn't get dizzy today. Managed to get a lot of work done and my mouth doesn't get dried up at night, and bowel movement is back to natural. I hope this keeps up and we found out exactly what is wrong.
>
> Irony is that at the end of 2010 I sensed my pressure pill was too high so my endo told me to buy a blood pressure machine and keep a record. He reduced my pill from 360 to 240 and I was fine. Went for my physical and my primary care physician was alarmed and upset that it had been lowered, saying even he has to have 360 mg, so raised it and I just gave in. Six months later in June of 2011 I had my first vertigo attack. You know the rest of the story. I hope we've solved my problem.

There is something terribly wrong with Jane's last correspondence. Her doctor raised her blood pressure medication based on *his* dosage. How is that logical? Jane is 4'10" and barely weighs 100 pounds. Could the Verapamil be affecting her doctor too?

In October 2012, the vertigo returned, milder, and she threw up again. The logical next step was to continue lowering her Verapamil dosage, and her gerontologist again lowered it from 240 mg to 120 mg.

Jane wrote:

> Thyroid affects personality and I'm in a "fight with everybody" stage. I fought with colleagues and even made one cry before I was first diagnosed years ago. My medication makes me very nasty in my dealing with people. I've lost a number of friends this way over the years. Sometimes people take things the wrong way—not what I intended.

Reading the above, I suggested that maybe her T3 dose was too high, and perhaps a reduction in T3 and raise in T4 might work better. High thyroid levels are known to cause irritability, quarrelsomeness, impatience, and sometimes, an explosive rage.[47] This can be observed, firsthand, in a few thyroid patients who leave furious comments on websites with thyroid articles that they do not agree with. Many of these patients maintain their Free T3 levels above the reference range, and their posts are angry, often written in all caps. There is sometimes a hysterical, screaming, condescending tone to their posts, as if what they think is 100% *right*, and the article is 100% *wrong*. It has been my experience that one cannot even start a rational discussion with someone in this frenzied state, and Jane's comments confirm that.

Jane had also mentioned that her short-term memory had disappeared; she might lay something down one minute, and then not recall where she'd laid it the next. Memory can also be negatively impacted by too much thyroid hormone; it results in hyperthyroid dementia.[48]

Unfortunately, Jane's endocrinologist was out-of-town, so no changes were made to her thyroid medications, and she continued to take 88 mcg T4 + 10 mcg T3. However, the reduction in her blood pressure medication was the right move. She reported feeling better, having more energy, and accomplishing more. She finally had enough energy to clean her house, organize the important papers, and toss out some of the junk. She felt more normal and wasn't afraid to go out.

In November 2012, Jane wrote:

> *Not having to cope with vertigo and vomiting takes a load off my mind. I suddenly feel like I've been freed from a terrible ordeal. I'm feeling more normal now and not afraid to go out or travel by myself. I'm almost certain now that I was overmedicated for my blood pressure. Imagine I dropped from 360 to 240 to 120mg. I lost over a year of my life. I haven't had an attack of vertigo, dizziness, nausea and vomiting for a while.*

Later that November, Jane wrote:

> *Happy Thanksgiving! I'm so happy, I'm not dizzy and vomiting anymore! Hope I'm not rejoicing too soon.*

In December, she realized she had indeed rejoiced too soon. Although she hadn't been dizzy for a month and a half, she sometimes felt tired and decrepit. Her blood pressure remained the same even though the dose had been lowered considerably. She went shopping at her local drug store one day, and her worst fears came true. She got dizzy in the store, took an anti-nausea pill, but it didn't help. She went to a corner of the store away from customers, hoping things would improve, but they only got worse and she started vomiting. She realized she couldn't drive home, and had to ask a stranger to call her son to take her home. Still, at two months, this had been the longest stretch between vomiting episodes, which had been as frequent as every other day at one point.

After this episode, Jane reported napping regularly every day because she felt so tired. I knew that being overmedicated can cause tiredness[49] as much as being undermedicated. Also, the fact that she had another vomiting episode probably meant that her cortisol was still too low, and too much thyroid hormone will lower cortisol. Vomiting is a symptom of Addison's disease, where there is little to no cortisol. Cortisol keeps blood sugar stable, and prevents hypoglycemia. When Jane confirmed that this last vomiting episode happened around lunchtime, when her stomach was empty, I knew she needed to lower her T3 dosage. Her doctor agreed to change her dosage from 88 mcg T4 + 10 mcg T3, to 100 mcg T4 + 5 mcg T3.

Jane started the new dosage in mid-December. In January 2013, she reported that her energy level was improving. In fact, she is starting her garden all over again; she loves her fresh peas and tomatoes. She is also actively helping out with some legal issues in the family business, which she had basically dropped out of, when her health became so poor.

After about a month on this new dosage, she reports:

> *Anyway, I'm not dizzy or vomiting anymore, my walking is more stable, and in the whole process, my stool went from a 1 to a 3 [hard pellets to a sausage on the Bristol stool scale] which is perfectly normal now. I had noticed the change in my stool and also skin tension. I had horrible sagging skin under my jaw and now it tightened up and isn't so bad. So physically I am aware of improvements probably due to my metabolism, but it is good to read articles that clarify my observations. Most people think I am 80 and surprised to learn I am 86 and can still walk. By the way, my balance in walking has improved remarkably. I used to be very unsteady. I think we're on the right track.*

In mid-January, new labs were run to see where her levels were on her new dose. She took her thyroid medication that morning, as the nurse instructed, before heading to the lab for the blood draw. As shown in Figure 3-8, her Free T3 tested above the reference range at 128%, even though her Total T3 was within the reference range. Free T3 levels are known to spike after taking any medication with T3 (including desiccated thyroid),[50] and because her blood was drawn within hours of her Cytomel dose, this spike is reflected in her lab results. Because of her very high Free T3 and a TSH < .07 uIU/mL, her endocrinologist told her that she could continue at her current dose of 100 mcg T4 + 5 mcg T3, but that she may eventually develop heart problems, which could lead to a stroke. He said she could continue to feel normal on this dosage, but that is the choice she has to make. I asked Jane about some of her current symptoms and she wrote:

> *My heels used to be real dry but they are fine now. I used to wonder why they were so bad. My stool is fine. My skin doesn't sag so much. My pulse rate is usually in the 70's and 80's, but I'm getting some high blood pressure readings that taper down by noon.*

Jane certainly didn't want a stroke, so she stopped the Cytomel, which meant she was back to 100 mcg T4, her original dose 30 years ago, which she claims she had felt fine on for years until she started taking Actonel, the osteoporosis drug.

In addition to the thyroid labs, two additional tests were run: an FSH (Follicle Stimulating Hormone) came back high and over the reference range, which is expected in post-menopausal women, which Jane is. My guess is that her endocrinologist was checking to see if she had any pituitary function at all, because her TSH, another pituitary hormone, is almost non-existent. The high FSH levels suggest that she does have a working pituitary. Her doctor had already checked her FSH in 2008, and it was high and over the reference range back then too.

The second hormone tested was morning cortisol, which tested at 17.9 (6.0-25.0 ug/dl), or 63% in the reference range. The last time her cortisol had been tested was shortly after her ER visit when she was throwing up and unable to walk normally. It measured 9% in the reference range then. The current cortisol level is much better and the lowering of her Verapamil dose (which lowers cortisol) appears to have been the right move.

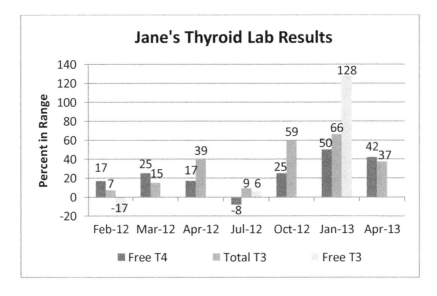

Figure 3-8. The addition of Cytomel starting in March 2012 brought Jane's T3 levels up.

In late January Jane wrote:

> *By the way, I couldn't do a tai chi balancing on one foot and was surprised I could do it again now. I guess thyroid affects your balance too.*

February 2013:

> *Lowering my blood pressure med and increasing my thyroid med has done wonders for me. Haven't had an attack for almost 2 months. If it goes beyond that I can safely say we finally got it diagnosed. I feel free to go out again instead of being jailed at home.*

By the end of February, about a month after dropping the 5 mcg of T3, Jane started getting high blood pressure readings, such as 177/116 mmHg. Both low and high thyroid levels can cause high blood pressure.[51] When the diastolic (bottom) number becomes high, that is a sign that thyroid levels are too low. In fact, there's an inverse relationship between T3 levels and diastolic dysfunction. The lower the T3 levels, the more severe the diastolic dysfunction and higher the B-type natriuretic peptide (BNP) levels (a marker of heart failure).[52]

The next day (February 26, 2013):

Guess what? After almost 3 months without a dizzy spell, I got a violent case of vertigo, nausea, vomiting and diarrhea at about 6:30 this evening. It was like the first attack I had. I was so sick it is amazing that I could still manage by myself. It went on for more than an hour. I was so miserable. But fortunately when it is over I am ok till the next episode.

My gerontologist said I don't need any tests, can't remember whether I told you or not. I think I'll have these episodes till the day I die. It is something I am going to have to live with.

Just took my blood pressure and it was like the other day. Top and bottom numbers are high again.

Since Jane had no vertigo episodes while taking Cytomel, but they restarted after she stopped the Cytomel, Jane went back to her 5 mcg of Cytomel, but split the pill, taking half in the morning after breakfast, and the remaining half after dinner. Five days later, she had a visit with her gerontologist:

Saw him today and he said my blood pressure readings were not a problem and accepted the fact that I needed T3 since I got sick a month after I stopped Cytomel. He sorta feels like I do that if I go past 4 months without an attack that essentially the problem has been solved since I am essentially back to normal and don't have to be escorted to the doctor's office like I used to. I'm able to get around on my own. It was a very routine visit. Do many people have the same problem I have? Why isn't it accepted as a thyroid problem? My case alone proves T3 is a problem for some, why isn't it accepted?

A few days later:

You told me to ask for testing T3 years ago but my endocrinologists simply dismissed it. You even gave me a paper for them to read. So I had to go through all the tests to prove that there was nothing wrong with me and then asked for an alternative med. I wasted time, money and exposure to all kinds of x-rays and more than 1-1/2 years of suffering before I got the test and alternative med. My energy level is very good now and I've proven I think beyond a shadow of a doubt that I really need T3.

Late March 2013:

> *Before I couldn't sleep at night and now I sleep ok but I am so tired during
> the day I have to take a nap and can't seem to get started on my taxes.
> Blood pressure is ok. Why am I so tired now? It may be just old age cause
> I walk like all the old ladies now. My short term memory is really horrible.*

In April, Jane had another set of thyroid labs run. Because her TSH was still suppressed at < .07 uIU/mL, her endocrinologist again recommended cutting her dose, in spite of the fact that her Free T4 was only 42% in the reference range, and her Total T3 was 37% in the reference range. Jane knew that she needed her T3, which meant the only thing she could consider lowering was her Synthroid dosage of 100 mcg. Her Free T4 tested at 1.4 ng/dL, which is a value many believe to be optimal. But given that Jane had complained about being tired lately, had memory problems, and was having trouble formulating sentences when she called me, it seemed that it might be worth trying out a slightly lower dose, as a trial. Fatigue, memory problems, and cognitive problems can be signs of overmedication.[53] So she dropped her T4 down to 88 mcg. The next time I talked to her she did seem more coherent, so it appears that 88 mcg T4 + 5 mcg T3 is a better dose for her.

Due to another vomiting and vertigo episode later in the year, Jane added just 2.5 mcg more T3 to her dose, so that she took 88 mcg once in the morning, plus 2.5 mcg T3 before breakfast, in the afternoon, and at bedtime. This appears to be the best dose for her so far, and she was fine for a solid three months with no attacks. Then, for whatever reason, her Cytomel was changed to generic liothyronine. A month after the change she had another vomiting and vertigo episode. When she felt sick for two days in a row, she had her prescription changed back to Cytomel and the episodes stopped. This highlights an important point—that some generics don't work as well as the name brands for some patients. Finding the optimal dose means not only trying out different doses, but different brands of thyroid hormones.

Conclusion

Jane's case shows how difficult it is to find an optimal dose, since TSH can't be used as a guideline. Her endocrinologist runs a Total or Free T3, but references ranges are so broad that it's hard to say what dose is appropriate for Jane without looking at other signs and symptoms. Jane has now joined many other thyroid patients who insist that T3 *must* be a part of their daily thyroid medication. For her, just 5 mcg of T3 made the difference between being incapacitated with vertigo and vomiting, to being functional and productive.

Jane has been undermedicated on thyroid hormone for many years and has suffered greatly, all because of the TSH rule that declares a patient overmedicated if their TSH is too low, and because T3 was considered unnecessary. Glomerular filtration rate (kidney function) and carbon dioxide levels (respiration rate) are standard tests in a comprehensive metabolic panel. They were both flagged for being outside of the reference range (low GFR and high CO_2) and suggest severe hypothyroidism, yet they were never addressed. It may be that no one knows the correlation of these values to low thyroid hormone levels. High cholesterol is another marker for low thyroid levels and was also ignored; this inverse relationship was recognized almost a century ago. Where did this knowledge go? A study published in 1939 analyzed cholesterol levels before and after desiccated thyroid hormone treatment in 29 hypothyroid patients. Cholesterol levels decreased in 100% of the cases. A 100% trend in a variable is a very clear case of cause and effect. In some cases, cholesterol levels dropped more than 50% after taking 1-2 grains of desiccated thyroid. One patient's cholesterol dropped from 680 mg/dL to 336 on only 1 grain. When thyroid hormone was stopped in four patients, their cholesterol started rising again, confirming the inverse relationship between thyroid hormone and cholesterol.[54] Some people have high cholesterol because they have a thyroid hormone deficiency; no one really has a statin deficiency.

The effect of various pharmaceutical drugs on thyroid and other related hormones was also not understood by the prescribing doctors. Both Actonel (a bisphosphonate osteoporosis drug) and Verapamil (a calcium channel blocker blood pressure medication) somehow interfered with Jane's thyroid hormone dose and started a downward spiral of side effects, because no one was aware of any possible interaction. Unfortunately, this may be more common than anyone would like to admit, and patients may have to become responsible for checking into these interactions themselves. Even more disturbing, however, is the fact that all the drugs prescribed were for ailments that can be *caused* by low thyroid levels. As stated earlier, high cholesterol, high blood pressure, and even osteoporosis[55] can be caused by low thyroid levels, especially insufficient T3. Jane may not have needed these drugs if she had just been prescribed some T3 in the first place.

When Jane's vertigo and vomiting became chronic, none of her doctors believed her low thyroid levels could be involved, even though lab tests flagged her Free T3 levels as below the reference range. Instead, she was sent for multiple tests which were paid for by Medicare and her secondary insurance, and she was subjected to multiple x-rays and injected with dyes. Her health care insurance summary for 2011 (when her vertigo began) lists charges to a rheumatologist, ER, pathologist, gastroenterologist, surgeon, cardiologist, radiologist, ophthalmologist, otolaryngologist, endocrinologist, primary care physician, hospital outpatient services, and audiologist. She added a gerontologist and physical therapist in 2012. Procedures performed were an upper GI endoscopy biopsy, upper GI contrast x-ray, drain joint/bursa, EKG, brain CT, brain MRI, ear microscopy exam, hearing test, echo exam of abdomen, and EKG with Doppler. None of the results of these medical tests resulted in a change in her thyroid treatment. She was only able to try a small dose of T3 because she begged her endocrinologist for it. The rationale for adding T3 was already there, in a simple blood test that had been performed *before* any of these additional tests were ordered.

Jane is fortunate that her medical bills have been covered by Medicare and her secondary insurance, so her out-of-pocket costs are minimal. Still, the costs to her insurance companies are nothing to sneeze at, and the ER visit alone is billed at over $5,000, though that is probably quite a bit more than what was actually paid by the insurance companies. Health care costs are said to be spiraling out of control, and yet, Jane's case illustrates that some of these costs were unnecessary, and were caused by undertreated hypothyroidism. How much does one prescription for Cytomel (T3) or desiccated thyroid cost compared to the numerous tests and office visits with all the specialists? The current treatment paradigm for thyroid hormone replacement leaves much to be desired; dosing by TSH simply does not work and many medical dollars could be saved if this erroneous paradigm were overturned.

Key points

- Low thyroid levels can cause heart abnormalities, a slow heart rate, and fainting.
- Salt craving may be a sign of hypothyroidism.
- Autoimmune diseases tend to run in families.
- Actonel, a bisphosphonate for osteopenia, may cause hypothyroid side effects.
- TSH stimulates T4 to T3 conversion; likewise, lack of TSH will limit conversion.
- Being low in thyroid hormone may feel identical to being high in thyroid hormone because excess norepinephrine is secreted when hypothyroid.
- High cholesterol is a sign of low thyroid levels.
- Statins may cause nosebleeds, leg weakness, frozen joints, visual problems, and dementia.
- Calcium channel blocker blood pressure medications may not be the right choice for thyroid patients, because they lower cortisol.
- Food intake negatively affects T4 absorption.
- ACE inhibitor blood pressure medications may cause a chronic cough in some patients along with a loss of taste.
- Bisphosphonates like Actonel can negatively impact vision.
- Surgery can induce the low-T3 syndrome and cause temporary cognitive dysfunction.
- TSH is not a good indicator of healthy thyroid levels. Low GFR, high cholesterol, and high CO_2 may be caused by low thyroid levels.
- Subclinical hyperthyroidism, or a suppressed TSH with normal T4 and T3 levels, may be temporary and usually does not lead to true hyperthyroidism. Many patients just have a subnormal TSH, but others later test with a normal TSH.
- TSH levels fluctuate daily and seasonally.
- Pharmaceutical drugs may interfere with any stage of thyroid production. Calcium channel blockers may inhibit TRH which inhibits TSH which inhibits thyroid hormone production and T4 to T3 conversion.
- In Jane's case, FT4 and Total T3 show no correlation whatsoever to her TSH. Her TSH has been suppressed while her FT4 has always been in the lower half of the reference range.
- Lowering Jane's thyroid medication did not raise her TSH, but did make her feel worse.
- Unbalanced, uncoordinated walking has been seen in severe hypothyroidism.
- Both hyper and hypothyroidism can cause reversible dementia.
- Vitamin C supports the adrenal glands which produce cortisol, Vitamin D is beneficial against autoimmunity and cancer, and selenium helps T4 to T3 conversion.

- Nausea, dizziness, vertigo, and vomiting have been documented in severely hypothyroid patients.
- Flat, scoop-like fingernails (koilonychia) can be a sign of hypothyroidism.
- A sweet tooth may be a sign of hypoglycemia, which can be caused by low cortisol.
- Thyroid hormone raises cortisol clearance, so too much thyroid hormone may result in low cortisol.
- High thyroid levels may cause irritability, quarrelsomeness, impatience, and sometimes, an explosive rage.
- Memory can be affected by too much thyroid hormone; it can cause hyperthyroid dementia.
- Tiredness is a symptom of both under and overmedication on thyroid hormone.
- Bowel movements reflect thyroid levels: constipation and hard pellets are signs of hypothyroidism, diarrhea a sign of hyperthyroidism. A healthy bowel movement exits in a sausage shape.
- High blood pressure, especially a high diastolic (bottom) number, may be a sign of hypothyroidism.

---

[1] Trachtenberg, Eduardo, et al. "Hypothyroidism and severe neuropsychiatric symptoms: a rapid response to levothyroxine." *Revista Brasileira de Psiquiatria* 34.4 (2012): 501-502.

[2] Schoenmakers, N., W. E. De Graaff, and R. H. J. Peters. "Hypothyroidism as the cause of atrioventricular block in an elderly patient." *Netherlands Heart Journal* 16.2 (2008): 57-59.

[3] Liamis, George, Haralampos J. Milionis, and Moses Elisaf. "Endocrine disorders: causes of hyponatremia not to neglect." *Annals of medicine* 43.3 (2011): 179-187.

[4] Tomer, Yaron. "Genetic susceptibility to autoimmune thyroid disease: past, present, and future." *Thyroid* 20.7 (2010): 715-725.

[5] Huang, Jian-bo, et al. "Chemosensitization role of endocrine hormones in cancer chemotherapy." *Chinese Medical Journal* 126.1 (2013): 176.

[6] Derry, David. "Breast Cancer and Iodine : How to Prevent and How to Survive Breast Cancer." Trafford Publishing, 2001.

[7] Fraunfelder, FW Rick. "Keep Alert for These Drug-Related Adverse Effects." Ophthalmology Management. October 2011.

[8] Ikeda, Tadasu, et al. "Effect of thyrotropin on conversion of T4 to T3 in perfused rat liver." *Life sciences* 38.20 (1986): 1801-1806.

[9] Wysowski, Diane K. "Reports of esophageal cancer with oral bisphosphonate use." *New England Journal of Medicine* 360.1 (2009): 89-90.

[10] Coulombe, Pierre, Jean H. Dussault, and Peter Walker. "Catecholamine metabolism in thyroid disease. II. Norepinephrine secretion rate in hyperthyroidism and hypothyroidism." *Journal of Clinical Endocrinology & Metabolism* 44.6 (1977): 1185-1189.

[11] Mills, I., et al. "Effect of thyroid status on catecholamine stimulation of thyroxine 5'-deiodinase in brown adipocytes." *American Journal of Physiology-Endocrinology And Metabolism* 256.1 (1989): E74-E79.

[12] Tan, Zaldy S., and Ramachandran S. Vasan. "Thyroid function and Alzheimer's disease." *Journal of Alzheimer's Disease* 16.3 (2009): 503-507.

[13] DeMartino, G. N., and A. L. Goldberg. "A possible explanation of myxedema and hypercholesterolemia in hypothyroidism: control of lysosomal hyaluronidase and cholesterol esterase by thyroid hormones." *Enzyme* 26.1 (1981): 1.

[14] Rodine, Robert J., et al. "Statin induced myopathy presenting as mechanical musculoskeletal pain observed in two chiropractic patients." *The Journal of the Canadian Chiropractic Association* 54.1 (2010): 43.

[15] Evans, Marcella A., and Beatrice A. Golomb. "Statin-Associated Adverse Cognitive Effects: Survey Results from 171 Patients." *Pharmacotherapy: The Journal of Human Pharmacology and Drug Therapy* 29.7 (2009): 800-811.

[16] Lando, Howard M., and Kenneth D. Burman. "Two cases of statin-induced myopathy caused by induced hypothyroidism." *Endocrine Practice* 14.6 (2008): 726-731.

[17] Fommei, Enza, and Giorgio Iervasi. "The role of thyroid hormone in blood pressure homeostasis: evidence from short-term hypothyroidism in humans." *Journal of Clinical Endocrinology & Metabolism* 87.5 (2002): 1996-2000.

[18] Davies, Eleanor, C. J. Kenyon, and R. Fraser. "The role of calcium ions in the mechanism of ACTH stimulation of cortisol synthesis." *Steroids* 45.6 (1985): 551-560.

[19] Kumari, Meena, et al. "Cortisol secretion and fatigue: associations in a community based cohort." *Psychoneuroendocrinology* 34.10 (2009): 1476-1485.

[20] Antonios, Tarek FT, and Graham A. MacGregor. "Angiotensin converting enzyme inhibitors in hypertension: potential problems." *Journal of Hypertension* 13 (1995): S11.

[21] Bach-Huynh, Thien-Giang, et al. "Timing of levothyroxine administration affects serum thyrotropin concentration." *Journal of Clinical Endocrinology & Metabolism* 94.10 (2009): 3905-3912.

[22] Karl, Michael, et al. "Hypocortisolemia in Graves hyperthyroidism." *Endocrine Practice* 15.3 (2009): 220-224.

[23] Kubo, Shin-ichi, et al. "Isolated Adrenocorticotropic Hormone Deficiency: An Autopsy Case of Adrenal Crisis: A Case Report." *The American journal of forensic medicine and pathology* 18.2 (1997): 202-205.

[24] Fraunfelder, FW Rick, and FT Fritz Fraunfelder. "American Academy of Ophthalmology Course Title: Drug-Related Adverse Effects of Clinical Importance to the Ophthalmologist November 2012." (2012).

[25] Mafrica, Federica, and Vincenzo Fodale. "Thyroid function, Alzheimer's disease and postoperative cognitive dysfunction: a tale of dangerous liaisons?" *Journal of Alzheimer's Disease* 14.1 (2008): 95-105.

[26] Lo, Joan C., et al. "Increased prevalence of subclinical and clinical hypothyroidism in persons with chronic kidney disease." *Kidney international* 67.3 (2005): 1047-1052.

[27] Ladenson, Paul W., Paul D. Goldenheim, and E. Chester Ridgway. "Prediction and reversal of blunted ventilatory responsiveness in patients with hypothyroidism." *The American journal of medicine* 84.5 (1988): 877-883.

[28] Abrams, Jeffrey J., and S. M. Grundy. "Cholesterol metabolism in hypothyroidism and hyperthyroidism in man." *Journal of lipid research* 22.2 (1981): 323-338.

[29] Mathew, Vivek, et al. "Myxedema coma: a new look into an old crisis." *Journal of thyroid research* 2011 (2011).

[30] Vadiveloo, Thenmalar, et al. "The Thyroid Epidemiology, Audit, and Research Study (TEARS): the natural history of endogenous subclinical hyperthyroidism." *Journal of Clinical Endocrinology & Metabolism* 96.1 (2011): E1-E8.

[31] Sviridonova, Marina A., et al. "Clinical Significance of TSH Circadian Variability in Patients with Hypothyroidism." *Endocrine Research* 38.1 (2013): 24-31.

32 Maes, M., et al. "Components of biological variation, including seasonality, in blood concentrations of TSH, TT3, FT4, PRL, cortisol and testosterone in healthy volunteers." *Clinical endocrinology* 46.5 (1997): 587-598.

33 Sawin, Clark T., et al. "Low serum thyrotropin (thyroid-stimulating hormone) in older persons without hyperthyroidism." *Archives of internal medicine* 151.1 (1991): 165.

34 Geras, Elizabeth, Mario J. Rebecchi, And Marvin C. Gershengorn. "Evidence that stimulation of thyrotropin and prolactin secretion by thyrotropin-releasing hormone occur via different calcium-mediated mechanisms: studies with verapamil." *Endocrinology* 110.3 (1982): 901-906.

35 Abrahamson, Martin J., Patricia J. Wormald, and Robert P. Millar. "Neuroendocrine regulation of thyrotropin release in cultured human pituitary cells." *Journal of Clinical Endocrinology & Metabolism* 65.6 (1987): 1159-1163.

36 Madi, Deepak, Basavaprabhu Achappa, and Abhishek Gupta. "Doctor I Am Swaying-An Interesting Case of Ataxia." *Journal of Clinical and Diagnostic Research* (2012): 1.

37 Ghosh, Amitabha. "Endocrine, metabolic, nutritional, and toxic disorders leading to dementia." *Annals of Indian Academy of Neurology* 13.Suppl2 (2010): S63.

38 Patak, P., H. S. Willenberg, and S. R. Bornstein. "Vitamin C is an important cofactor for both adrenal cortex and adrenal medulla." *Endocrine research* 30.4 (2004): 871-875.

39 Dutta, Deep, and Sujoy Ghosh. "Vitamin D and thyroid: Autoimmunity and cancer." *Thyroid Research and Practice* 10.1 (2013): 1.

40 Gärtner, Roland. "Selenium and thyroid hormone axis in critical ill states: an overview of conflicting view points." *Journal of Trace Elements in Medicine and Biology* 23.2 (2009): 71-74.

41 Sweet, Chris, Abhishek Sharma, and George Lipscomb. "Unusual presentation of more common disease/injury: Recurrent nausea, vomiting and abdominal pain due to hypothyroidism." *BMJ Case Reports* 2010 (2010).

42 Gregoriou, Stamatis, et al. "Nail disorders and systemic disease-What the nails tell us." *Journal of Family Practice* 57.8 (2008): 509-514.

43 Torchinsky, Michael Y., Robert Wineman, and George W. Moll. "Severe Hypoglycemia due to Isolated ACTH Deficiency in Children: A New Case Report and Review of the Literature." *International Journal of Pediatrics* 2011 (2011).

44 Deane, Helen Wendler, and Roy O. Greep. "A cytochemical study of the adrenal cortex in hypo-and hyperthyroidism." *Endocrinology* 41.3 (1947): 243-257.

45 Arlt, Wiebke, and Bruno Allolio. "Adrenal insufficiency." *The Lancet* 361.9372 (2003): 1881-1893.

46 Ajish, T. P., and R. V. Jayakumar. "Geriatric thyroidology: An update." *Indian Journal of Endocrinology and Metabolism* 16.4 (2012): 542.

47 van der Dennen, Johan MG. "Clinical aggressology: Neuropathology and (violent) aggression." *abstract in Aggressive Behavior* 10.2 (1984): 175.

48 Ii, Yuichiro., et al. "[Transient dementia during hyperthyroidism of painless thyroiditis. A case report]." *Rinsho shinkeigaku= Clinical neurology* 43.6 (2003): 341.

49 Li, Zhong-ke, and Bo Xu. "Misdiagnosis Analysis of 31 Cases of Atypical Hyperthyroidism." *Clinical Misdiagnosis & Mistherapy* 2 (2011): 040.

50 Saravanan, P., et al. "Twenty-four hour hormone profiles of TSH, Free T3 and free T4 in hypothyroid patients on combined T3/T4 therapy." *Experimental and clinical endocrinology & diabetes* 115.04 (2007): 261-267.

[51] Mazza, A., et al. "Arterial hypertension and thyroid disorders: What is important to know in clinical practice?" *Annales d'endocrinologie*. Vol. 72. No. 4. Elsevier Masson, 2011.

[52] Selvaraj, Senthil, et al. "Association of serum triiodothyronine with B-type natriuretic peptide and severe left ventricular diastolic dysfunction in heart failure with preserved ejection fraction." *The American journal of cardiology* 110.2 (2012): 234-239.

[53] Tran, Anh, et al. "The many faces of hyperthyroidism in primary care." *Endocrine Abstracts*. Vol. 21. 2010.

[54] Gildea, E. F., E. B. Man, and J. P. Peters. "Serum lipoids and proteins in hypothyroidism." *Journal of Clinical Investigation* 18.6 (1939): 739.

[55] Varga, F., et al. "T3 affects expression of collagen I and collagen cross-linking in bone cell cultures." *Biochemical and biophysical research communications* 402.2 (2010): 180-185.

4

Ironman

You need to get more sleep Tony.

—Tony's high school chemistry teacher, after Tony would fall asleep in his afternoon class

Even though Tony is only in his early 20s, he has been fighting fatigue for a while. Looking at him, no one would ever think anything was wrong: he's tall, muscular, handsome, smart, and looks like a model. But what people can't see is that underneath it all, he is Ironman, but not in the way you'd think.

Hemochromatosis is a genetic condition where iron is retained within the body until it becomes excessive; it can damage major organs like the liver, heart, and the endocrine system, including the thyroid and pituitary gland. Because there are no telltale external signs, there is no way to determine if someone has this condition without specific iron lab tests. These people look completely normal, but slowly, over the years, their iron levels rise until they are toxic, unless blood is donated on a regular basis. Some men will exhibit skin color changes by the time they are in their 40s. Their skin may become metallic gray, bronze, or brown.[1] Woman with hemochromatosis don't usually exhibit symptoms until they stop having monthly menstrual periods. Liver disease, heart failure, and diabetes are some of the consequences of chronically high iron levels, because the iron accumulates and damages various organs.

As in infant in the late 1980s, Tony was prescribed daily multivitamins with iron, along with iron-fortified formula. This was standard practice for all infants to prevent iron deficiency anemia.[2] The first time his iron levels were ever checked, he was almost 24 years old. His complaints were joint pain and profound fatigue, and he was having trouble just getting out of bed every day. Lab work revealed that his total serum iron and percent saturation were both over the reference range, and his ferritin, a measure of stored iron, was 204 ng/mL (20-345), which is technically normal. Ferritin values in the thousands have been reported by others, but a value over 200 combined with the other over range lab values is suspicious for hemochromatosis.

When Tony was a senior in high school, a bloodmobile visited, and he and his friends all donated blood, curious to see what their blood types were. When Tony realized the blood bank gave out freebies for each donation, he donated a couple more times that year before heading off to college, where he donated one more time. Those chance donations may have added years to his life, though he didn't realize it at the time.

When Tony's total iron and percent saturation labs came back flagged as over the reference range, he was tested for the two most common hereditary hemochromatosis (HH) gene mutations, and was found to be heterozygous for the H63D mutation. This means that he has only one copy of this particular iron loading gene. Because HH is considered a recessive disorder, Tony would need to have two copies (homozygous) to fully express the gene. He obviously got this gene from one of his parents, but since both parents have normal iron lab tests, one parent is simply a carrier, also with only one copy of the gene. Tony does not have the other common HH gene, C282Y. There are other known gene mutations, but they are not as common, so not routinely tested for. These other genes can be more problematic than the more well-known HH gene mutations he was tested for.

Tony's ancestors were the Scots, and there's a case study of a man of Scottish descent who was also heterozygous for the same H63D mutation, yet suffered from severe iron overload. Three mutations in his transferrin receptor 2 gene were identified as the problem.[3] Another man of Scot-Irish descent (yes Tony has Irish blood too) was also heterozygous for the H63D mutation, yet also loaded iron. His mutation was in the ferroportin gene.[4] Tony has not been tested for these particular gene mutations, and there are even more that have been identified.

Iron loading can easily be kept in check with regular blood donations (phlebotomy), and that's exactly what Tony did when his iron lab tests came back high. Just one donation brought all his high results back into the normal range, but of course, they will rise again over time. Currently, it's looking like he can maintain his iron levels within the reference range by donating blood every six months.

High iron levels can damage the endocrine system, and many of Tony's symptoms are those of someone with low thyroid function. However, his initial Thyroid Stimulating Hormone (TSH) test, which is typically used to diagnose hypothyroidism, was completely normal at 1.84 (0.4-4.5 mIU/L). TSH is made in the pituitary gland and the pituitary can be damaged by high iron levels. Magnetic Resonance Imaging (MRI) of the pituitary gland of a man with hemochromatosis showed iron deposition in the pituitary. All his pituitary hormones were found to be low, resulting in a diagnosis of hypogonadism.[5] In other words, this man's pituitary hormones were not accurate gauges of his hormone levels, because pituitary hormones should rise, to stimulate hormone production, when actual hormones levels are low. Measurement of the actual hormones revealed the true hormone deficiencies.

From looking at him, you'd think Tony has a working thyroid—he's not overweight, he has a full head of hair, and he's certainly not too brain fogged, since he went to college on full scholarships, although he did complain about attention issues while studying. But aching joints, swollen knees at times,[6] inflamed gums, enlarged tonsils,[7] occasional dark circles under his eyes, general fatigue, and restless sleep have plagued him since high school. His blood glucose (non-fasting) tested below the reference range, which could be a hypothyroid indicator.[8] Thyroglobulin antibodies and an ANA (antinuclear antibody) screen were also positive, which means there is some autoimmunity going on in his body. He has female relatives with both Graves' disease and Hashimoto's, the two autoimmune thyroid diseases. Mini-physicals from the blood bank donations in the past show low normal cholesterol (124-142 mg/dL), low body temperatures (96-97° where 98.6° is normal) and a slow pulse (60-70 beats per minute). Cholesterol is made in the liver and the liver is often damaged in hemochromatosis patients. Low body temperature and a slow pulse are both signs of hypothyroidism.

Because of Tony's numerous symptoms, his doctor prescribed 25 mcg levothyroxine or T4. While it seems plausible that this would *raise* Tony's total thyroid levels, it actually *lowered* them because of the TSH feedback loop. TSH is the signal that tells the thyroid to produce hormone. Thyroid hormone levels in the blood are sensed by the hypothalamus and pituitary gland, which then adjust their signals up or down to trigger either more or less production from the thyroid gland. Since there was now an additional 25 mcg of T4 available in the blood, his body assumed he didn't need to produce as much thyroid hormone, and Tony's TSH decreased slightly. Because TSH also stimulates T4 to T3 conversion,[9] the additional T4 hurt more than it helped, because it lowered his TSH, which then lowered his Total T4 and Free T3, as shown in Figure 4-1.

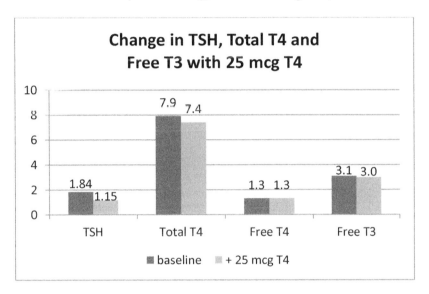

Figure 4-1. A dose of 25 mcg T4 effectively lowered most thyroid levels. For simplicity's sake, all values are plotted on one graph, but the vertical axis represents different units for each value. The units are mIU/L for TSH, mcg/dL for Total T4, ng/dL for Free T4, and pg/mL for Free T3. Baseline refers to Tony's first set of labs, before he was on any prescription thyroid hormone.

These lab results suggest that any further raises in T4 would only result in a lower TSH, and consequently, lower overall thyroid levels, until his dose became high enough to completely suppress his TSH. At that point, all his thyroid hormone would come from his prescription dose. Over the next year, various combinations were tried until he reached a maintenance dose of 1 grain of desiccated thyroid + 75 mcg T4. This is equivalent to 113 mcg T4 + 9 mcg T3, which is very close to what is secreted by the average thyroid gland (100 mcg T4 + 10 mcg T3[10]). Tony's final dose seems very reasonable based on average thyroid gland output, and not excessive in any way. In fact, this dose gives him a Total T4 identical to what he initially produced on his own, as shown in Figure 4-2. The difference though, is that he now has much more T3 in his system (see Figure 4-3), and many of his symptoms have improved: he falls asleep easier, his sleep is deeper, he sleeps 8-9 hours per day instead of 12, he has more energy throughout the day, his blood sugar has risen into the normal range, and his grades are back to As instead of the Bs and Cs they had dropped to. He also seems more talkative and upbeat than he was a year ago when he complained of depression, which is another hypothyroid symptom.[11]

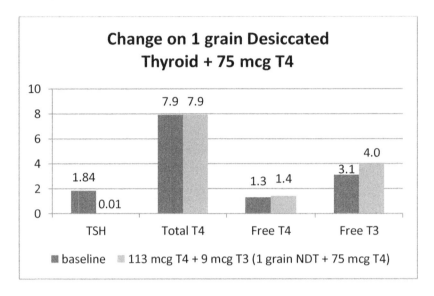

Figure 4-2. A dose of 1 grain of desiccated thyroid + 75 mcg of T4 suppressed TSH to nearly zero. However, actual thyroid hormone values are still well within the reference range. In fact, the total T4 value is unchanged from his original baseline labs, but the Free values have risen. For simplicity's sake, all values are plotted on one graph, but the vertical axis represents different units for each value. The units are mIU/L for TSH, mcg/dL for Total T4, ng/dL for Free T4, and pg/mL for Free T3.

Figure 4-2 illustrates some important points. There are four different types of hormone values depicted on that graph. TSH is a pituitary hormone, not a thyroid hormone, and Tony's has decreased drastically, and is now below the reference range. TSH normally has an inverse relationship to thyroid hormone levels: a high TSH implies hypothyroidism and a low TSH implies hyperthyroidism. Tony's TSH decreased from a level that is considered "normal" to one that is considered hyperthyroid. Yet the four measures of the actual thyroid hormones (Free T3, Total T3, Free T4, and Total T4) are still within the reference range, and certainly nowhere near what would be considered hyperthyroid, as shown in Figure 4-4. Tony does not exhibit hyperthyroid symptoms at this dose. At a recent blood bank donation, his blood pressure was 120/80 mm Hg, his pulse was 72 beats per minute, and his temperature (a morning donation) was 98.2°F. The TSH has become suppressed because it is reacting to the T3 in the desiccated thyroid dose. Even though a dose of 9 mcg T3 (what is found in his 1 grain dose) is hardly excessive, the hypothalamus and pituitary sense the T3, and have downregulated his TSH; at 0.01, it is almost zero. A "normal" TSH and thyroid hormone levels where the patient feels well seem to be mutually exclusive goals when T3 is supplemented! In fact [see Chapter 25, the TSH & T3 Dilemma], studies prove that it is nearly impossible to have both a normal TSH and healthy T3 levels at the same time when thyroid hormone is supplemented. If TSH is normal, then T3 is lower than normal; if T3 is normal, then TSH is lower than normal. This case illustrates what hundreds of thousands of thyroid patients on internet forums have reported—that TSH becomes suppressed whenever T3 is added,[12] but the patient does not feel hyperthyroid—they finally feel well!

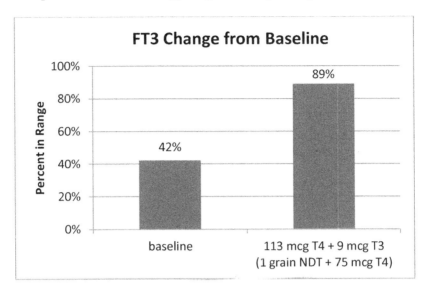

Figure 4-3. Tony's Free T3 levels, expressed as a percent in range, have more than doubled on the prescription thyroid hormones. Tony felt fatigued at the initial baseline levels and has more energy at the new levels, even though the baseline levels were still well within the reference range.

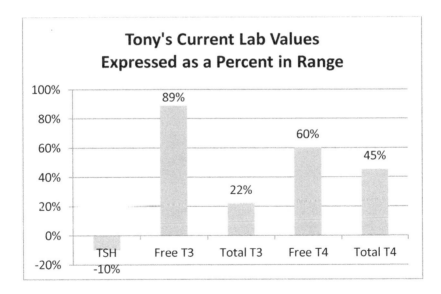

Figure 4-4. Tony's current lab values expressed as a percent in range show that only TSH, a pituitary hormone, is flagged as out of the reference range. It is low, which implies he is hyperthyroid, but he has no hyperthyroid symptoms, and his actual thyroid hormone levels are all within the reference range.

Key points

- Hemochromatosis or iron loading is a silent disease that can cause organ and endocrine damage if left untreated.
- When total iron, percent saturation, and ferritin are all high, further genetic testing should be performed.
- Donating blood is the standard treatment to reduce ferritin/iron levels. Once normal ferritin levels are reached, some patients may still need to donate blood monthly, others only once a year.[13]
- Not all gene mutations that cause iron loading are routinely tested for. In these cases, iron, percent saturation, and ferritin should be monitored and phlebotomy performed as needed.
- Iron can damage the pituitary gland, so pituitary hormones like TSH, Follicle Stimulating Hormone (FSH), Luteinizing Hormone (LH), and Adrenocorticotropic hormone (ACTH) may be lower than they should be. Therefore, the actual hormones should be tested and treated if low: thyroid, testosterone, cortisol, etc.
- A "normal" TSH does not rule out hypothyroidism, especially if there are multiple hypothyroid symptoms.
- Because of the TSH feedback loop, it is very difficult to "supplement" thyroid hormone, and most will do better with full replacement that includes some T3.
- Once T3 is added, TSH usually becomes suppressed and cannot be used to adjust the dose.

[1] Deal, J. E., T. M. Barratt, and M. J. Dillon. "Dermatologic Features." *Genetic Skin Disorders* 93.60 (2010): 308.

[2] Moy, R. J. D. "Iron fortification of infant formula." *Nutrition Research Reviews* 13.2 (2000): 215-228.

[3] Lee, Pauline L., and James C. Barton. "Hemochromatosis and Severe Iron Overload Associated with Compound Heterozygosity for *TFR2* R455Q and Two Novel Mutations *TFR2* R396X and G792R." *Acta haematologica* 115.1-2 (2006): 102-105.

[4] Lee, Pauline L., et al. "*SLC40A1* c. 1402G→ A Results in Aberrant Splicing, Ferroportin Truncation after Glycine 330, and an Autosomal Dominant Hemochromatosis Phenotype." *Acta haematologica* 118.4 (2007): 237-241.

[5] Wlazlo, N., W. Peters, and B. Bravenboer. "Hypogonadism in a patient with mild hereditary haemochromatosis." *The Netherlands journal of medicine* 70.7 (2012): 318.

[6] McLean, Robert M., and David N. Podell. "Bone and joint manifestations of hypothyroidism." *Seminars in arthritis and rheumatism*. Vol. 24. No. 4. WB Saunders, 1995.

[7] Khasanov, C. A., and V. N. Kirsanov. "[Clinical features and surgical treatment of chronic tonsillitis in patients with thyroid diseases]." *Vestnik otorinolaringologii* 5 (1996): 34-36.

[8] McDaniel, Huey G., et al. "Carbohydrate metabolism in hypothyroid myopathy." *Metabolism* 26.8 (1977): 867-873.

[9] Ikeda, Tadasu, et al. "Effect of thyrotropin on conversion of T4 to T3 in perfused rat liver." *Life sciences* 38.20 (1986): 1801-1806.

[10] Bunevičius, Robertas, et al. "Effects of thyroxine as compared with thyroxine plus triiodothyronine in patients with hypothyroidism." *New England Journal of Medicine* 340.6 (1999): 424-429.

[11] Hage, Mirella P., and Sami T. Azar. "The link between thyroid function and depression." *Journal of thyroid research* 2012 (2011).

[12] Appelhof, Bente C., et al. "Combined therapy with levothyroxine and liothyronine in two ratios, compared with levothyroxine monotherapy in primary hypothyroidism: a double-blind, randomized, controlled clinical trial." *Journal of Clinical Endocrinology & Metabolism* 90.5 (2005): 2666-2674.

[13] Bacon, Bruce R., et al. "Diagnosis and management of hemochromatosis: 2011 Practice Guideline by the American Association for the Study of Liver Diseases." *Hepatology* 54.1 (2011): 328-343.

5

Winning the Battle Against Graves' Disease

If you have RAI, you'll be done with all this!

—an endocrinologist

Lucy, now in her 60s, has battled episodes of Graves' disease since she was 45-years-old. Graves' is an autoimmune disease that results in hyperthyroidism, or an overactive thyroid gland, and tends to run in families. Before Lucy was born, her mother was treated for thyroid cancer with a thyroidectomy and radioactive iodine (RAI), and then given prescription thyroid hormone. Only a couple of years later, she became pregnant with Lucy. Lucy remembers her mother as chronically ill, mentally unstable, and basically psychotic. Her mother suffered from chronic debilitating migraines and severe arthritis, which might have explained her foul mood and violent outbursts. Thyroid hormone's effect on the brain and behavior is often overlooked, but too much or too little thyroid hormone can cause profound changes, from paranoid delusions, to rage, to complete stupor.[1]

Lucy remembers her mother taking her to an endocrinologist when she was a teenager and being diagnosed with "adolescent goiter." She had always been a skinny kid, but after taking the little white pills that she was prescribed, she gained weight and felt depressed and fatigued. She only took the pills for six months or so, because she was shipped off to boarding school not long after that, and the prescription was never refilled. She was never skinny again.

Lucy graduated from high school and started college in the late 60s, during the hippie era. Pot and LSD were readily available and helped her forget her miserable childhood. After a while, Lucy felt mentally unstable, so she dropped out of college. She spent nearly three years in intense psychotherapy (without drugs) where she learned how to be a "normal human being," something she had not learned growing up. She does not remember any hyperactive (Graves') symptoms during this period in her life, and feels that her emotional instability at the time was the result of growing up with a psychotic mother. The counseling finally addressed that, and it was a turning point in her life.

She traveled, had her first child abroad at 23 on her own, then came back home, settled down, and got a job as a restaurant cook. At 31, she married a wonderful man, and they eventually had two more children. They recently celebrated their 33rd wedding anniversary.

When her youngest was 6-years-old, Lucy began teaching cooking part-time in adult education. She added catering and culinary events to her accomplishments over the next 20 years while continuing to teach. In her early 40s, she attended culinary school to round out her education in the cooking industry, and at age 53, she opened her own culinary event and catering business.

Lucy had her first episode of Graves' disease when she was 45. She was attending culinary school, and just when she should have been graduating, many stressful family matters culminated, including her father's death from Alzheimer's. Unfortunately, his funeral was in another state, and Lucy was in the process of selling her home and purchasing a new one. She was not there for the closing or the move, which meant her husband and kids were in charge. Anyone who has ever moved from one residence to another, with kids, knows how stressful this is. It can be months before everything is unpacked and accessible again. Since Lucy hadn't even been there for the move, she returned to a new home that was completely unfamiliar. Many studies have implicated stress as a trigger for Graves' disease.[2]

In addition, her father's death meant an estate needed to be settled, but he had remarried, and his new wife was not the least bit cooperative with Lucy. Her stress was over the top and she could feel it: her heart rate was elevated, her hands trembled, she couldn't sleep, and she was angry and fatigued. Her doctor tested her Thyroid Stimulating Hormone (TSH) and it was close to zero, a hyperthyroid sign, so she was referred to an endocrinologist.

A radioactive iodine (RAI) uptake test confirmed she had Graves' disease. Her endocrinologist offered RAI treatment, which would destroy Lucy's thyroid, so that she would no longer be hyperthyroid. She would then become hypothyroid instead, and have to take replacement thyroid hormone for the rest of her life. Because she saw firsthand what RAI did to her mother, Lucy refused the RAI. Intuitively, she knew that her thyroid gland itself was not the *cause* of overproduction. Constant stimulation from Graves' antibodies is the problem, and is thought to be responsible for other Graves' symptoms like Thyroid Eye Disease (TED), which looks like bulging eyes. The ideal treatment is one that reduces Graves' antibodies, and RAI is actually the least effective method for that, compared with anti-thyroid drugs and surgery.[3] In fact, RAI sometimes worsens the antibodies and can worsen TED.[4] RAI has even induced TED in patients who had no previous TED symptoms.[5] Anti-thyroid drugs and thyroidectomies offer better odds of remission. The thyroid gland is not the only organ that takes up iodine; radioactive iodine treatment can damage other organs and result in decreased saliva secretion, decreased tear secretion, radiation-induced pneumonitis (lung inflammation), ovarian and testicular dysfunction, and increased risk of secondary tumors.[6] As time passed, Lucy became more convinced that RAI was a barbaric and unnecessary treatment. In fact, she authored a short piece entitled "Top 20 reasons NOT to have RAI" that can still be found on a Graves' disease internet forum.

So how did Lucy deal with her hyperthyroid symptoms? Her husband happened to be an herbalist, and the Chinese herbal medicines he gave her brought her symptoms down to a manageable level. She was still somewhat hyperthyroid, though not nearly as bad as before the herbs. But she relapsed when she went on a long vacation to Italy and had to forgo her daily boiled herbal potions. Her hyperthyroid symptoms became severe and upon her return to the U.S., she started on Tapazole, a pharmaceutical anti-thyroid medication designed to lower thyroid levels. A daily dose of Tapazole kept her hyperthyroid symptoms in check for 17 years, from 1994 – 2011. She started Tapazole at 30 mg per day, but as her thyroid levels quickly dropped, she had to reduce her dose down to 20 mg, then 10 mg, then 5 mg. But even 5 mg of Tapazole caused a drastic reduction in her thyroid hormone levels. A 2.5 mg dose allowed her thyroid to produce some hormone, but any additional stress resulted in a hyperthyroid relapse. For Lucy, 5 mg seemed to be the smallest effective dose, but even this dose left her with very low thyroid levels and the resulting brain fog and physical misery. Sleeping was difficult because her hips and legs were in pain. She had problems breathing at night, gained a lot of weight, and was quite miserable.

Lucy tried to wean off Tapazole several times over those years, but was never successful, because her hyperthyroid symptoms always returned. Tapazole kept her symptoms in check, and in 2003 she started her own culinary event and catering business, building a 2,400 square foot warehouse kitchen in 2004. During her first three years in business, she did everything including mopping her commercial kitchen, cleaning the hood etc., so Graves' never stopped her from achieving her goals.

Around 2008, she joined a Graves' internet group and learned about modified block and replace, where anti-thyroid drugs like Tapazole are taken in conjunction with levothyroxine. Anti-thyroid drugs limit thyroid production and lower the antibodies, but are so effective they usually make the patient profoundly hypothyroid. To counter that, levothyroxine (T4) is prescribed to bring the patient's thyroid levels up into the normal range. The patient's thyroid hormones (Free T3 and Free T4) are monitored, and the levothyroxine dose is adjusted to keep these levels about mid-range, or wherever the patient feels best. The TSH level cannot be used to adjust the dose in a person with Graves', because the TSH is generally always close to zero, whether the patient's Free T3 and Free T4 are high and above the reference range, or low and below the range.[7] This is because Graves' antibodies affect the thyroid gland's TSH Receptors, usually resulting in constant stimulation, which is why thyroid hormone continues to be produced. In a normal person, TSH levels rise and fall in response to the T3 and T4 levels in the bloodstream. When thyroid levels are low, TSH should rise, which signals the thyroid to make more hormone. A TSH near zero tells the thyroid that no more hormone should be made. Since patients with active Graves' have a TSH near zero, the feedback loop *is* working—the pituitary is not producing TSH (not asking for any more thyroid hormone to be made). However, thyroid hormone continues to be produced because of Graves' antibody stimulation, not TSH stimulation.

For Lucy, 5 mg of Tapazole and 25 mcg of Levoxyl (a brand of T4) kept her thyroid levels fairly stable. But every fall season, for some unknown reason, she became more hyperthyroid and had to raise her Tapazole and lower her T4 dose. But as soon as fall turned to winter, she had to readjust her doses back to what they were previously. In spite of her Free T3 and Free T4 levels being in the "normal" range with this protocol, she developed classic hypothyroid metabolic symptoms: her cholesterol rose to 321 mg/dL (below 200 is desirable), and her weight continued to increase, in spite of valiant efforts on her part to lose weight, including following a low carb diet. These symptoms suggest that her thyroid levels were too low. Even though her Free T4 was usually mid-range or higher, her Free T3 over the years was usually in the bottom half of the range. Free T3 is the thyroid lab value that most correlates with hypothyroid or hyperthyroid symptoms.[8] TSH and Free T4 have very poor correlation to symptoms; someone can have a normal TSH and Free T4, and yet be hypothyroid with symptoms such as weight gain, feeling cold, constipation, etc., as Lucy's case illustrates.

Lucy learned about Low Dose Naltrexone (LDN) in June 2011 from an LDN internet group and found another doctor to prescribe it for her. LDN is a prescription substance that, for some patients, lowers autoimmune antibodies considerably, sometimes to the point of remission.[9] While some patients experience vivid dreams or insomnia when starting LDN, Lucy doesn't recall anything disturbing, and her sleep was not affected. She did feel a little under the weather during the first month, but feels fine now. And she is not as sick as often. After only six months on LDN, she could tell that her Graves' symptoms were improving, and gradually weaned off her drugs, first reducing the Levoxyl, and then the Tapazole, until she had totally weaned off both drugs by December 2011. Intuitively, she knew she didn't need either one anymore. Lab tests for the Graves' antibodies, both TRAb (TSH Receptor antibodies) and TSI (Thyroid Stimulating Immu-noglobulin), confirmed that her levels were now well within the reference range. She had her usual autumn flare-up the following year and went back on 5 mg Tapazole for a few days, weaning down to 2.5 mg and then completely off again within a couple of weeks. She continues to take 3 mg of LDN daily. She reserves the Tapazole for those stressful occasions when her Graves' flares up, and then only needs low doses for a limited time period.

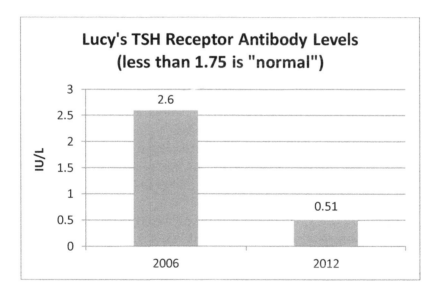

Figure 5-1. Lucy's TSH Receptor antibody levels have greatly decreased over the years with the help of medications like Tapazole and Low Dose Naltrexone.

Lucy's successful culinary event and catering business celebrated its 10th anniversary in 2013. She launched the business while taking Tapazole for the Graves' disease she has dealt with since 1994. She still has a brief relapse every fall, but manages to work through it. The addition of LDN has made a world of difference in managing her Graves' and she is confident she made the right decision when she chose not to have RAI or a thyroidectomy. In fact, after two years on LDN, Lucy reports that her goiter has shrunk and her endocrinologist believes it is now half the size it was at its peak. His notes estimate it was 80-85 grams at one point, and is now down to 40-45 grams. It has slowly diminished in size just over the last year.

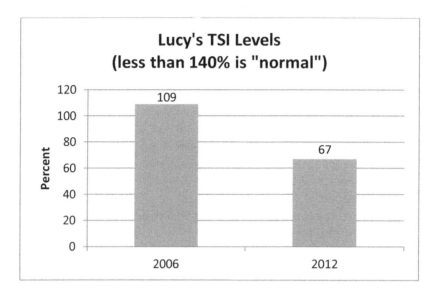

Figure 5-2. Lucy's TSI levels have also decreased significantly. TSI indicates how strong or potent the antibodies are. Lower is always better.

Key points

- Thyroid hormone excess or deficiency can cause profound changes in behavior, from paranoid delusions, to rage, to complete stupor.
- Stress may be one trigger for Graves' disease.
- RAI is not the only treatment option for Graves' disease.
- Graves' symptoms are caused by the Graves' antibodies, not the thyroid gland itself; RAI is less effective than anti-thyroid drugs or thyroidectomy for reducing the Graves' antibodies.
- RAI can result in decreased saliva and tear secretion, lung inflammation, ovarian and testicular dysfunction, and increased risk of secondary tumors.
- RAI can induce or worsen Thyroid Eye Disease (TED).
- If the Graves' antibodies can be reduced back to normal levels, the thyroid gland may resume normal production.
- TSH cannot be used to adjust a Graves' patient's dose; TSH is generally always close to zero because of TSH Receptor antibodies.
- Anti-thyroid drugs can be used long-term, at low doses.
- Modified block and replace, where levothyroxine is used in conjunction with anti-thyroid drugs, is one option for managing Graves'.
- LDN may reduce Graves' antibodies in some patients.

[1] Davis, Anthony T. "Psychotic states associated with disorders of thyroid function." *The International Journal of Psychiatry in Medicine* 19.1 (1989): 47-56.

[2] Kostoglou-Athanassiou, I., A. Gkountouvas, and P. Kaldrymides. "Stressful life events and Graves' disease." *Endocrine Abstracts*. Vol. 29. 2012.

[3] Laurberg, Peter, et al. "TSH-receptor autoimmunity in Graves' disease after therapy with anti-thyroid drugs, surgery, or radioiodine: a 5-year prospective randomized study." *European Journal of Endocrinology* 158.1 (2008): 69-75.

[4] Träisk, Frank, et al. "Thyroid-associated ophthalmopathy after treatment for Graves' hyperthyroidism with antithyroid drugs or iodine-131." *Journal of Clinical Endocrinology & Metabolism* 94.10 (2009): 3700-3707.

[5] Vannucchi, G., et al. "Graves' orbitopathy activation after radioactive iodine therapy with and without steroid prophylaxis." *Journal of Clinical Endocrinology & Metabolism* 94.9 (2009): 3381-3386.

[6] Kiani, Javad, et al. "Evaluation of glucose tolerance in methimazole and radioiodine treated Graves' patients." Int J Endocrinol Metab 8.3 (2010): 132-7.

[7] Brokken, Leon JS, Wilmar M. Wiersinga, and Mark F. Prummel. "Thyrotropin receptor autoantibodies are associated with continued thyrotropin suppression in treated euthyroid Graves' disease patients." Journal of Clinical Endocrinology & Metabolism 88.9 (2003): 4135-4138.

[8] Baisier, W. V., J. Hertoghe, and W. Eeckhaut. "Thyroid insufficiency. Is TSH measurement the only diagnostic tool?" Journal of Nutritional and Environmental Medicine 10.2 (2000): 105-113.

[9] Whitaker, Julian. "Low-Dose Naltrexone: A Miracle Drug for Immune Challenges." Dr. Julian Whitaker's Health & Healing. 22.6 (2012):1-3.

PART II:

FACTS EVERY DOCTOR AND

PATIENT SHOULD KNOW

6

Adrenal Dysfunction (Low Cortisol) and the Side Effects of Hydrocortisone Supplementation

There is no connection between the thyroid and adrenal glands.

—common misconception of many medical professionals

The adrenal glands

The adrenal glands are small glands above the kidneys that produce both cortisol and noradrenaline, along with some other hormones. When the thyroid gland does not produce enough thyroid hormone for the body's needs, the adrenals compensate by releasing cortisol[1] and noradrenaline[2] to give the body energy. Blood sugar and blood pressure are often low in hypothyroid patients, and cortisol counteracts both problems.[3] Lack of thyroid hormone will lower the heart rate while noradrenaline will raise the heart rate. Patients with rapid heart rates and high blood pressure may actually be hypothyroid, but instead of being prescribed thyroid hormone, they are often prescribed beta blockers for their symptoms. Unfortunately, the patient does not have a beta blocker deficiency; they have a thyroid deficiency.[4]

Cortisol has a natural circadian rhythm and should be highest at waking and lowest at bedtime. People with low thyroid function often have adrenal dysfunction, with cortisol levels that are either too high or low overall, or high at some times and low at others. When someone has high cortisol at night, they have a hard time falling asleep and often suffer from insomnia.[5] Someone with low cortisol, on the other hand, is often fatigued and unable to withstand any stress.[6]

Adrenal fatigue, adrenal insufficiency, adrenal dysfunction, and hypoadrenia are the terms used to describe low adrenal function and the resulting low cortisol. *Adrenal fatigue* is the term most commonly used by patients, though it is not recognized by the medical profession and has no insurance billing code. The term *adrenal insufficiency* is found in medical literature and is often used interchangeably with the condition called Addison's disease, where little to no cortisol is produced because the adrenal glands have been destroyed by tuberculosis, autoimmune disease, or other conditions.[7] Addison's disease is a form of *primary adrenal insufficiency*, where the adrenal gland itself is damaged and thus cannot secrete the necessary hormone. The adrenal glands produce cortisol in response to signals from the hypothalamus and pituitary gland. Head injuries can damage the pituitary gland, resulting in what is called *secondary adrenal insufficiency*, or damage may be to the hypothalamus, resulting in what is called *tertiary adrenal insufficiency*. Women who suffer major blood loss during childbirth may end up with pituitary damage in a condition known as Sheehan's syndrome. Unrelenting stress can also affect the adrenal glands. If the adrenal gland, hypothalamus or pituitary are not functioning, cortisol must be taken for life to replace the essential missing hormone.

Lack of cortisol can be fatal and is called an *adrenal crisis*; it can be triggered by infections, strenuous physical activity, surgery, or emotional distress.[8] Those with Addison's are usually quite thin. Cushing's is the opposite state, where the adrenals over-produce cortisol. Cushing's patients are usually quite heavy, with a moon face and buffalo hump (hump on the backside of their neck).

Some hypothyroid patients appear to have Addison's; their saliva cortisol labs show a flat-lined pattern at the bottom of the reference range all day, yet they have never had tuberculosis, nor do they have adrenal antibodies. Their adrenals are not producing what they should because of a lack of thyroid hormone. They have what is called *relative adrenal insufficiency*. There are animal studies that show an effect on the thyroid gland after an adrenalectomy (removal of the adrenal glands), and other studies that show an effect on the adrenal glands after a thyroidectomy (removal of the thyroid gland), so the two glands are definitely interrelated. In one study, rats were given anti-thyroid drugs like carbimazole or methimazole; these drugs are used to lower thyroid levels in Graves' patients.[9] The rat's adrenal glands atrophied when hypothyroid. The adrenal cortex actually shrank in size, especially the zona fasciculata, which is where cortisol is produced. As expected, blood cortisol levels were lower in these hypothyroid rats. Interestingly, Brewer's yeast, which is high in B vitamins and selenium, appeared to have a protective effect on the adrenal gland, somewhat offsetting the methimazole-induced atrophy.[10] Thyroidectomized dogs exhibited the same effect—their cortisol levels dropped significantly only seven days post-thyroidectomy. Their adrenocortical function was restored after they were given levothyroxine.[11] Adrenalectomies for Cushing's syndrome patients have worsened autoimmune hypothyroidism.[12] These studies illustrate that thyroid hormone is essential for adrenal health and vice versa.

When a hypothyroid patient is started on thyroid hormone, cortisol levels must be high enough to handle the influx of thyroid hormone, because thyroid hormone raises metabolism, which results in increased cortisol clearance. If the body cannot produce the amount of cortisol needed for the higher metabolism, it can result in a fatal adrenal crisis. While a true adrenal crisis is rare, low cortisol symptoms including fatigue, weight loss, low blood pressure, dizziness, nausea, vomiting, and body tanning (or hyperpigmentation) are more common. Blood chemistry may show hyponatremia (low sodium) and hyperkalemia (high potassium).[13]

How Cortisol is Produced

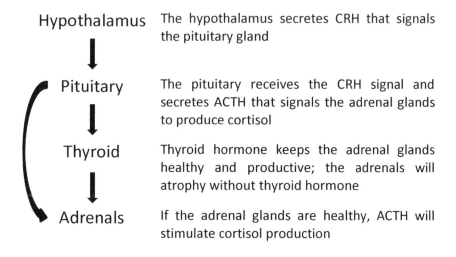

Figure 6-1. The hypothalamus, pituitary, and thyroid must all be healthy and functional for cortisol to be produced by the adrenal glands. This is referred to as the HPT (hypothalamus-pituitary-thyroid) axis. A malfunction in any gland in this process and lack of the appropriate signal will result in low cortisol production. If the adrenal glands are damaged, it is called primary adrenal insufficiency. If the pituitary is damaged and cannot produce adrenocorticotropic hormone (ACTH), it is called secondary adrenal insufficiency. If the hypothalamus is damaged and cannot produce corticotropic-releasing hormone (CRH), it is called tertiary adrenal insufficiency.

Because so many seeking help on thyroid internet forums have low cortisol symptoms, they are often advised to take hydrocortisone before they start on thyroid hormone so they don't experience an adrenal crisis. However, most of these people do not have true Addison's disease, which means they may just have sluggish adrenal glands caused by low thyroid hormone levels. The addition of thyroid hormone may "reactivate" their adrenal glands to produce cortisol again. Anecdotal testimonies suggest that it is the lack of triiodothyronine (T3, the active thyroid hormone) over many years that makes the adrenal glands sluggish. Studies on thyroidectomized rats show that hypothyroidism induces adrenal insufficiency, which becomes progressively worse with time. Initially, only the pituitary hormone that stimulates cortisol production, adrenocorticotropic hormone (ACTH), is decreased, but with time, the hypothalamus hormone that stimulates the pituitary, corticotropic-releasing hormone (CRH), also drops.[14] The rats appear to suffer from primary, secondary, and tertiary adrenal insufficiency, even though lack of thyroid hormone was the original cause. This illustrates the difficulty in diagnosing the cause of relative adrenal insufficiency.

The thyroid gland primarily produces two thyroid hormones: thyroxine (T4) and T3. T4 can also convert to T3, adding to the total T3 content in the body. T3 has a circadian rhythm and peaks in the human body around 4 a.m., about 90 minutes after Thyroid Stimulating Hormone (TSH) peaks.[15] TSH stimulates T4 to T3 conversion in the liver,[16] which means TSH is essential for someone who only takes T4. Patients who have no TSH to stimulate conversion may provide T3 overnight by taking a small bedtime dose of T3. Cortisol also has a circadian rhythm and is lowest around midnight, starts to rise around 3 a.m., and is highest around 8:30 a.m.[17] The rise in cortisol after T3 peaks suggests that T3 is what gives the adrenals the energy they need at that hour to produce cortisol. Patients taking a dose of T3 before waking have reported improved cortisol levels, and some that were taking hydrocortisone have been able to wean off.

Thyroidectomized animal studies show that low thyroid levels lead to low cortisol levels. To correct low thyroid levels, thyroid hormone must be administered. However, thyroid hormone replacement can trigger an adrenal crisis if cortisol levels are insufficient. How can this vicious circle be broken? Instead of taking hydrocortisone, the adrenals can be supported with various vitamins, herbs, and supplements, and thyroid hormone should be raised *slowly*. Vitamins A, B, and C are found in high concentrations in the adrenal glands and can be supplemented.[18] There are also adrenal glandular supplements that people have used successfully. Thyroid hormone and corticosteroid binding globulin (CBG) have an inverse relationship. As thyroid levels rise, CBG drops, resulting in more free cortisol circulating in the bloodstream.[19] Cortisol is released from CBG as body temperature rises, and body temperature correlates positively with thyroid levels. Therefore, raising thyroid levels can naturally raise cortisol levels.[20] Any increases must be done slowly—weekly thyroid increases may be too much and do not give the body time to adjust. There are people who are so sensitive that they can only raise 1/4 grain of desiccated thyroid or 12.5 mcg of T4 every 12 weeks. Taking smaller amounts of T3 throughout the day (including bedtime), instead of once a day, will also give all organs, including the adrenals, a more steady supply of energy to perform their function. A dose of T3 before waking will mimic normal thyroid function and may also stimulate morning cortisol production. Anecdotal testimonies say that there is an optimal time before waking when the T3 must be taken. This is determined by trial and error.

Side effects of hydrocortisone supplementation

Hydrocortisone supplementation to treat adrenal fatigue is not risk-free and people using hydrocortisone (on thyroid internet forums) have reported some serious side effects such as:

- osteoporosis[21]
- glaucoma (which can lead to blindness)[22]
- weight gain ("buddha belly")[23]
- immune suppression (which can lead to fungal infections[24] and resistance to some cancer treatments[25])
- cardiovascular disease/hypertension[26]
- diabetes[27]
- insomnia[28]
- inability to tolerate *any* stress, which can lead to a fatal adrenal crisis.[29]

Anyone on the hydrocortisone protocol must learn how to "stress dose," or manually provide the hydrocortisone needed for any stress, since the body becomes completely dependent on external dosing. In the same way that thyroid medications with T3 (desiccated thyroid and Cytomel) suppress TSH, hydrocortisone suppresses the ACTH feedback loop, which would normally stimulate natural cortisol production. It is also impossible to supplement just a little hydrocortisone, because even small amounts turn off natural production. A medical alert bracelet/necklace/card should be carried at all times by anyone on hydrocortisone replacement, because the ACTH feedback loop does not work while on this protocol. If someone cannot provide the required increased hydrocortisone for the stress, it can be fatal. More than one person on this protocol has ended up in the emergency room from high blood pressure and/or a high heart rate (when combined with the T3-only protocol). People on hydrocortisone (HC) can have low cortisol symptoms in conjunction with physical signs of high cortisol because manual dosing creates high cortisol levels shortly after a dose, but low cortisol levels just before the next dose. It is extremely difficult to replicate natural cortisol production, or to mimic an automatic ACTH feedback loop. People should be aware of the risks before embarking on this protocol.

The proponents of this protocol say that hydrocortisone side effects don't occur at physiological doses, only at excessive pharmaceutical doses. But how is physiological defined? Maybe what is physiological for one person is an overdose for another. In one study of primary or secondary adrenal insufficient patients, those on hydrocortisone doses greater than 30 mg/day had a lower Quality of Life score than those on lower daily doses.[30] In another study of primary or secondary adrenal insufficient patients, the dosing schedule that brought the highest proportion of simulated patients within physiological cortisol targets was 10 + 5 + 5 mg at 0730, 1200 and 1630 hours, respectively. However, even with this regimen, about 54%, 44% and 32% of patients remained over- or under-treated when compared to the physiological ranges at 0800, 1600 and 2400 h, respectively.[31] These high percentages of being over or underdosed on what is considered a physiological dose confirm what many patients on hydrocortisone report—that it is *extremely* difficult to manually dose hydrocortisone. This may explain the side effects many report.

In a study of 12 Addison's and 20 hypopituitary patients on replacement glucocorticoid therapy, 75% of the patients were found to be taking excessive doses when serum cortisol levels were correlated with 24-hour urine free cortisol excretion. In other words, while their serum cortisol levels were within the reference range, their 24-hour urine free cortisol levels were high, which meant their dose needed to be reduced. Their mean daily dose of hydrocortisone was reduced from 29.5 to 20.8 mg. This caused median osteocalcin (a protein involved with bone formation) to increase (which is good) from 16.7 to 19.9 micrograms/l.[32] Osteoporosis is a serious side effect of any glucocorticoid therapy, so patients should not be overmedicated.[21]

Patients on thyroid forums are advised to take HC to "rest" their adrenals, because hydrocortisone supplementation suppresses the HPA (hypothalamus-pituitary-adrenal) axis. Suppression occurs because of a process called transrepression (which HC does very well), but side effects like glaucoma and diabetes can be induced by a different mechanism called transactivation, where the HC activates genes involved in those conditions. Other side effects like osteoporosis seem to involve both transrepression and transactivation. So while patients may get the intended HPA effect of suppression, they may also unknowingly be putting themselves at risk for other serious side effects.[27] The concept of letting an organ "rest" is questionable. All organs "work," as needed, under stress; they aren't allowed to rest. A heart may beat only 70 beats per minute at rest, but it can easily rise to more than double that when someone exercises. The same concept applies to the lungs. Interestingly, heart and respiration rates are both slower in someone who is hypothyroid, because the organs don't have enough energy to perform at normal rates. The same analogy can be applied to the adrenal glands—they cannot provide the necessary cortisol because they lack the energy that should be supplied by the thyroid gland. It's analogous to running a 6-cylinder engine on only 4 cylinders. It still runs, but not as effectively as it should.

Hydrocortisone supplementation does not seem to work as it should when patients are on other pharmaceutical drugs like benzodiazepines, or any medication that treats anxiety and depression. These drugs probably work at some level on the HPA axis and cortisol levels,[33] creating unintended, conflicting reactions.[34] Also, if Lyme disease or some other underlying medical condition is present, taking hydrocortisone may exacerbate the condition because of its suppressive effect on the immune system.

Conclusion

The cause of adrenal insufficiency should be determined *before* any hydrocortisone is taken. Is it primary adrenal failure, or secondary, or tertiary, or are the adrenal glands just deprived of thyroid hormone? Has there been any recent overwhelming stress? Did the person ever have a head injury? If the cause is primary, secondary, or tertiary, cortisol replacement is for life, and the patient must learn to dose HC through trial and error. If the cause is relative adrenal insufficiency due to low thyroid levels or chronic stress, there's a chance that natural cortisol production can return once thyroid levels are brought up and the stress becomes more manageable. Because of the serious side effects, difficulty with multi-day dosing, and the impact on the quality of life,[35] hydrocortisone treatment should not be entered into lightly. Some have ended up worse than before they started any treatment.

Key points

- When thyroid hormone levels are insufficient, the adrenal glands produce cortisol and noradrenaline to compensate.
- Low thyroid levels often lead to adrenal dysfunction with high and/or low cortisol levels.
- Adrenal insufficiency can be caused by a damaged adrenal gland, or a head injury that damaged the hypothalamus or pituitary gland.
- Lack of cortisol can be fatal and is called an *adrenal crisis*; it can be triggered by infections, strenuous physical activity, surgery, or emotional distress.
- Lack of thyroid hormone can cause relative adrenal insufficiency.

- Thyroid hormone replacement cannot be started if cortisol levels are insufficient; it may trigger an adrenal crisis.
- Long-term hypothyroidism causes relative adrenal insufficiency and lowers ACTH, the pituitary hormone, and CRH, the hypothalamus hormone. Both hormones are needed to stimulate cortisol production.
- Both T3 and cortisol have a circadian rhythm, and taking some T3 before rising has successfully stimulated natural cortisol production in some patients.
- Thyroid hormone and corticosteroid binding globulin (CBG) have an inverse relationship. As thyroid levels rise, CBG drops, leaving more cortisol free.
- Cortisol is also released from CBG as body temperature rises, and body temperature correlates positively with thyroid levels. Therefore, raising thyroid levels can naturally raise cortisol levels.
- Some patients with sluggish adrenals can only raise their thyroid dose very slowly. They may have to hold a dose for 12 weeks, while most will stabilize on a dose in 6 weeks.
- Hydrocortisone supplementation has serious side effects: osteoporosis, glaucoma (which can lead to blindness), weight gain ("buddha belly"), immune suppression (which can lead to fungal infections and resistance to some cancer treatments), cardiovascular disease/hypertension, diabetes, insomnia, and inability to tolerate *any* stress.
- Because cortisol is an essential hormone, the patient must manually provide all cortisol needed by the body while on this protocol, especially when under stress. Failure to do so can result in a fatal adrenal crisis.
- People on hydrocortisone often exhibit both high and low cortisol symptoms because it's nearly impossible to replicate natural cortisol levels without the ACTH feedback loop, which becomes suppressed the minute any hydrocortisone is taken.
- The concept of "resting" the adrenal glands is questionable. All organs work as hard as they can, up to their limits, which may be determined by available thyroid energy.
- Pharmaceutical anti-anxiety drugs like benzodiazepines conflict with hydrocortisone replacement.
- Hydrocortisone has a suppressive effect on the immune system and may worsen underlying infections like Lyme disease.

---

[1] Fommei, Enza, and Giorgio Iervasi. "The role of thyroid hormone in blood pressure homeostasis: evidence from short-term hypothyroidism in humans." Journal of Clinical Endocrinology & Metabolism 87.5 (2002): 1996-2000.

[2] Christensen, Niels Juel. "Increased levels of plasma noradrenaline in hypothyroidism." Journal of Clinical Endocrinology & Metabolism 35.3 (1972): 359-363.

[3] Bajwa, Sukhminder Jit Singh, and Ravi Jindal. "Endocrine emergencies in critically ill patients: Challenges in diagnosis and management." Indian journal of endocrinology and metabolism 16.5 (2012): 722.

[4] Richards, A. M., et al. "Hypertension in hypothyroidism: arterial pressure and hormone relationships." Clinical and Experimental Hypertension 7.11 (1985): 1499-1514.

[5] Basta, Maria, et al. "Chronic insomnia and the stress system." Sleep medicine clinics 2.2 (2007): 279-291.

[6] Widmer, Isabelle E., et al. "Cortisol response in relation to the severity of stress and illness." Journal of Clinical Endocrinology & Metabolism 90.8 (2005): 4579-4586.

[7] Zelissen, Pierre MJ, Egbert JEG Bast, and Ronald JM Croughs. "Associated autoimmunity in Addison's disease." Journal of autoimmunity 8.1 (1995): 121-130.

[8] Hahner, Stefanie, et al. "Epidemiology of adrenal crisis in chronic adrenal insufficiency: the need for new prevention strategies." European Journal of Endocrinology 162.3 (2010): 597-602.

[9] Sarwar, Ghulam, and Sughra Parveen. "Carbimazole-induced hypothyroidism causes the adrenal atrophy in 10 days' prenatally treated albino rats." Journal of the College of Physicians and Surgeons–Pakistan: JCPSP 15.7 (2005): 383.

[10] Dehghani, Farzaneh, et al. "Protective effect of Brewer's yeast On Methimazole-Induced-Adrenal Atrophy (A stereological study)." The Tokai journal of experimental and clinical medicine 35.1 (2010): 34.

[11] Eik-Nes, Kristen, and Kenneth R. Brizzee. "Adrenocortical activity and metabolism of 17-hydroxycorticosteroids in thyroidectomized dogs." American Journal of Physiology--Legacy Content 184.2 (1956): 371-375.

[12] Russo, Laura, et al. "Exacerbation of autoimmune thyroiditis following bilateral adrenalectomy for Cushing's Syndrome." Thyroid 20.6 (2010): 669-670.

[13] Graves III, Leland, Robert M. Klein, and Anne D. Walling. "Addisonian crisis precipitated by thyroxine therapy: a complication of type 2 autoimmune polyglandular syndrome." Southern medical journal 96.8 (2003): 824-827.

[14] Johnson, Elizabeth O., et al. "Effects of short-and long-duration hypothyroidism on hypothalamic–pituitary–adrenal axis function in rats: In vitro and in situ studies." Endocrine 42.3 (2012): 684-693.

[15] Russell, Wanda, et al. "Free triiodothyronine has a distinct circadian rhythm that is delayed but parallels thyrotropin levels." Journal of Clinical Endocrinology & Metabolism 93.6 (2008): 2300-2306.

[16] Ikeda, Tadasu, et al. "Effect of thyrotropin on conversion of T4 to T3 in perfused rat liver." Life sciences 38.20 (1986): 1801-1806.

[17] Chan, Sharon, and Miguel Debono. "Review: Replication of cortisol circadian rhythm: new advances in hydrocortisone replacement therapy." Therapeutic advances in endocrinology and metabolism 1.3 (2010): 129-138.

[18] Lockwood, Julia E., and Frank A. Hsartman. "Relation of the Adrenal Cortex to Vitamins A, B1 and C." Endocrinology 17.5 (1933): 501-521.

[19] Dumoulin, Sonia C., et al. "Opposite effects of thyroid hormones on binding proteins for steroid hormones (sex hormone-binding globulin and corticosteroid-binding globulin) in humans." European journal of endocrinology 132.5 (1995): 594-598.

[20] Henley, D. E., and S. L. Lightman. "New insights into corticosteroid-binding globulin and glucocorticoid delivery." Neuroscience 180 (2011): 1-8.

[21] Weinstein, Robert S., et al. "Inhibition of osteoblastogenesis and promotion of apoptosis of osteoblasts and osteocytes by glucocorticoids. Potential mechanisms of their deleterious effects on bone." Journal of Clinical Investigation 102.2 (1998): 274.

[22] Tripathi, Ramesh C., et al. "Corticosteroids and glaucoma risk." Drugs & aging 15.6 (1999): 439-450.

[23] Meikle, A. Wayne. "A diagnostic approach to Cushing's syndrome." The Endocrinologist 3.5 (1993): 311-320.

[24] Lionakis, Michail S., and Dimitrios P. Kontoyiannis. "Glucocorticoids and invasive fungal infections." The Lancet 362.9398 (2003): 1828-1838.

[25] Herr, Ingrid, and Jesco Pfitzenmaier. "Glucocorticoid use in prostate cancer and other solid tumours: implications for effectiveness of cytotoxic treatment and metastases." The lancet oncology 7.5 (2006): 425-430.

[26] Wei, Li, Thomas M. MacDonald, and Brian R. Walker. "Taking glucocorticoids by prescription is associated with subsequent cardiovascular disease." Annals of Internal Medicine 141.10 (2004): 764-770.

[27] Schäcke, Heike, Wolf-Dietrich Döcke, and Khusru Asadullah. "Mechanisms involved in the side effects of glucocorticoids." Pharmacology & therapeutics 96.1 (2002): 23-43.

[28] Forss, M., et al. "Current practice of glucocorticoid replacement therapy and patient-perceived health outcomes in adrenal insufficiency-a worldwide patient survey." BMC Endocrine Disorders 12.1 (2012): 8.

[29] Shenker, Yoram, and James B. Skatrud. "Adrenal insufficiency in critically ill patients." American journal of respiratory and critical care medicine 163.7 (2001): 1520-1523.

[30] Bleicken, Benjamin, et al. "Influence of hydrocortisone dosage scheme on health-related quality of life in patients with adrenal insufficiency." Clinical endocrinology 72.3 (2010): 297-304.

[31] Simon, Nicolas, et al. "Pharmacokinetic evidence for suboptimal treatment of adrenal insufficiency with currently available hydrocortisone tablets." Clinical pharmacokinetics 49.7 (2010): 455-463.

[32] Peacey, Steven R., et al. "Glucocorticoid replacement therapy: are patients over treated and does it matter?" Clinical endocrinology 46.3 (1997): 255-261.

[33] Grottoli, S., et al. "Alprazolam, a benzodiazepine, does not modify the ACTH and cortisol response to hCRH and AVP, but blunts the cortisol response to ACTH in humans." Journal of endocrinological investigation 25.5 (2002): 420.

[34] Pompéia, Sabine, et al. "Acute benzodiazepine administration induces changes in homocysteine metabolism in young healthy volunteers." Progress in Neuro-Psychopharmacology and Biological Psychiatry 33.6 (2009): 933-938.

[35] Han, Thang S., et al. "Quality of life in adults with congenital adrenal hyperplasia relates to glucocorticoid treatment, adiposity and insulin resistance: United Kingdom Congenital adrenal Hyperplasia Adult Study Executive (CaHASE)." European Journal of Endocrinology 168.6 (2013): 887-893.

7

Asthma, Eczema, Allergies, Hives, and Yellow #5 (Tartrazine or E102)

FD&C Yellow No. 5 may be safely used for coloring foods (including dietary supplements) . . . [1]

—US Food & Drug Administration **food** regulation: no warning is required on food products, though yellow #5 must be listed as an ingredient

For prescription drugs for human use containing FD+C Yellow No. 5 that are administered orally, nasally, vaginally, or rectally, or for use in the area of the eye, the labeling . . . shall . . . bear the warning statement **"This product contains FD+C Yellow No. 5 (tartrazine) which may cause allergic-type reactions (including bronchial asthma) in certain susceptible persons.** *Although the overall incidence of FD+C Yellow No. 5 (tartrazine) sensitivity in the general population is low, it is frequently seen in patients who also have aspirin hypersensitivity." This warning statement shall appear in the "Precautions" section of the labeling.*[2]

—US Food & Drug Administration **drug** regulation: a yellow #5 warning is only required on prescription, but not over-the-counter drugs

A severe asthma attack can be fatal.[3] *The route of ingestion (food or drug) doesn't matter. Either can trigger a fatal asthma attack.*

—Barbara Lougheed, Tired Thyroid author

My asthma, eczema, allergies, and hives have greatly decreased in severity since I've reached a more optimal dose of thyroid hormone, *and* eliminated yellow #5 food color from my diet. I have Graves' disease, which is an autoimmune thyroid condition, so by definition, my immune system is dysfunctional. Insufficient thyroid hormone is a stress on the body, because there is not enough energy to keep all systems running smoothly. Taking enough thyroid hormone greatly relieves this stress, and for many Hashimoto's (autoimmune hypothyroid) patients, has caused their anti-thyroglobulin and anti-thyroid peroxidase antibodies to decline.[4] In other words, having adequate thyroid levels lessens the severity of immune dysfunction.

Asthma, low cortisol, and low thyroid levels

At one time, when my thyroid levels were too low, wheezing and breathing problems were something that plagued me every night after dinner, no matter what I ate. What was so confusing was that I could eat a can of soup at lunchtime and be ok, and then the next day, have the exact same flavor of soup before bed, and would end up wheezing. How could I be allergic to something one day, and not the next? It made no sense.

Cortisol, the hormone that deals with stress and inflammation, is highest in the morning and lowest at night, and this might explain why what was tolerated at lunch was not tolerated at night. One study found that asthmatic children with significantly lower cortisol levels at night had lower Forced Expiratory Volumes compared to controls.[5] Cortisol moderates inflammation in the body, including the lungs. Less cortisol results in more inflammation. Cortisol levels positively correlate with thyroid levels,[6] so it would be a reasonable hypothesis to say that low thyroid levels caused the low cortisol levels, and therefore, raising thyroid levels would raise cortisol, and asthma would disappear. This correlation has been observed by others, and one doctor noticed that once his asthma patients were placed on desiccated thyroid, their asthma symptoms showed dramatic improvement.[7] It certainly is true in my case. Could the asthma epidemic actually be a hypothyroidism epidemic in disguise?

Asthma is strongly correlated to low thyroid levels in several other studies as well. One study examined hypothyroid patients (who'd had a total thyroidectomy and then received radioactive iodine treatment for cancer) who had no previous pulmonary (lung) disease. There was a significant increase in non-specific bronchial reactivity in these non-asthmatic subjects when hypothyroid and untreated, than when treated with thyroid hormone.[8] Since these patients only developed bronchial reactivity after removal of their thyroid, it appears that thyroid hormone plays a role in healthy lung function. In another study, chronic bronchial asthma patients were given triiodothyronine (T3) daily for 60 days. Peak (air) flow increased in all patients, with an average increase of 25%.[9] A third study examined the effect of T3 for 30 days on children with bronchial asthma. These children were not considered to be hypothyroid based on symptoms, yet 30% were able to stop their anti-asthmatic medications while continuing the T3 treatment, and 13% reduced the amount of bronchodilators needed. All patients noted a significant improvement in pulmonary function tests.[10]

Thyroid function affects the respiratory system, and studies have shown that untreated hypothyroidism results in lower breathing measures, but no significant correlation could be found between serum thyroxine (T4), serum Thyroid Stimulating Hormone (TSH), and pulmonary parameters. This leaves T3 as the only variable that wasn't measured that could possibly show a correlation. Shortness of breath and weakness of both the inhalation and exhalation muscles are commonly reported in hypothyroid patients; replacement thyroid hormone significantly raised all breathing parameters.[11]

Yellow #5 food color (tartrazine or E102) gives me hives and eczema

Many eczema and hives attacks I experienced were caused by a food color called yellow #5, also known as tartrazine, or E102. It is found in many unrelated processed foods, which is why it was so difficult to figure out. Pickles, lime gelatin, macaroni and cheese, and chocolate mint cookies are hardly in similar food groups, but yellow #5 is found in all of these products. And yes, I have learned my lesson and now eat mostly whole foods from scratch. Dining out is still problematic, however, because there is really no way to tell if yellow #5 is in one of the ingredients used in a dish. I make a serious effort to avoid anything that's bright orange, yellowish, or light green though. I have even found yellow #5 in certain brands of toothpaste and vitamins, so even non-food items must be checked. Yellow #5 is also used to color topical lotions, which I cannot use because my skin reacts to it. Dishwashing detergents and liquid soaps may also contain yellow #5 and may cause a reaction in those who are highly sensitive. There is even a bright blue gel used for muscle pain relief (that contains yellow #5) that caused my skin to break out in a rash within minutes of application. My aching back became an aching back broken out in hives!

Yellow #5 reactions may be caused by a defect in the phase 2 liver detoxification process called sulfation. Sulfates (a molecule formed from sulfur, which is in a normal diet) should attach to salicylates (found in fruits), phenols (found in food dyes like yellow #5 and preservatives), hormones, neurotransmitters, and toxins, making them more soluble so they can eventually be cleared from the body via urine or feces. However, some of us have poor sulfation because:

1. We don't consume enough sulfur in our diet, which is the raw material for sulfates
2. Or we are low in the sulfite oxidase enzyme which converts sulfites to sulfates
3. Or we are low in the cofactors used by the sulfite oxidase enzyme, which are molybdenum and iron; Vitamin B12 levels may also be low
4. Or we are low in the phenol sulfotransferase enzyme (PST) that attaches sulfates to toxins in the sulfation process
5. Or there's a high copper/low zinc imbalance, which slows the transsulfuration pathway (from dietary sulfur to sulfate)

If the sulfation detoxification process is suboptimal, then food additives are not efficiently processed out, and a hives outbreak or an asthma attack results.[12] Since sulfate levels are presumed to be low, one way to increase the body's sulfate content is through magnesium sulfate baths (epsom salts), which provide sulfate through the skin. Molybdenum in low doses has been reported to help asthmatics who tend to be low in this trace mineral,[13] because it is part of the sulfite oxidase enzyme reaction that converts sulfites to sulfates.[14] In one patient, lack of the molybdenum cofactor was the problem, rather than a lack of the sulfite oxidase enzyme.[15] Vitamin B12 and molybdenum supplementation have reduced sulfite sensitivity in some patients.[16] Both molybdenum and zinc supplementation can lower copper levels and cause another imbalance such as anemia, so any supplementation should be carefully monitored. Asthmatics tend to react to sulfites, yellow #5, salicylates, and aspirin.[17] Ironically, epinephrine, which is used to treat life-threatening, allergic emergencies, is preserved with sodium metabisulfite.[18] Metabisulfite is found in most dental anesthetics too, so patients should always alert medical practitioners of their sensitivity.[19]

Molybdenum is also a component of aldehyde oxidase, an enzyme involved in metabolizing drugs and azo dyes, which yellow #5 is classified as.[20] Azo dyes are manufactured, synthetic colors and thus do not biodegrade readily. In fact, rivers and ground water in areas where azo dyes are produced suffer from severe contamination, and conventional, aerobic sewage treatments of wastewater are not 100% effective.[21] Because azo dyes are so difficult to break down, a whole industry has grown around cost-effective removal of these dyes from wastewater by photodegradation,[22] chemical catalytic oxidation,[23] or physical adsorption.[24] The textile industry produces a large part of this toxic industrial wastewater when it dyes fabrics, but the same dye is consumed daily in a diet comprised of processed foods. Unfortunately, many of these processed foods are marketed to children.

There is an interesting overlap of symptoms between asthmatic people who are sensitive to sulfites and autistics. Autistics tend to be low in the PST enzyme[25] and to have a high copper/low zinc ratio,[26] which is also found in asthmatics.[27] Yellow #5 reduces serum zinc levels in hyperactive children.[28] Researching this topic makes me wonder if a defective sulfation process is the cause of autism. Unless I overconsume sulfites, you would never know I had asthma. Sulfites are the trigger. Likewise, acetaminophen, mercury, and aluminum exposure often occur together when vaccinations are given, and any one of these may be the trigger; acetaminophen is primarily metabolized through sulfation.[29] Thimerosal, the mercury preservative found in some vaccinations, is a sulfur compound.

Aspirin, sulfites, and sulfur dioxide all make me wheeze, yellow #5 gives me hives and eczema, thimerosal in a flu shot gave me whole body hives, and a sulfa antibiotic sent me to the ER in what seemed like anaphylactic shock (I puffed up, turned blue, couldn't walk normally, shook like I had Parkinson's, felt so cold I needed 4 blankets but still shivered, BP dropped, etc.). Hypersensitivity to anticonvulsants and sulfa antibiotics has been noted in other thyroid patients, so anyone with a known thyroid condition might be wise to choose another type of antibiotic.[30] Beer is another major allergen for me, though I'm not sure how it fits in here. It made my throat swell so badly that I lost my voice for a week. Beer contains sulfites and sulfur dioxide, but it also contains hops, which is in no other food product I know of.

Sulfites, sulfur dioxide, sulfa antibiotics, thimerosal, and yellow #5 all contain a sulfur molecule. Sulfur is also naturally consumed in a normal diet, and two sulfur amino acids (methionine and cysteine) are derived from meat proteins. Five possible reasons for a suboptimal sulfation pathway were listed earlier. The remedy for #1, insufficient sulfur, could easily be fixed by increasing sulfur in the diet. But if the actual problem is #2, or insufficient conversion of sulfite to sulfate, then increasing sulfur intake would be one of the worst things to do, because it would just increase the amount of toxic sulfite produced that would be unable to convert to sulfate, creating a backlog of sulfite. Sulfur amino acids in our bodies follow a lengthy conversion pathway, and sulfites are naturally created at one point, followed by the final conversion to sulfates. Sulfites consist of an SO3 ion (sulfur with 3 oxygen atoms attached) and yellow #5 has two SO3 ions in its chemical structure.[31] Does yellow #5 metabolize and liberate two sulfite molecules that cannot be metabolized by those with poor sulfation? Is this why yellow #5 causes asthma and hives, which is the same reaction that sulfites cause?[32] Sulfites were banned by the U.S. Food & Drug Administration in 1986 due to some fatal adverse reactions. Yet yellow #5 is still in our food and drug supply, even though reactions ranging from systemic anaphylaxis, severe asthma, urticaria (hives), and mild rhinitis (runny nose) have been reported.[33]

There's a case study of an individual who was known to be sensitive to sulfites and sulfa drugs, who then developed hypersensitivity to taurine and the artificial sweetener acesulfame potassium. Sulfites, taurine and acesulfame potassium all contain SO_3. The subject is also allergic to thiuram mix (used in the manufacture of rubber products) and thimerosal, both sulfur containing compounds, as well as to various food products.[34]

My skin has now been completely normal for over a decade, and I attribute that to two things: a more optimal thyroid dose, and the elimination of yellow #5 products from my life. This is a complete turnaround from the whole body, burning, itching, dermographic hives that plagued me 24/7 when I was unknowingly consuming yellow #5 on a daily basis through various products. I was also only taking levothyroxine at the time, and now take both levothyroxine and desiccated thyroid, which more closely replicates normal thyroid gland output. The itching was always most intense at night, when cortisol, our natural anti-inflammatory hormone, is lowest, which meant I also got little sleep. Talk about crabby! I believe optimal thyroid levels improve the sulfation pathway, because they raise the rate of metabolism. In a hypothyroid patient, toxins would remain in the body longer simply because all systems in the body are sluggish, including detoxification. It's possible adequate thyroid levels also raise the threshold amount that invokes a reaction, since the quantities that cause reactions have such a broad range. The highest amount of aspirin that produced a response in susceptible subjects was 415 times greater than the smallest amount. For yellow #5 the highest amount was 260 times greater.[17] I know I have had small amounts of sulfites without a reaction (balsamic vinegar!) now that I'm on a higher thyroid dose. Some studies have noted a correlation between chronic urticaria (hives) and autoimmune thyroiditis. Some patients have had dramatic improvement (their hives stopped) once they were placed on thyroid hormone (levothyroxine).[35] A second study achieved the same results: levothyroxine treatment resulted in remission, and when the levothyroxine was stopped, the hives returned.[36]

Conclusion

Some people live with chronic asthma, eczema, and hives, and can only control them with pharmaceutical drugs that don't really eliminate the outbreaks, but only help to lower the symptoms so they're tolerable. I was lucky that my condition was corrected by the elimination of yellow #5 food color and sulfites from my diet, and the addition of some T3 to my thyroid dose. I knew I could not tolerate sulfites by the time I was eight years old, when I had my first wheezing episode after eating too many dried apricots, which contain sulfur dioxide as a preservative. I had noticed slight wheezing when I'd eaten them previously, so that last full-blown asthma attack confirmed that I shouldn't eat dried apricots. I later reacted to wine, beer, and yellow #5, so the connection became quite clear.

The association with hypothyroidism is more subtle, and while I think a lot of patients would have an improvement in their symptoms if they were given thyroid hormone, it's extremely difficult to prove that someone really is hypothyroid, because the Thyroid Stimulating Hormone (TSH) screening test usually returns a "normal" result. I once asked someone on an asthma forum, "Do you have trouble with your weight, are your hair and eyebrows thin, is your cholesterol high, are your hands and feet cold, skin dry, brain foggy?" Her response? "Yeah I have all of that . . . it also doesn't necessarily equate to having hypothyroid though." I couldn't believe her response. And then I found out why she thought the way she did—she's a nurse, which means she's been *taught* that her "normal" TSH rules out hypothyroidism.

In my opinion, anyone who has chronic hives or asthma should have full thyroid tests run, which includes much more than just a TSH. If they react to aspirin, wine, or beer, they should also consider looking into the elimination of sulfites and yellow #5 from their diet. Sulfites are found naturally in some foods, so it's a difficult detective game, but the end result, freedom from hives and asthma, is worth it.

Key points

- The hypothyroid state is a stress on the body. Thyroid hormone replacement has caused Hashimoto's antibodies to decline in some patients.
- Low thyroid levels may cause a decrease in cortisol levels, which means there is less of the body's natural anti-inflammatory hormone. This may be one way that low thyroid levels can lead to asthma.
- Studies on hypothyroid patients show a weakness in both the inhalation and exhalation muscles, and patients report feeling short of breath.
- T3 has been shown to have a positive effect on breathing parameters in chronic bronchial asthma patients.
- Yellow #5 food color can cause asthma, hives, and eczema in some people.
- Yellow #5, sulfites, sulfur dioxide, and sulfa antibiotics all contain sulfur, and a faulty sulfation detoxification pathway may be to blame for reactions to these substances.
- Sulfites are used as preservatives in some medications and anesthetics, so all medical personnel, including dentists, should be notified of this sensitivity.
- Yellow #5 is an artificial azo dye which is extremely difficult to degrade; materials and chemical engineers have created processes to remove it from wastewater, yet it is legally in our food supply in the U.S.
- Asthmatics and autistics both have a high copper/low zinc ratio.
- More than one study has reported the elimination of hives with thyroid hormone replacement.

[1] Code of Federal Regulations, Title 21 – Food & Drugs, Chapter 1 – Food & Drug Administration, Department of Health & Human Services, Subchapter A – General, Part 74 - Listing of Color Additives Subject to Certification, Subpart A—Foods, § 74.705, FD&C Yellow No. 5.   http://www.accessdata.fda.gov/scripts/cdrh/cfdocs/cfcfr/CFRSearch.cfm?fr=74.705 accessed 9/27/13

[2] Code of Federal Regulations, Title 21 – Food & Drugs, Chapter 1 – Food & Drug Administration, Department of Health & Human Services, Subchapter A – General, Part 74 - Listing of Color Additives Subject to Certification, Subpart B—Drugs, § 74.1705, FD&C Yellow No. 5.   http://www.accessdata.fda.gov/scripts/cdrh/cfdocs/cfcfr/CFRSearch.cfm?fr=74.1705 accessed 9/27/13

[3] Birda, J. Andrew, and A. Wesley Burksa. "Food allergy and asthma." Primary Care Respiratory Journal 18.4 (2009): 258-265.

[4] Aksoy, Duygu Yazgan, et al. "Effects of prophylactic thyroid hormone replacement in euthyroid Hashimoto's thyroiditis." Endocrine journal 52.3 (2005): 337-343.

[5] Landstra, Anneke M., et al. "Role of serum cortisol levels in children with asthma." American journal of respiratory and critical care medicine 165.5 (2012).

[6] Dumoulin, Sonia C., et al. "Opposite effects of thyroid hormones on binding proteins for steroid hormones (sex hormone-binding globulin and corticosteroid-binding globulin) in humans." European journal of endocrinology 132.5 (1995): 594-598.

[7] Dr. David Derry Answers Reader Questions. Brought to you by Mary Shomon, Your Thyroid Guide. Topic: Asthma and Thyroid Hormone. Accessed 9/26/13. http://thyroid.about.com/library/derry/bl10.htm

[8] Wieshammer, Siegfried, et al. "Effects of hypothyroidism on bronchial reactivity in non-asthmatic subjects." Thorax 45.12 (1990): 947-950.

[9] Ismail, A. A., E. Shalaby, and I. Gadalla. "Effect of triiodothyronine on bronchial asthma II." The Journal of asthma research 14.3 (1977): 111.

[10] Khalek, Karima Abdel, et al. "Effect of triiodothyronine on cyclic AMP and pulmonary function tests in bronchial asthma." Journal of Asthma 28.6 (1991): 425-431.

[11] Bassi, Roopam, et al. "Effect Of Thyroid Hormone Replacement On Respiratory Function Tests In Hypothyroid Women." Pak J Physiol 8.2 (2012).

[12] Juhlin, Lenmart. "Incidence of intolerance to food additives." International journal of dermatology 19.10 (1980): 548-551.

[13] Ziying, Han, et al. "Study on the Contents of Ten Kinds of Necessary Trace Elements in Serum of Sufferers from Allergic Asthma." CNKI Journal 09 (1996).

[14] Ranguelova, Kalina, Marcelo G. Bonini, and Ronald P. Mason. "(Bi) sulfite Oxidation by Copper, Zinc-Superoxide Dismutase: Sulfite-Derived, Radical-Initiated Protein Radical Formation." Environmental health perspectives 118.7 (2010): 970.

[15] Johnson, Jean L., et al. "Molybdenum cofactor deficiency in a patient previously characterized as deficient in sulfite oxidase." Biochemical medicine and metabolic biology 40.1 (1988): 86-93.

[16] Bold, Justine. "Considerations for the diagnosis and management of sulphite sensitivity." Gastroenterology and Hepatology from bed to bench 5.1 (2011).

[17] Corder, Elizabeth H., and C. Edward Buckley III. "Aspirin, salicylate, sulfite and tartrazine induced bronchoconstriction. Safe doses and case definition in epidemiological studies." Journal of clinical epidemiology 48.10 (1995): 1269-1275.

[18] Smolinske, Susan C. "Review of parenteral sulfite reactions." Clinical Toxicology 30.4 (1992): 597-606.

[19] Dooms-Goossens, A., et al. "Local anesthetic intolerance due to metabisulfite." Contact Dermatitis 20.2 (1989): 124-126.

[20] Hartmann, Tobias, et al. "The impact of single nucleotide polymorphisms on human aldehyde oxidase." Drug Metabolism and Disposition 40.5 (2012): 856-864.

[21] Stolz, A. "Basic and applied aspects in the microbial degradation of azo dyes." Applied Microbiology and Biotechnology 56.1-2 (2001): 69-80.

[22] Gupta, Vinod K., et al. "Removal of the hazardous dye—tartrazine by photodegradation on titanium dioxide surface." Materials Science and Engineering: C 31.5 (2011): 1062-1067.

[23] Beach, Evan S., et al. "Fe-TAML/hydrogen peroxide degradation of concentrated solutions of the commercial azo dye tartrazine." Catalysis Science & Technology 1.3 (2011): 437-443.

[24] Mishra, Ashish Kumar, T. Arockiadoss, and S. Ramaprabhu. "Study of removal of azo dye by functionalized multi walled carbon nanotubes." Chemical Engineering Journal 162.3 (2010): 1026-1034.

[25] O'Reilly, B. A., and R. H. Waring. "Enzyme and sulphur oxidation deficiencies in autistic children with known food/chemical intolerances." Journal of Orthomolecular Medicine 8 (1993): 198-198.

[26] Faber, Scott, et al. "The plasma zinc/serum copper ratio as a biomarker in children with autism spectrum disorders." Biomarkers 14.3 (2009): 171-180.

[27] El-Kholy, M. S., et al. "Zinc and copper status in children with bronchial asthma and atopic dermatitis." The Journal of the Egyptian Public Health Association 65.5-6 (1990): 657.

[28] Ward, Neil I., et al. "The influence of the chemical additive tartrazine on the zinc status of hyperactive children-a double-blind placebo-controlled study." Journal of Nutritional and Environmental Medicine 1.1 (1990): 51-57.

[29] Seneff, Stephanie, Robert M. Davidson, and Jingjing Liu. "Empirical data confirm autism symptoms related to aluminum and acetaminophen exposure." Entropy 14.11 (2012): 2227-2253.

[30] Gupta, Abhya, et al. "Drug-induced hypothyroidism: the thyroid as a target organ in hypersensitivity reactions to anticonvulsants and sulfonamides." Clinical Pharmacology & Therapeutics 51.1 (1992): 56-67.

[31] Ngah, Wan Saime Wan, Noorul Farhana Md Ariff, and Megat Ahmad Kamal Megat Hanafiah. "Preparation, characterization, and environmental application of crosslinked chitosan-coated bentonite for tartrazine adsorption from aqueous solutions." Water, Air, and Soil Pollution 206.1-4 (2010): 225-236.

[32] Vally, Hassan, N. L. A. Misso, and V. Madan. "Clinical effects of sulphite additives." Clinical & Experimental Allergy 39.11 (2009): 1643-1651.

[33] Miller, Klara. "Sensitivity to tartrazine." British medical journal (Clinical research ed.) 285.6355 (1982): 1597.

[34] Stohs, Sidney J., and Mark JS Miller. "A Case Study Involving Allergic Reactions to Sulfur-Containing Compounds Including, Sulfite, Taurine, Acesulfame Potassium and Sulfonamides." Food and Chemical Toxicology (2013).

[35] Bangash, Shahid A., and Sami L. Bahna. "Resolution of chronic urticaria and angioedema with thyroxine." Allergy and asthma proceedings. Vol. 26. No. 5. OceanSide Publications, Inc, 2005.

[36] Rumbyrt, Jeffrey S., Joel L. Katz, and Alan L. Schocket. "Resolution of chronic urticaria in patients with thyroid autoimmunity." Journal of allergy and clinical immunology 96.6 (1995): 901-905.

8

Autoimmunity, Autism, and Asthma May be Triggered by Acetaminophen, Amalgams, or Aluminum

The continued use of dental amalgam as a restorative material does not pose a health hazard to the nonallergic patient.

—Debatable statement by the American Dental Association, 2012 Current Policies[1]

When the body senses foreign pathogens, such as bacteria or viruses, a healthy immune system will form antibodies against the pathogens so they won't harm the body. In autoimmune diseases, healthy tissues in the body are attacked, and antibodies to the tissues themselves (as opposed to a bacteria) develop. Hashimoto's thyroiditis (hypothyroid) and Graves' disease (hyperthyroid) are autoimmune thyroid diseases. In Hashimoto's disease, the thyroid gland is attacked and antibodies to thyroid peroxidase (TPO) and thyroglobulin (Tg) are formed. TPO is an enzyme and thyroglobulin is a protein found within the thyroid gland; both are involved in the production of thyroid hormones. In Graves' disease, antibodies are formed against the Thyroid Stimulating Hormone (TSH) Receptor, the site that receives the signal from TSH to produce more thyroid hormone. Why do some people contract an autoimmune disease, when others don't, when both are exposed to the exact same environment? The answer may lie in genetic differences, specifically, genetic detoxification enzyme deficiencies.

This chapter goes into technical detail because more and more people are having genetic testing done, and the exact names of the enzymes and genes at work may be useful to them. Hopefully, readers will recognize some of their own genetic variations.

Genetics

Autoimmune conditions tend to run in families,[2] and studies on twins prove there is a genetic component to autoimmune thyroid disease. In fact, about 75% of the symptoms can be attributed to genetics. However, since identical twins can express different symptoms, about 25% must be caused by other external factors; cigarette smoking and infection with the bacterium *Yersinia enterocolitica* are two documented causes.[3]

Specific genes are associated with autoimmune thyroid disease—HLA-DR3 was the first gene found to be associated with both Graves' disease and Hashimoto's thyroiditis in the 1980s. Research continues to identify more genes associated with thyroid auto-immunity disorders: immune regulation genes (CD40, CTLA-4, PTPN22) and polymor-phisms (genetic variations) in the thyroglobulin and the TSH Receptor genes have also been identified.[4]

Detoxification enzymes

Molecules that are foreign to the body (xenobiotics) are metabolized and eliminated from the body by enzymes in two phases. Elimination is either through urine or feces, and the molecule must be water soluble to be eliminated. The process of converting a xenobiotic to a water soluble compound happens in two phases. In the first phase, B vitamins and other cofactors react with the xenobiotic to create an intermediate metabolite that is more water soluble than the original fat soluble toxin.[5] These phase I enzymes, also called cytochrome P450 enzymes (CYPs), are found primarily in the liver, but can also be found in the intestine, brain, kidney, placenta, lung, adrenal gland, pancreas, skin, mammary gland, uterus, ovary, testes and prostate. CYP enzymes located outside of the liver play an important role in the local metabolism of toxins.[6] The phase I enzymes are key to the metabolism of drugs, environmental noxious agents, food components, etc., and other lipid-derived substrates, such as prostaglandins, fatty acids and steroids (the sex hormones).

Some enzyme reactions are not beneficial—a few CYPs transform pro-carcinogens into ultimate carcinogens. In other words, our own enzymes convert a xenobiotic into a true carcinogen. Based on genetic variations in enzyme activity, people can be classified as poor metabolizers (reduced/zero enzyme metabolic activity), extensive metabolizers (normal enzyme capacity), and ultrarapid metabolizers (higher-than-normal metabolic activity). Poor metabolizers would be exposed to xenobiotics for a longer period of time, which may explain the reactions they experience. Genetic variations in different phase I enzymes (flavoprotein monooxygenase, amine oxidases, xanthine oxidase, and others) have been identified. Many of the enzymes express differently by race, meaning that whites, blacks, and Asians metabolize different substances at different rates.[7]

In phase II, conjugating enzymes transform the intermediate metabolite into a truly water soluble compound that can then be excreted in urine or feces. The cofactors for these processes are amino acids that come from the diet. Sulfur amino acids, for example, are essential for the processing of acetaminophen.[8] Sulfur is found primarily in meat proteins, but is also present in cruciferous vegetables and garlic and onions.[9] In some cases, it is not that the amino acid is lacking, but defective transformation pathways are preventing the transformation of the intermediate metabolite. Sulfation, for example, is a phase II enzyme process that requires sulfates, which are (normally) readily created from sulfur.

Phase II enzymes include:

- catechol-O-methyl transferases (COMT)
- epoxide hydrolases (EPH)
- glutathione S-transferases (GST)
- N-acetyltransferases (NAT)
- DT-diaphorase or NAD(P)H:quinone oxidoreductase (NQO) or NAD(P)H:menadione oxidoreductase (NMOR)
- sulfotransferases (SULT)
- and UDP-glucuronosyltransferases (UGT)[10]

Methylation is a phase II process involving COMT that thyroid patients may be familiar with, since methylation mutations have been reported on thyroid forums. GSTs are involved in the detoxification of chemotherapeutic agents, insecticides, herbicides, carcinogens, and by-products of oxidative stress. SULTs process drugs such as acetaminophen, chemical carcinogens, hormones, bile acids, neurotransmitters such as dopamine, peptides, and lipids.[11] UGTs help metabolize drugs, chemical toxicants, carcinogens, phytochemicals, etc. and endogenous compounds such as steroids (sex hormones), bilirubin, thyroid hormones, bile acids, fatty acids, prostaglandins, and retinoic acid.

Phase I reactions generate reactive oxygen species (ROS) as a normal byproduct of cellular metabolism: superoxide anion-radical, hydrogen peroxide, lipid peroxides, and others. High ROS levels can be damaging and these must be reduced to non-toxic levels by antioxidant enzymes such as superoxide dismutase (SOD), catalase, glutathione peroxidase, and peroxiredoxins. Non-enzymatic antioxidants such as a reduced form of glutathione (GSH), uric acid, ascorbic acid, ceruloplasmin, and others also help neutralize these free radicals. Enzyme deficiencies at any stage of detoxification (phase, I, II, or free radical neutralization) are implicated in many diseases.

The potency of a toxin and the duration of exposure will determine toxicity. Even a healthy person with a full complement of enzymes will not be able to withstand high levels of a toxin for a long period of time—that's how poisons work. Likewise, a genetic aberration or deficiency of any of the enzymes will lead to incomplete detoxification, or excessive generation of toxic by-products. The toxicity of a substance can affect multiple organs or just specific tissues. *Idiopathic Environmental Intolerances* (IEI) is the term used to describe several syndromes with similar symptoms. Amalgam disease (from dental mercury fillings), multiple chemical sensitivity, fibromyalgia, chronic fatigue syndrome, sick building syndrome, electric hypersensitivity, irritable bowel syndrome, and Persian Gulf War veteran syndrome all have overlapping symptoms: muscular weakness and fatigue, confusion and memory loss, depression, anxiety, panic disorders, respiratory distress, chronic bronchitis and asthma, gastrointestinal tract malfunction, and joint pains. Interestingly, these same symptoms have also been reported by hypothyroid patients.

Amalgam disease (sensitivity to mercury)

On thyroid forums, patients are often advised to avoid mercury. There is no question that mercury is poisonous to humans.[12] But what about the low doses found in dental fillings (amalgams)? Is mercury really a problem for hypothyroid patients? Can it cause thyroid autoimmunity? Should all thyroid patients have their mercury fillings replaced?

Human mercury exposure is primarily from two sources: dental amalgams and sea-food. Occupational exposure and multiple vaccinations (containing thimerosal) can also contribute to the total mercury load. Dental amalgams give off inorganic elemental or metallic mercury vapor, while fish from contaminated waters contain organic (methyl and dimethyl) mercury.[13] Dental amalgams outgas mercury vapor, which can then be absorbed through the lungs and transported throughout the body. Autopsies show mercury deposits in multiple organs, including the brain, thyroid, and pituitary gland.[14] In fact, there's a positive correlation between the mercury concentration in these glands and the number of amalgams. In other words, the more dental fillings the person had, the higher the mercury concentration in the thyroid and pituitary glands. Both the pituitary and thyroid work together to regulate thyroid output, therefore damage to either gland will affect thyroid function and output.

In the 1980s, an American dermatologist observed that certain susceptible, highly sensitive patients developed a variety of illnesses after their teeth were filled with mercury amalgams. When the fillings were removed, their health improved. In one patient, eczema that had been present for 30 years disappeared after his fillings were removed. Different people presented with different symptoms, but the list of illnesses that improved or completely disappeared when mercury fillings were removed included inter-stitial cystitis, Lyme disease, immune dysfunction, extreme sensitivity to inhalants (particle and vapors) and ingestants (food and chemicals), asthma, dyslexia, and epilepsy.[15] This doctor is convinced that the chemically sensitive and the mercury sensitive are actually the same group, and that they suffer from genetic enzyme deficiencies that prevent toxins from being flushed from the body. Because of these deficiencies, this group of people tends to be hypersensitive (intolerant) to sulfites, monosodium glutamate, and aspirin. A true allergy would reveal antibodies to the offending substance in the blood, but many who are hypersensitive do not have these antibodies. Their reactions are caused by enzyme deficiencies and would best be labeled a sensitivity instead of an allergy. True mercury allergy is low, but mercury sensitivity is more common.

Thyroid antibodies (anti-thyroid peroxidase (anti-TPO) and anti-thyroglobulin (anti Tg) antibodies) decreased significantly after dental amalgams were removed from patients who were hypersensitive to inorganic mercury.[16] While all test subjects were considered to have autoimmune thyroiditis because of positive anti-TPO and anti-Tg antibodies, not all subjects reacted positively to inorganic mercury in the MELISA test for metal allergies and hypersensitivity. This test measures the reactivity of white blood cells to various metals. Those who tested positive were considered hypersensitive and reported intolerance to other metal objects such as earrings, jean buttons, watches, and intrauterine devices. They also reported chronic fatigue, depression, and sleep disturbances, all common symptoms in hypothyroid patients. Both thyroid antibodies and mercury reactivity decreased after amalgam removal, which suggests an immunological rather than toxicological effect of the amalgams in these particular patients. In other words, these patients were exhibiting a response more in line with an allergy or sensitivity to mercury, rather than mercury poisoning.

In general, autoimmune thyroiditis is thought to have multiple causes, from genetic predisposition, to physical and chemical triggers, to infectious agents. Metal allergies (most commonly mercury and nickel) have been pinpointed as triggers, but so have infectious agents such as *Helicobacter pylori* (the bacterium that causes ulcers). Likewise, infection with the bacterium *Yersinia enterocolitica* (which may cause fever and bloody diarrhea) has been shown in patients with Graves's thyrotoxicosis. In one study, removal of mercury amalgams in those who were mercury sensitive improved the health of about 70% of the patients. In some patients harboring *Helicobacter pylori*, successful treatment of the bacteria eliminated the infection and autoimmunity. This study concluded that amalgam removal may be beneficial if the patient shows signs of having a mercury allergy or sensitivity.[17]

Enzyme deficiencies and disease

While I have not been formally tested, I have many of the symptoms listed for chemical sensitivity. I react to aspirin (related to my yellow #5 food color sensitivity that causes hives), nickel (cheap earrings make my ears itch), thimerosal (this mercury preservative in contact lens solutions makes my eyes bloodshot; flu shots give me hives), and sulfites (make me wheeze). I also have an autoimmune condition (Graves' thyroid disease), and suffer from atopy, better known as the "allergic triad" of eczema, asthma, and hay fever. I am definitely allergic to cats and oak pollen, and a runny nose confirms the results of a pinprick allergy test. Genetic enzyme deficiencies were mentioned as the possible root cause of these types of reactions. These enzyme processes are supposed to remove toxins, but if they don't, then the toxins could build up to toxic levels, and cause many of the reactions common to hypersensitive individuals like me.

Systemic lupus erythematosus (SLE) is an inflammatory autoimmune disease that appears in the genetically susceptible from environmental triggers such as ultraviolet irradiation (sunlight), organic solvents, petrochemicals, organic and inorganic xenobiotics, infections, and sex hormones–both exogenous (supplemented) and endogenous (natural). Lupus can also develop after treatment with cyclosporine chemotherapy and is then referred to as drug-induced SLE. Polymorphisms (genetic variations) of GSTM1, a phase II enzyme, are associated with lupus.[18]

Vitiligo, a disease where skin loses some of its pigment, is another condition associated with other autoimmune conditions such as thyroiditis, diabetes mellitus, adrenal insufficiency, psoriasis, systemic lupus erythematosus, etc. Vitiligo can be triggered by contact with phenols/quinones (found in foods and chemicals), psychological stress, trauma, and viral diseases, but it also has a genetic component. A polymorphism in the GSTP1 gene, a phase II enzyme, shows association with vitiligo.[19]

Even cancer may result from suboptimal detoxification pathways. An increased risk of breast cancer was found for women with the UGT1A6_19_GG polymorphism.[20] UGTs are one of the phase II enzymes involved in detoxification of the sex hormones. In another study of women with breast tumors, the expression of three different CYPs, or phase I enzymes, was significantly reduced (nearly 80%) in the tumors compared to normal breast tissue. At the same time, expression of COMT, a phase II enzyme, was nearly seven times higher in breast tumors. The decreased expression of the phase I enzymes means estradiol may not be metabolized efficiently, resulting in prolonged exposure to estradiol, which could be a risk factor for breast cancer.[21]

Asthma may result from a polymorphism of Glutathione S-transferase M1 (GSTM1), a phase II enzyme, which regulates stress-activated asthma. Those with an active GSTM1 gene will display bronchoconstriction at a lower threshold of allergens than asthmatics without the GSTM1 gene.[22]

Catalase is an antioxidant enzyme that neutralizes free radicals that are generated during the phase I process. It may be absent or only present at reduced levels in disease states, and it can also be inactivated by xenobiotics. Catalase levels also decrease with age, and may contribute to anemia, atherosclerosis, tumors, and type 2 diabetes as well as eye disorders, cataracts and macular degeneration.[23] Catalase polymorphisms are implicated in vitiligo and lupus.

Glutathione peroxidase is another antioxidant enzyme that aids in neutralizing free radicals generated during phase I detoxification. Glutathione peroxidase levels that are either higher or lower than normal have been found in patients with vitiligo, lupus, and chronic fatigue syndrome.

Is autism caused by detoxification enzyme deficiencies?

Enzyme deficiencies are implicated in autism. Autistics tend to be low in the phase II phenol-sulphotransferase-P enzyme that metabolizes phenols and amines. Without sufficient levels of this enzyme, autistics are unable to fully metabolize foods and chemicals that contain phenols, such as berries, olive oil, chocolate, BHT (a preservative), and salicylic acid (aspirin). Inability to metabolize amines means that neurotransmitters such as serotonin, dopamine, and noradrenaline could build up, negatively affecting the brain. The unusual reactions of autistics to drugs (sedatives have the opposite effect) may also be explained by the low levels of this enzyme.[24]

Acetaminophen (or paracetamol) could induce autism in newborns due to faulty enzyme processing. Acetaminophen should be metabolized in the liver by the phase II enzyme processes, sulfation and glucuronidation, which transform it for excretion. But newborns have immature detoxification pathways, so they cannot fully metabolize the acetaminophen. Newborns with low birth weight have reduced glucuronidation capacity, and this has been associated with autism. Sulfation pathways in autistic children are also abnormal, which means they cannot process the acetaminophen through sulfation either. Instead, the CYP or phase I pathway produces a toxic, highly reactive metabolite, n-acetyl-p-benzoquinoneimine (NAPQI), which is inactivated with glutathione. But once glutathione is depleted, the reactive metabolite can cause oxidative stress, immune system activation, and asthma. It has been observed that both autistic children and their mothers have abnormal glutathione metabolism. Maternal preeclampsia (high blood pressure) has been associated with an increased risk of having a child with autism spectrum disorder. Some studies show women who used acetaminophen during the third trimester of pregnancy had an increased risk of preeclampsia. Finally, pregnant women have a naturally lower sulfation capacity, which further lowers their ability to metabolize acetaminophen.[25]

Acetaminophen is often given after newborn circumcisions for pain management. Prior to the 1990s, circumcisions were usually performed without any pain medications. In the mid-1990s, guidelines suggested a first dose of acetaminophen two hours before the procedure, and then additional doses every 4-6 hours for the first 24 hours. A newborn male with immature detoxification pathways could receive 5-7 doses of acetaminophen after circumcision. Newborn females are obviously not subjected to these procedures, and this may explain why autism is 4.6 times higher in males compared to females, if acetaminophen use is the triggering event.

High doses of acetaminophen have caused acute liver failure, which has been fatal. When my son was a toddler, acetaminophen was recommended for teething, any fever, and after every vaccination, to relieve his "discomfort." Acetaminophen is commonly prescribed for fever relief, even though there is no real evidence that fever itself is harmful.[26] In fact, the high temperature from a fever may be the body's way of killing off viruses. In animal experiments, preventing a rise in temperature often resulted in higher mortality.[27] Yet there was never any warning given to us that acetaminophen could be toxic when too much was taken, or when given repeatedly in "normal" doses. There are case studies where parents inadvertently overdosed their children, after giving them a dose every four hours, as the directions stated.[28] Parents were sometimes unaware that acetaminophen was also an ingredient in the cough and cold medications they were simultaneously giving their child, which resulted in a higher total daily intake than recommended. Deaths have occurred due to liver or kidney failure.

Autism cases have risen considerably since the 1980s, which coincides with the rise in acetaminophen use after the Centers for Disease Control (CDC) warned against giving aspirin to children because it could induce a condition called Reye's syndrome.[29] Children are given multiple vaccinations before they are two years old: the diphtheria, tetanus, and acellular pertussis (DTaP) vaccine is given at ages two, four, and six months, with a fourth shot between 15 and 18 months. This DTaP vaccine is said to cause the most fever and pain, and acetaminophen is the standard remedy. The measles-mumps-rubella (MMR) vaccine is given between 12 and 15 months of age. For convenience, the MMR is often given with the DTaP at 15 months. Autistic children were eight times more likely to have gotten sick after the MMR vaccine compared to controls, and six times more likely to have been given acetaminophen for their symptoms.[30] While it would seem plausible that the vaccines may be responsible for the rising number of autism cases, it doesn't explain the fact that there are more cases of autism at birth. On closer examination, it turns out that the CDC now recommends flu shots (which contain thimerosal, a mercury preservative) to all pregnant women,[31] and acetaminophen is recommended by doctors for fever and pain during pregnancy.[32] This means drug exposure begins before birth. Drugs used to induce labor may also be a risk factor.[33] Other toxins that are now commonplace in our environment may be a factor too, since mothers of autistics were also shown to have disturbed detoxification enzyme processes.

Thimerosal (found in some, but not all vaccines) is believed by many to be the cause of autism that appears a few months after MMR vaccines. Yet according to the U.S. Food and Drug Administration (FDA) website on vaccines, the MMR vaccine has never contained thimerosal.[34] Another study hypothesizes that autistic children are instead unable to metabolize the aluminum present in some vaccines, and the acetaminophen given afterwards. Aluminum is added to vaccines as an adjuvant; in other words, the presence of aluminum encourages the immune system to create antibodies to the antigen in the vaccine.[35] However, there is no aluminum in the MMR vaccine, though it is in four other vaccinations that may be given simultaneously with the MMR vaccine at 15 months, as shown in Table 8-1.[36] An analysis of the U.S. Center for Disease Control Vaccine Adverse Events Reporting System (VAERS) database revealed that use of the word *autism* steadily increased in the late 1990s when thimerosal was being phased out, aluminum in vaccines became more prevalent, and the number of required vaccinations increased.[37] The hepatitis B vaccine, given at birth and then twice more before age two, contains both aluminum and mercury. Male newborns vaccinated with the hepatitis B vaccine prior to 1999 had a threefold higher risk for autism compared to boys who were not vaccinated.[38] It may be that the accumulated load of aluminum, mercury, and acetaminophen from multiple vaccinations reaches a threshold and triggers autism after 15 months, in those born with phase II sulfation and glucuronidation enzyme deficiencies.

U.S. Recommended Immunization Schedule
from Birth to 15 Months in 2012

		Age in Months					
	Birth	1	2	4	6	15	
Hepatitis B	Al		Al		Al		Total
Rotavirus			X	X	X		vaccines
Diphtheria, tetanus, pertussis			Al	Al	Al	Al	with
Haemophilus influenzae type b			Al	Al	Al	Al	aluminum
Pneumococcal			Al	Al	Al	Al	by 15
Inactivated poliovirus			X	X	X		months
Influenza					X		
Measles, mumps, rubella						X	
Varicella						X	
Hepatitis A						Al	
Number of Shots with Aluminum	1		4	3	4	4	16

Table 8-1. A sample vaccination schedule for an infant born in the US in 2012.[39] The shots that contain aluminum are represented with an "Al" in the table. Other scheduled shots are noted with an "X." Note that there is some leeway in this schedule. For example, the MMR shot can be given at 12 or 15 months, and the DTaP at 15 or 18 months, but for the sake of convenience, both shots are often administered in one office visit. There are 25 vaccinations given during this early developmental period, and 16 of these shots contain aluminum.

There is strong evidence that vaccinations trigger the development of certain autoimmune diseases. Professor Yehuda Shoenfeld, founder and head of the Zabludowicz Center for Autoimmune Diseases at the Sheba Medical Center in Israel, noticed that four conditions: siliconosis (from silicone implants), Gulf War syndrome (GWS), macrophagic myofasciitis syndrome (MMF), and post-vaccination phenomena were all linked with previous exposure to an adjuvant. Patients also presented with similar clinical symptoms, even though they were not exposed to the same adjuvant. In 2011, Professor Shoenfeld suggested these similar conditions should be given the name ASIA, for Autoimmune (Autoinflammatory) Syndrome Induced by Adjuvants. Chronic stimulation of the immune system by adjuvants leads to the release of inflammatory cytokines (cell signaling molecules), which eventually leads to severe fatigue, poor sleep, myalgias (muscle pain), and arthralgias (joint pain).[40] The adjuvants associated with ASIA are squalene (Gulf War syndrome), aluminum hydroxide (postvaccination phenomena and macrophagic myofasciitis), and silicone (siliconosis). Mineral oil, guaiacol and iodine gadital are also associated with ASIA.[41]

While aluminum is not in every vaccine, it is in quite a few, including the new GARDASIL, which is now being given to teenagers to protect against diseases caused by the Human Papillomavirus (HPV).[42] Aluminum is a confirmed neurotoxin that can affect the brain and central nervous system, especially in its early developmental stages.[43] Unfortunately, that is when it is given, in repeated, frequent doses, to infants in western countries. Table 8-1 shows that 16 vaccinations containing aluminum are given to infants in the U.S. by the time they are 15 months old.

Other conditions that show a link to aluminum adjuvant vaccines are arthritis, type I diabetes mellitus, multiple sclerosis, systemic lupus erythematosus, chronic fatigue syndrome, and autism spectrum disorders. Vaccines themselves could induce autoimmune diseases; they contain antigens along with adjuvants that upregulate the immune system, which triggers the activation of autoreactive T (immune) cells. When more than one antigen is introduced at the same time (the standard immunization schedule gives multiple vaccines at once), or exposure to the antigen is repeated often (every few months is standard), stimulation to the immune system will be high for an extended period, resulting in a magnified inflammatory response, which creates the perfect environment for autoimmunity.[44]

Gut health

The gastrointestinal tract has two basic functions: to absorb nutrients, and to prevent the penetration of dangerous pathogens. It consists of an external anatomical barrier, and an internal immunological barrier. Healthy gut microorganisms (microbiome), a mucous layer, and an intestinal epithelial layer are found in the outer anatomical barrier. Immune cells are found in the deeper inner barrier; they respond to pathogens and provide immune tolerance.[45] A change in the gut microbiota or damage to the epithelial layer would lead to increased intestinal permeability, which would affect the inner immune barrier and could lead to immune dysfunction and autoimmunity. The microbiome may play a role in inflammatory bowel disease, celiac disease, psoriasis, rheumatoid arthritis, type I diabetes, and multiple sclerosis. Diet, antibiotics, microbe-microbe interactions, and host genetics affect the microbiome, and a disruption can lead to dysbiosis (an imbalance in the natural gut microbiota).[46]

The gut of a newborn is colonized shortly after birth; the gut microbiota in a newborn from vaginal delivery differs from that of a newborn delivered through caesarean section. Likewise, whether the infant is fed breast milk or formula also affects the microbiome. In both cases, direct physical contact with the mother establishes a more normal microbiota.[47] Intestinal microbiota is highly individual and similar in identical twins and others that are genetically related.[48]

There are several diseases that show an association with altered intestinal microbiota: Crohn's disease, ulcerative colitis, irritable bowel syndrome, *Clostridium difficile* infection, colorectal cancer, allergy/atopy, celiac disease, Type 1 diabetes, Type 2 diabetes, and obesity all have multiple studies supporting the correlation. Association is not proof of causality, but there is a definite difference in the microbiota of patients with these conditions when compared to healthy individuals.[49]

Fecal Microbiota Transplantation (FMT) is a way to recreate a healthy intestinal microbiota in those with chronic diseases. Also called intestinal microbiota transfer or fecal bacteriotherapy, it has been successfully used to treat *Clostridium difficile* infections (CDI). A healthy donor provides the microbiota that repopulates the patient's gut, and it has been successful approximately 90% of the time. Antibiotics are often initially prescribed for CDI, but they suppress not only the pathogen, but the protective microbiota, so the patient is never really "cured" with antibiotics. Recurrences and complications (including death) are common with antibiotic therapy, whereas cases of recurrent CDI have been cured with only one FMT treatment.[50]

Infectious causes of autoimmunity

Several infectious agents show an association with autoimmune thyroid diseases. A protozoa (*Toxoplasma gondii*) has been implicated in both Hashimoto's thyroiditis and Graves' disease.[51] The bacteria *Helicobacter pylori* and *Yersinia enterocolitica* are possible triggers for Hashimoto's or Graves', respectively.[52] HHV-6, the human herpes virus, may be a trigger for Hashimoto's thyroiditis.[53] The hepatitis C virus is associated with autoimmunity.[54] There is even a case of autoimmune hyperthyroidism (Hashitoxicosis) developing after infection with *Bartonella henselae*, more commonly known as cat scratch disease.[55]

Chemical causes of autoimmunity

Clusters of people living near toxic waste sites have developed lupus, which suggests that ongoing chemical exposure can overwhelm the phase II detoxification enzyme systems and trigger autoimmunity. Women who were GSTM1 deficient or had altered GSTP1 binding sites were more likely to develop lupus at an earlier age if they lived near hazardous waste sites.[56] The GST enzymes should break down organic compounds such as DDT pesticides and petroleum byproducts.

A woman went for a hair straightening treatment and was told that the product to be used was formaldehyde free. This was important because she'd had previous reactions to formaldehyde. The hair is normally washed after treatment, but because it was closing time, she was sent home and told to leave it in till her next appointment. She developed diarrhea, vomiting, total body flushing and low-grade fever a few days later. She finally washed her hair eight days after the treatment and felt a burning sensation on her scalp. She had sores and bald spots on her scalp similar to chemical burns. She felt she couldn't breathe in the shower, and then developed a chronic nosebleed which continued for months. She lost 25 pounds over the next three months and was unable to eat, did not have bowel movements for 2 to 3 weeks at a time, and was hospitalized for intermittent bloating and abdominal pain. Her entire body turned bright red whenever she took a shower. She developed tachycardia and total body tingling up to 15 times a day. She tested positive for Anti-Nuclear Antibodies (ANA) and was eventually diagnosed with an unclassified autoimmune disease based on multiple organ impairment and peripheral neuropathy, anemia, joint and muscle pain, fever, flushing, weakness, amenorrhea, fatigue and weakness.[57]

Drug induced autoimmunity

Statins, which are prescribed to reduce cholesterol, may induce a form of autoimmune myopathy (muscle weakness) in some patients. Autoantibodies are formed against an enzyme that statins target, 3-hydroxy-3-methylglutaryl-coenzyme A reductase (HMGCR). These antibodies are also found in some autoimmune myopathy patients without statin exposure.[58]

Other pharmaceutical drugs have induced autoimmune hepatitis,[59] lupus,[60] vasculitis,[61] interstitial lung disease, multiple sclerosis,[62] and thrombocytopenia.[63] Drugs are foreign metabolites to the body, and must be processed out by detoxification enzymes. Those who are deficient in certain enzymes may be more susceptible to these auto-immune diseases.

Conclusion

Not everyone has an autoimmune disease, though most of us live in similar environments. Genetics appear to be the overriding factor, and those of us with genetic detoxification enzyme deficiencies appear to be at greatest risk. Those of us with multiple allergies and sensitivities are probably deficient in several detoxification enzymes, so anything perceived as a foreign compound or xenobiotic remains in our system far longer than it should. The number of xenobiotics in our food and environment today is staggering and may be a major factor in the rising number of autoimmune cases today.

While some of the compounds in vaccinations appear to be perceived by the body as xenobiotics, it would be unwise, in my opinion, for everyone to shun vaccinations. Vaccinations have eradicated several once common diseases, and this progress would be lost if vaccinations stopped. Children today are also placed in daycare at an early age, which would be a perfect breeding ground for epidemics if no one was vaccinated. There have been several fatal cases of the flu this year, and none of the cases had received a flu shot. Would those people still be with us if they'd had a shot? Everyone will have to do their own risk/benefit analysis and make their own decision regarding shots for themselves.

Autism spectrum cases in the United Stated and the United Kingdom are 9-12 times higher than the rates in Iceland and Finland.[36] What do they do differently? The first vaccination in these Nordic countries is not given until the infant is three months old. In contrast, U.S. infants receive seven shots by the time they are only two months old (beginning on the day of birth), and five of these contain aluminum. Giving the first vaccination when the child is older, after the child's detoxification pathways have a chance to develop, would be wiser. Is it really necessary to vaccinate all newborns for Hepatitis B at birth? What are the chances of a newborn catching this disease, which is transmitted through the blood, semen, or other body fluids of an infected person? A newborn can catch hepatitis B at birth if the mother is infected, but it seems that it would be safer to test the mother than risk inducing autism in a newborn. Studies show a strong correlation of autism to acetaminophen usage. Therefore, it would seem wise for all pregnant mothers and newborns to avoid acetaminophen.

Adults have had negative reactions to vaccinations too (Gulf War syndrome). Screening tests should be devised to tell when someone is a risky candidate for a vaccination. The last time I had a flu shot I broke out in whole body hives, and my reaction to thimerosal in contact lens solutions should have been the clue that I should not be injected with any mercury containing compound. The only screening question I was asked was, "are you allergic to eggs?" and I'm not. Cheap earrings make my ears itch, which suggests I am sensitive to metals. Aluminum adjuvant vaccines would therefore not be a good idea for me either. Since the rates of autism are continuing to rise, and a strong case can be made that aluminum is the trigger, vaccine manufacturers should be looking into alternative adjuvants.

A healthy gut is the first line of defense against incoming pathogens, and establishing a healthy microbiome in a newborn should be a priority. Because the microbiome of a newborn's gut is established shortly after birth, women should be encouraged to breastfeed for as long as possible to help establish a natural flora. Antibiotics should also not be dispensed so readily, without confirmation that the illness is truly bacterial and not viral (antibiotics are ineffective against viruses).

While none of us has any control over the genes we inherit, we can do our best to avoid further health problems by limiting our contact with xenobiotics found in our food and environment.

Key points

- Genetic predisposition, detoxification enzyme deficiencies, drugs, vaccinations, infections, and chemical exposure are just a few of the triggers for autoimmunity.
- Enzyme deficiencies at any stage of detoxification (phase I, II, or free radical neutralization) are implicated in many diseases.
- Detoxification enzymes metabolize xenobiotics, or foreign compounds, such as drugs, pesticides, and carcinogens, and eliminate them from the body through feces and urine.

- Detoxification enzyme deficiencies lead to illnesses such as amalgam disease (from dental mercury fillings), multiple chemical sensitivity, fibromyalgia, chronic fatigue syndrome, sick building syndrome, electric hypersensitivity, irritable bowel syndrome, and Persian Gulf War veteran syndrome.

- Lupus, vitiligo, cancer, and asthma may all result from polymorphisms in phase II enzymes.

- Mercury is poisonous, but not everyone is "sensitive" to it. Those who are may develop autoimmunity and extreme sensitivity to inhalants (particle and vapors) and ingestants (food and chemicals) from dental amalgams.

- Autistics are low in a phase II enzyme (phenol-sulphotransferase-P), which prevents them from fully metabolizing certain foods and chemicals.

- Acetaminophen (or paracetamol) may induce autism in newborns with impaired sulfation and glucuronidation phase II detoxification processes.

- Aluminum in some vaccines may induce autism.

- The cumulative exposure to mercury, aluminum, and acetaminophen may reach a threshold that triggers autism after 15 months in children in the U.S. By then, 25 vaccinations have been given, 16 of which contain aluminum.

- Conditions associated with aluminum adjuvant vaccines are arthritis, type I diabetes mellitus, multiple sclerosis, systemic lupus erythematosus, chronic fatigue syndrome, and autism spectrum disorders.

- Vaccines may trigger autoimmune diseases because they contain antigens along with adjuvants that upregulate the immune system. Multiple antigens and repeated exposure overstimulate the immune system, which creates the perfect environment for autoimmunity.

- A healthy gut is the first line of defense against incoming pathogens, and establishing a healthy microbiome in a newborn should be a priority. Breast-feeding should be encouraged for as long as possible and antibiotics limited, if possible.

- The microbiome may play a role in inflammatory bowel disease, celiac disease, psoriasis, rheumatoid arthritis, type I diabetes, and multiple sclerosis.

- Fecal Microbiota Transplantation (FMT) may help restore a healthy microbiome to those with poor gut health.

- Various viruses and bacteria are associated with autoimmune disease.

- Chemicals in our environment can trigger autoimmune disease.

[1] American Dental Association, Current Policies, Adopted 1954-2012, http://www.ada.org/sections/about/pdfs/doc_policies.pdf accessed 11/29/13

[2] Cárdenas-Roldán, Jorge, Adriana Rojas-Villarraga, and Juan-Manuel Anaya. "How do autoimmune diseases cluster in families? A systematic review and meta-analysis." *BMC medicine* 11.1 (2013): 73.

[3] Brix, Thomas Heiberg, and Laszlo Hegedüs. "Twin studies as a model for exploring the aetiology of autoimmune thyroid disease." *Clinical endocrinology* 76.4 (2012): 457-464.

[4] Eschler, Deirdre Cocks, Alia Hasham, and Yaron Tomer. "Cutting edge: the etiology of autoimmune thyroid diseases." *Clinical reviews in allergy & immunology* 41.2 (2011): 190-197.

[5] Liska, D. J. "The detoxification enzyme systems." *Altern Med Rev* 3.3 (1998): 187-98.

[6] Pavek, Petr, and Zdenek Dvorak. "Xenobiotic-induced transcriptional regulation of xenobiotic metabolizing enzymes of the cytochrome P450 superfamily in human extrahepatic tissues." *Current drug metabolism* 9.2 (2008): 129-143.

[7] Korkina, L., et al. "The chemical defensive system in the pathobiology of idiopathic environment-associated diseases." *Current drug metabolism* 10.8 (2009): 914-931.

[8] Pujos-Guillot, Estelle, et al. "Therapeutic paracetamol treatment in older persons induces dietary and metabolic modifications related to sulfur amino acids." *Age* 34.1 (2012): 181-193.

[9] Nimni, Marcel E., Bo Han, and Fabiola Cordoba. "Are we getting enough sulfur in our diet." *Nutr Metab (Lond)* 4 (2007): 24.

[10] Xu, Changjiang, Christina Yong-Tao Li, and Ah-Ng Tony Kong. "Induction of phase I, II and III drug metabolism/transport by xenobiotics." *Archives of pharmacal research* 28.3 (2005): 249-268.

[11] Gamage, Niranjali, et al. "Human sulfotransferases and their role in chemical metabolism." *Toxicological Sciences* 90.1 (2006): 5-22.

[12] Sarikaya, Sezgin, et al. "Acute mercury poisoning: a case report." *BMC emergency medicine* 10.1 (2010): 7.

[13] Bernhoft, Robin A. "Mercury toxicity and treatment: a review of the literature." *Journal of environmental and public health* 2012 (2011).

[14] Guzzi, Gianpaolo, et al. "Dental amalgam and mercury levels in autopsy tissues: food for thought." *The American journal of forensic medicine and pathology* 27.1 (2006): 42-45.

[15] Zamm, Alfred. "Dental Mercury: A Factor that Aggravates and Induces Xenobiotic Intolerance." *Journal of Orthomolecular Medicine* 6.2 (1991).

[16] Sterzl, Ivan, et al. "Removal of dental amalgam decreases anti-TPO and anti-Tg autoantibodies in patients with autoimmune thyroiditis." *Neuroendocrinology letters* 27 (2006): 25-30.

[17] Hybenova, Monika, et al. "The role of environmental factors in autoimmune thyroiditis." *Neuroendocrinol. Lett* 31 (2010): 283-289.

[18] Zhang, Jufeng, et al. "Association of GSTT1, GSTM1 and CYP1A1 polymorphisms with susceptibility to systemic lupus erythematosus in the Chinese population." *Clinica Chimica Acta* 411.11 (2010): 878-881.

[19] Minashkin, Mikhail M., et al. "Possible contribution of GSTP1 and other xenobiotic metabolizing genes to vitiligo susceptibility." *Archives of dermatological research* (2012): 1-7.

[20] Justenhoven, Christina, et al. "The UGT1A6_19_GG genotype is a breast cancer risk factor." *Frontiers in genetics* 4 (2013).

[21] Zhao, Ya-Nan, et al. "Relative imbalances in the expression of catechol-O-methyltransferase and cytochrome P450 in breast cancer tissue and their association with breast carcinoma." *Maturitas* 72.2 (2012): 139-145.

[22] Hoskins, Aimee, et al. "Asthmatic Airway Neutrophilia after Allergen Challenge Is Associated with the Glutathione S-Transferase M1 Genotype." *American journal of respiratory and critical care medicine* 187.1 (2013): 34-41.

[23] Terlecky, Stanley R., Jay I. Koepke, and Paul A. Walton. "Peroxisomes and aging." *Biochimica et Biophysica Acta (BBA)-Molecular Cell Research* 1763.12 (2006): 1749-1754.

[24] O'Reilly, B. A., and R. H. Waring. "Enzyme and sulphur oxidation deficiencies in autistic children with known food/chemical intolerances." *Journal of Orthomolecular Medicine* 8 (1993): 198-198.

[25] Bauer, Ann Z., and David Kriebel. "Prenatal and perinatal analgesic exposure and autism: an ecological link." *Environmental Health* 12.1 (2013): 41.

[26] Obu, Herbert A., et al. "Paracetamol use (and/or misuse) in children in Enugu, South-East, Nigeria." *BMC pediatrics* 12.1 (2012): 103.

[27] Kluger, Matthew J., et al. "Role of fever in disease." *Annals of the New York Academy of Sciences* 856.1 (1998): 224-233.

[28] Shivbalan, So, Malathi Sathiyasekeran, and Kuruvilla Thomas. "Therapeutic misadventure with paracetamol in children." *Indian journal of pharmacology* 42.6 (2010): 412.

[29] Centers for Disease Control and Prevention. CDC study shows sharp decline in Reye's Syndrome among U.S. children. Accessed 8/11/2013. http://www.cdc.gov/media/pressrel/r990506.htm

[30] Good, Peter. "Did acetaminophen provoke the autism epidemic." *Altern. Med. Rev* 14 (2009): 364-372.

[31] Summary Recommendations: Prevention and Control of Influenza with Vaccines: Recommendations of the Advisory Committee on Immunization Practices—(ACIP)—United States, 2013-14. Accessed on 9/28/13: http://www.cdc.gov/flu/professionals/acip/2013-summary-recommendations.htm

[32] Thiele, K., et al. "Acetaminophen and pregnancy: short-and long-term consequences for mother and child." *Journal of reproductive immunology* 97.1 (2013): 128.

[33] Gregory, Simon G., et al. "Association of Autism With Induced or Augmented Childbirth in North Carolina Birth Record (1990-1998) and Education Research (1997-2007) Databases Autism and Induced or Augmented Childbirth Autism and Induced or Augmented Childbirth." *JAMA pediatrics* 167.10 (2013): 959-966.

[34] U.S. Food and Drug Administration. Vaccines, Blood & Biologics: Thimerosal in Vaccines. Accessed 7/19/2013. http://www.fda.gov/BiologicsBloodVaccines/SafetyAvailability/VaccineSafety/UCM096228

[35] Kuroda, Etsushi, Cevayir Coban, and Ken J. Ishii. "Particulate Adjuvant and Innate Immunity: Past Achievements, Present Findings, and Future Prospects." *International reviews of immunology* 32.2 (2013): 209-220.

[36] Tomljenovic, Lucija, and Christopher A. Shaw. "Do aluminum vaccine adjuvants contribute to the rising prevalence of autism?" *Journal of Inorganic Biochemistry* 105.11 (2011): 1489-1499.

[37] Seneff, Stephanie, Robert M. Davidson, and Jingjing Liu. "Empirical data confirm autism symptoms related to aluminum and acetaminophen exposure." *Entropy* 14.11 (2012): 2227-2253.

[38] Gallagher, C. M., and M. S. Goodman. "Hepatitis B vaccination of male neonates and autism diagnosis, NHIS 1997-2002." *Journal of toxicology and environmental health. Part A* 73.24 (2010): 1665.

[39] Centers for Disease Control and Prevention. Recommended Immunization Schedules for Persons Aged 0 Through 18 Years — United States, 2012. Accessed 7/24/13. http://www.cdc.gov/mmwr/preview/mmwrhtml/mm6105a5.htm

[40] Shoenfeld, Yehuda. "Video Q&A: what is ASIA? An interview with Yehuda Shoenfeld." *BMC medicine* 11.1 (2013): 118.

[41] Vera-Lastra, Olga, et al. "Autoimmune/inflammatory syndrome induced by adjuvants (Shoenfeld's syndrome): clinical and immunological spectrum." *Expert review of clinical immunology* 9.4 (2013): 361-373.

[42] USPPI, Patient Information about GARDASIL®, issued April 2011. Accessed 8/11/2013. http://www.merck.com/product/usa/pi_circulars/g/gardasil/gardasil_ppi.pdf

[43] Shaw, C. A., and L. Tomljenovic. "Aluminum in the central nervous system (CNS): toxicity in humans and animals, vaccine adjuvants, and autoimmunity." *Immunologic research* (2013): 1-13.

[44] Tomljenovic, Lucija, and C. A. Shaw. "Mechanisms of aluminum adjuvant toxicity and autoimmunity in pediatric populations." *Lupus* 21.2 (2012): 223-230.

[45] Lopetuso, Loris R., Saleem Chowdhry, and Theresa T. Pizarro. "Opposing functions of classic and novel IL-1 family members in gut health and disease." *Frontiers in immunology* 4 (2013).

[46] Fung, Irene, et al. "Do Bugs Control Our Fate? The Influence of the Microbiome on Autoimmunity." *Current allergy and asthma reports* 12.6 (2012): 511-519.

[47] Mulle, Jennifer G., William G. Sharp, and Joseph F. Cubells. "The Gut Microbiome: A New Frontier in Autism Research." *Current psychiatry reports* 15.2 (2013): 1-9.

[48] Turnbaugh, Peter J., et al. "A core gut microbiome in obese and lean twins." *Nature* 457.7228 (2008): 480-484.

[49] de Vos, Willem M., and Elisabeth AJ de Vos. "Role of the intestinal microbiome in health and disease: from correlation to causation." *Nutrition reviews* 70.s1 (2012): S45-S56.

[50] Bakken, Johan S., et al. "Treating *Clostridium difficile* Infection With Fecal Microbiota Transplantation." *Clinical Gastroenterology and Hepatology* 9.12 (2011): 1044-1049.

[51] Tozzoli, R., et al. "Infections and autoimmune thyroid diseases: parallel detection of antibodies against pathogens with proteomic technology." *Autoimmunity Reviews* 8.2 (2008): 112-115.

[52] Pordeus, V., et al. "Infections and autoimmunity: a panorama." *Clinical reviews in allergy & immunology* 34.3 (2008): 283-299.

[53] Caselli, Elisabetta, et al. "Virologic and immunologic evidence supporting an association between HHV-6 and Hashimoto's thyroiditis." *PLoS pathogens* 8.10 (2012): e1002951.

[54] Vergani, Diego, and Giorgina Mieli-Vergani. "Autoimmune manifestations in viral hepatitis." *Seminars in immunopathology*. Vol. 35. No. 1. Springer-Verlag, 2013.

[55] Chiuri, Rosa Maria, et al. "Bartonella henselae Infection Associated with Autoimmune Thyroiditis in a Child." *Hormone research in paediatrics* 79.3 (2013): 185-188.

[56] Karlson, Elizabeth W., et al. "Effect of glutathione S-TRANSFERASE polymorphisms and proximity to hazardous waste sites on time to systemic lupus erythematosus diagnosis: Results from the roxbury lupus project." *Arthritis & Rheumatism* 56.1 (2007): 244-254.

[57] Dahlgren, James, et al. "Case Report: Autoimmune Disease Triggered by Exposure to Hair Straightening Treatment Containing Formaldehyde." *Open Journal of Rheumatology and Autoimmune Diseases*, 3 (2013): 1-6.

[58] Mohassel, Payam, and Andrew L. Mammen. "Statin-associated autoimmune myopathy and anti-HMGCR autoantibodies: A review." *Muscle & nerve* (2013).

[59] Bjornsson, Einar, et al. "Drug-induced autoimmune hepatitis: Clinical characteristics and prognosis." *Hepatology* 51.6 (2010): 2040-2048.

[60] Katz, Uriel, and Gisele Zandman-Goddard. "Drug-induced lupus: an update." *Autoimmunity reviews* 10.1 (2010): 46-50.

[61] Jarrett, Stephen J., et al. "Anti-tumor necrosis factor-alpha therapy-induced vasculitis: case series." *The Journal of rheumatology* 30.10 (2003): 2287-2291.

[62] Ramos-Casals, Manuel, et al. "Autoimmune diseases induced by biological agents: a double-edged sword?." *Autoimmunity reviews* 9.3 (2010): 188-193.

[63] Aster, Richard H., and Daniel W. Bougie. "Drug-induced immune thrombocytopenia." *New England Journal of Medicine* 357.6 (2007): 580-587.

9

Blood Tests to Diagnose a
Thyroid or Hormone Imbalance

Your TSH is normal, so you're not hypothyroid;
would you like an anti-depressant instead?

—what patients report their doctors say

Laboratories offer several different tests that measure thyroid hormones. Some of them are direct measures of actual thyroid hormones, others are calculated (inferred) measurements. Since direct measures are available, it really makes no sense that inferred measures are even used today. When a patient has hypothyroid symptoms, a primary care physician will often request a "thyroid panel," thinking it will give them a variety of thyroid tests that clearly show whether a patient is either normal or hypothyroid. Unfortunately, this is not an "either or" proposition, and there are shades of hypothyroidism, just like many other conditions. Most patients have "normal" results.

T3 uptake and the Free T4 Index (FTI or T7) are some of the inferred measures still used today. T3 uptake does not actually measure T3, but T3's binding ability, based on the amount of thyroid binding globulin (TBG) available. T3 uptake and Total T4 are then used to calculate a Free T4 Index, which is an estimate of Free T4. Since Free T3 and Free T4 tests already exist, it doesn't make much sense to use these calculated, estimated tests. TBG is altered by high estrogen levels, liver or kidney disease, heparin, antibiotics, aspirin, and other conditions, which could affect the calculation of either T3 uptake or the Free T4 Index. Because the results of these tests can be misleading, the following tests are recommended instead:

Lab tests (recommended)

- Free T3 (FT3 or Free triiodothyronine - not part of a "thyroid panel" and must be requested; not to be confused with Total T3)
- Free T4 (FT4 or Free thyroxine)
- Total T4
- Reverse T3

- TSH (Thyroid Stimulating Hormone)
- TPO (Thyroid Peroxidase) antibodies
- Tgab (Thyroglobulin) antibodies
- TSI (Thyroid Stimulating Immunoglobulin) **or** TSab (Thyroid Stimulating antibodies) if Graves' hyperthyroidism is suspected; either test is fine, some labs offer TSI, others TSab
- TRab (TSH Receptor antibodies) **or** TBII (Thyrotropin Binding Inhibitory Immunoglobulin) antibodies - if Graves' hyperthyroidism is suspected; either test is fine, some labs offer TRab, others TBII
- Full iron panel (includes serum iron, iron binding capacity, and % saturation)
- Ferritin (not included in the full iron panel and must be requested separately)
- CBC or Complete Blood Count (includes RBC, hemoglobin, hematocrit, MCH)
- Vitamin D3
- Vitamin B12
- Lipid panel (includes cholesterol, triglycerides)
- Comprehensive Metabolic Panel (includes fasting glucose, sodium, potassium)
- Morning cortisol (24-hr saliva labs are preferred because multiple samples are necessary to determine if a daily cortisol rhythm is abnormal; however, a blood sample gives at least one reading)
- Estradiol (for both men and women; women should test on day 19-21 of their cycle, or 5-7 days after ovulation)
- Progesterone (for both men and women; women should test on day 19-21 of their cycle, or 5-7 days after ovulation)
- Total testosterone (for both men and women)
- SHBG (Sex Hormone Binding Globulin) for both men and women

Why test reverse T3?

When reverse T3 is hundreds of points over the reference range, it is a marker for a serious disease, and the cause needs to be investigated. The medical term for this condition is *non-thyroidal illness*, because normal thyroid conversion is altered by the disease state. The disease state causes T4 to convert to rT3 (an inactive metabolite) instead of to T3 (the active thyroid hormone).[1] The thyroid itself has not gone bad (as in autoimmune thyroid disease), and in fact, may return to normal function if the disease state can be successfully treated.

The absolute value of reverse T3 (whether it is within or above the reference range) is what matters, not a rT3 ratio. The rT3 ratio is a contrived calculation that can give misleading information.

The difference between *Free* and *Total* T3 and T4

A healthy thyroid produces mostly T4 and small amounts of T3,[2] so the most important thyroid blood test is the total T4, because that test will indicate if there is even enough thyroid hormone to work with. Free T4 (FT4) can be artificially elevated from certain drugs like aspirin,[3] diuretics, or heparin, so it is important to measure the total T4 to get an accurate picture of thyroid levels. Critical illness, multiple medications, late pregnancy, and genetic binding variations are situations where *total* T4 and T3 measurements may give a better indication of thyroid status than *free* T3 and T4.[4] During an acute illness, the fall in the totals is much more pronounced than the fall in the free levels, which is why it's important to measure both total and free T4.[5]

Free T3 (FT3) is the next most important thyroid blood test because if that lab result is on the low end while total T4 is mid-range or higher, it suggests improper conversion. If poor conversion is suspected, factors that impede conversion like low selenium,[6] low ferritin,[7] etc. should be corrected. An unhealthy liver may also be a factor, because the majority of conversion is performed in the liver.[8]

Free T4 would be the next thyroid blood test to examine, to see whether it correlates to the total T4 level. Sometimes there is an excess of thyroid hormone binding proteins, leading to a low Free T4, even though there is ample total T4.[9] This could be caused by high thyroxine binding globulin which is caused by high estrogen levels, pregnancy, or some illnesses. Oftentimes the Free T4 can be close to mid-range, but the total T4 will show the true picture of a deficit, since it will be below mid-range. Free T4 is usually measured in a laboratory in one of two ways: by liquid chromatography tandem mass spectrometry, or by immunoassay. The validity of immunoassay methods has been questioned, because FT4 correlates with albumin and thyroxine binding globulin when measured by immunoassay, which means the accuracy of the test is dependent on an uncontrolled variable. This suggests that the results may not accurately reflect true FT4 levels,[10] and why a Total T4 should always be used to confirm thyroid status. Most commercial laboratories have websites that describe the methodology used for each test.

Total T3 is not as good a yardstick of healthy levels as Free T3, because it is the unbound or free part that exerts the biological effect. Free T3 levels correlate better with symptoms. My Free T3 has been over range (121%) while Total T3 was at 75% of range. Symptoms indicated I was on too much T3, not too little. Another patient also presented with a Free T3 over range (110%), but a Total T3 at only 41% of range. His SHBG was also over range, which suggests that T3 levels were too high, not low, since SHBG rises as T3 rises.[11]

A study of 832 hypothyroid patients showed that 24 hour urine Free T3 had the highest inverse correlation with clinical symptoms. In other words, the higher the urine Free T3, the lower the symptoms and vice versa. Urine Free T3 is not influenced by binding globulins and correlated well with the severity of eight clinical hypothyroid symptoms: fatigue, depression, coldness, headache, muscle cramps, constipation, arthritis, and Achilles tendon reflex. Serum T4, Free T4, and TSH often had no correlation to these symptoms, which makes their use questionable.[12]

Free T3 was the strongest (based on statistical analysis) and only independent predictor of mortality (the lower the FT3, the higher the chance of mortality) in another study in an intensive care unit (ICU). Individually, Total T3, Total T4, Free T4, TSH and reverse T3 (rT3) could not predict the patient's outcome. Interestingly, rT3 levels were similar in survivors and non-survivors. Most of these patients had cardiovascular or pulmonary disease, and 19% (91/480) of them died. Only 3.54% of them had a TSH that registered as abnormally high (a hypothyroid indicator) upon admittance to the ICU, even though FT3 was below the reference range in the majority (54.38%) of patients.[13] TSH is obviously not a good indicator of health if these patients had a "normal" TSH but were in ICU (Figure 9-1).

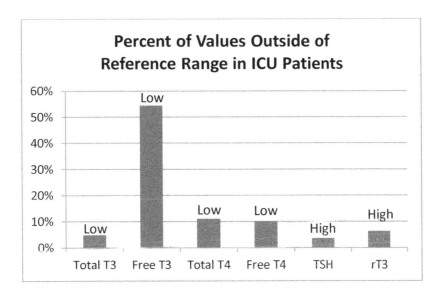

Percent of Values Outside of Reference Range in ICU Patients

Figure 9-1. The percentages were calculated from 480 ICU patients in the study (59.79% male; mean age 71.71 ± 15.52 years). The only lab value that was outside of the normal reference range for more than half the patients was Free T3.

Another study of healthy men in Finland compared the same thyroid lab results over 14 months to see if there was any correlation with colder temperatures. Again, only Free T3 showed a statistically significant correlation with severe cold, being lowest in February and highest in August. Serum Total T3, Total T4, Free T4, rT3, and urinary T4 were basically unchanged throughout the year. Urinary T3 displayed an inverse relationship with serum T3, being significantly higher in winter than in summer, which indicates higher clearance or usage of the hormone by the body over the colder months. Interestingly, TSH did not show any correlation to the thyroid hormone levels, but did change throughout the year, with a peak in December, when sunlight is lowest.[14]

Oddly, Free T3 is not routinely measured in someone being tested for hypothyroidism. It must be specifically requested and is not on most lab forms; TSH and T4 or FT4 are what are usually ordered, even though TSH levels often do not reflect thyroid levels, and T4 is not as biologically active as T3. Many have decent (mid-range) T4 levels with multiple hypothyroid symptoms, and the root problem only becomes apparent when Free T3 is examined.

Lab results reflect when the last dose was taken

Thyroid medications that contain T3 (such as desiccated thyroid or Cytomel) cause a peak in Free T3 levels a few hours after ingestion (42% rise within the first 4 hours), and then a decline until the next dose. Even T4 medications like Synthroid or levothyroxine cause a small bump in thyroid levels a few hours after a dose (16% rise in Free T4 with no change in free T3).[15] This peak and trough of the Free T3 level can greatly affect lab results, depending on when the labs are drawn relative to the last dose. For example, I take my desiccated thyroid four times a day: between 5-7 a.m., around noon before lunch, around 5:30 p.m. before dinner, and around 11 p.m. before bedtime, and then test in the morning around 9 a.m. If I don't take my morning dose on the day of testing, it would result in a lower lab result than what my body normally experiences on a daily basis, because it is about 10 hours after my last dose, when I normally dose closer to every 5-6 hours during a normal day. I also have no idea how high my Free T3 peaks, since I am measuring a trough (low point). If my lab results showed me at the top of the reference range even after this long delay, my peak levels may actually be above the range, and could be a cause for concern.

Thyroid lab work could also be done later in the day, 5-6 hours after the last dose, or at a time midway between doses to see where the Free T3 falls in the reference range then. This should give a lab result between the peak and trough levels. I've recently started taking my early morning dose and then testing around 11 a.m., or right before my next dose, to get a more accurate gauge of what my trough levels are. They are significantly higher than a 9 or 10 a.m. reading without a morning dose, and explain some of my other abnormal lab values. While many thyroid groups advise patients *not* to take their thyroid hormone the morning of testing, my results show this gives a lower than normal FT3 reading than what I normally experience throughout the day, which can then lead to incorrect dosing adjustments. For me, a ½ grain morning dose of desiccated thyroid had my FT3 significantly over the reference range 6 hours after my dose, so I've dropped back to ¼ grain every 6 hours and raised my T4 dose to compensate for the change.

Taking a lower dose more often will cause smaller peaks and troughs. All lab tests are only guidelines though, and symptoms should always trump labs when adjusting doses, because lab tests are never performed in identical conditions. Variables that can affect the results are the time elapsed since the last dose, length of time the sample sits before it's analyzed, the temperature the sample sits in, etc. The patient's condition also varies between tests, and what they ate last, how much they slept the night before, and how stressed they feel can all affect the results. Lab results also only measure serum levels from a blood draw, not what goes on at the cellular level. Total T4 and Total T3 are more reliable (because of testing methodology) in terms of test consistency from one laboratory to the next, compared to Free T3 and Free T4, which have shown wide variability in results. In fact, some tests are more accurate for either high or low values, but not both, because of inherent test limitations.[16]

Thyroid hormone levels, in excess, will affect other lab test results. These can be used to confirm whether a dose is too high. Total cholesterol may become low,[17] while glucose, triglycerides, sex hormone binding globulin (SHBG),[18] calcium, and alkaline phosphatase[19] may become elevated. The last three markers correlate with hyperthyroidism and bone loss, and should not be ignored. The hyperthyroid state (too much T3 or T4, not a low TSH) causes osteoporosis, which is why doctors are so wary of prescribing too much T3.[20] Cortisol, free testosterone and DHEA values may also fall below normal when too much thyroid hormone is taken.[21] This is one of the drawbacks of the T3-only protocol. The high T3 levels reduce cortisol and sex hormones, which patients must then replace manually. It is analogous to straightening out a table with one leg that's too long, by trying to adjust all the other legs to match.

Conclusion

The comprehensive list of lab tests should give an indication of *why* someone feels unwell. Some patients are suffering from an autoimmune thyroid disease, and the antibody tests will reveal that. Others may be anemic, or have Anemia of Chronic Disease, or adrenal or pituitary problems, which some of the other tests will reveal. In any case, the TSH test only gives limited information; certainly not enough to draw any firm conclusions. Patients should insist on full testing if they do not feel well.

Key points

- Because Free T3 correlates most with symptoms, it should be requested when thyroid labs are run, even if it's not on a standard "thyroid panel."
- Total T4 is not useless; Free T4 is sometimes artificially inflated due to testing methodology, some drugs, or critical illness.
- High levels of reverse T3 may indicate a serious non-thyroidal illness, which is not always a hypothyroid condition.
- Testing for Graves' disease should include two separate types of tests, because they measure two different things: 1) either TSI or TSab *and* 2) either TRab or TBII.
- Lab tests should *not* be done within four hours of a dose. On the other hand, because T3 has a half-life of about a day, testing nearly 24 hours after a dose will give an artificially low reading.
- When a thyroid dose is too high, glucose, triglycerides, SHBG, calcium, and alkaline phosphatase may become elevated, while total cholesterol, cortisol, free testosterone, and DHEA may decrease
- The TSH test only gives limited information; certainly not enough to draw any firm conclusions about thyroid status.

---

[1] Pappa, Theodora A., Apostolos G. Vagenakis, and Maria Alevizaki. "The nonthyroidal illness syndrome in the non-critically ill patient." *European journal of clinical investigation* 41.2 (2011): 212-220.

[2] Sapin, R., and J. L. Schlienger. "Thyroxine (T4) and tri-iodothyronine (T3) determinations: techniques and value in the assessment of thyroid function]." *Annales de biologie clinique*. Vol. 61. No. 4. 2003.

[3] Lim, Chen-Fee, et al. "Drug and fatty acid effects on serum thyroid hormone binding." *Journal of Clinical Endocrinology & Metabolism* 67.4 (1988): 682-688.

[4] Stockigt, Jim R. "Measurements of Thyroxine and Triiodothyronine." *Thyroid Function Testing*. Springer US, 2010. 85-107.

[5] Warner, Maria H., and Geoffrey J. Beckett. "Mechanisms behind the non-thyroidal illness syndrome: an update." *Journal of Endocrinology* 205.1 (2010): 1-13.

[6] Pizzulli, Antonio, and Alireza Ranjbar. "Selenium deficiency and hypothyroidism." *Biological Trace Element Research* 77.3 (2000): 199-208.

[7] Hess, Sonja Y., and Michael B. Zimmermann. "The effect of micronutrient deficiencies on iodine nutrition and thyroid metabolism." *International journal for vitamin and nutrition research* 74.2 (2004): 103-115.

[8] Mansourian, Azad Reza. "Disorders: An Overview on Liver Dysfunction and Hypothyroidism." *Pakistan Journal of Biological Sciences* 16.23 (2013): 1641-1652.

[9] Bartalena, L., et al. "Measurement of serum free thyroid hormone concentrations: an essential tool for the diagnosis of thyroid dysfunction." *Hormone Research in Paediatrics* 45.3-5 (1996): 142-147.

[10] van Deventer, Hendrick E., et al. "Inverse log-linear relationship between thyroid-stimulating hormone and free thyroxine measured by direct analog immunoassay and tandem mass spectrometry." *Clinical chemistry* 57.1 (2011): 122-127.

[11] Sanyal, Triranjan, et al. "Gynaecomastia as the initial presentation of thyrotoxicosis." *Indian journal of endocrinology and metabolism* 16.Suppl 2 (2012): S352.

[12] Baisier, W. V., J. Hertoghe, and W. Eeckhaut. "Thyroid insufficiency. Is TSH measurement the only diagnostic tool?" *Journal of Nutritional and Environmental Medicine* 10.2 (2000): 105-113.

[13] Wang, Feilong, et al. "Relationship between thyroid function and ICU mortality: a prospective observation study." *Critical Care* 16.1 (2012): R11.

[14] Hassi, Juhani, et al. "The pituitary-thyroid axis in healthy men living under subarctic climatological conditions." *Journal of endocrinology* 169.1 (2001): 195-203.

[15] Saravanan, P., et al. "Twenty-four hour hormone profiles of TSH, Free T3 and free T4 in hypothyroid patients on combined T3/T4 therapy." *Experimental and clinical endocrinology & diabetes* 115.04 (2007): 261-267.

[16] Grebe, Stefan KG, and George J. Kahaly. "Laboratory Testing in Hyperthyroidism." *American Journal of Medicine* 125.9 (2012): 2.

[17] Cachefo, A. N. A., et al. "Hepatic lipogenesis and cholesterol synthesis in hyperthyroid patients." *Journal of Clinical Endocrinology & Metabolism* 86.11 (2001): 5353-5357.

[18] Hoppé, Emmanuel, et al. "Sex hormone-binding globulin in osteoporosis." *Joint Bone Spine* 77.4 (2010): 306-312.

[19] Dhanwal, Dinesh Kumar. "Thyroid disorders and bone mineral metabolism." *Indian journal of endocrinology and metabolism* 15.Suppl2 (2011): S107.

[20] Smith, Steven R., et al. "Triiodothyronine increases calcium loss in a bed rest antigravity model for space flight." *Metabolism* 57.12 (2008): 1696-1703.

[21] Kollind, M., and K. Carlström. "Ovarian ultrasound and ovarian and adrenal hormones before and after treatment for hyperthyroidism." *Gynecologic and obstetric investigation* 54.1 (2002): 50-55.

10

Cofactors for Thyroid Metabolism:
Iron, Cortisol, Selenium,
Iodine, Zinc, Vitamin A

Your serum Iron is low so you should take iron supplements.

—Dangerous advice to someone who has
Anemia of Chronic Disease

Iron Deficiency Anemia

Low iron, or more specifically, low ferritin, is one of the most overlooked causes of low thyroid function. Ferritin tends to be low in those who are hypothyroid and high in those who are hyperthyroid.[1] Ferritin is the stored form of iron that is used by the cells and tends to be a better measure of available iron levels than serum iron. Iron is a component of multiple enzymes that are used to generate energy; in fact, performance times of endurance athletes decreased in those who were iron deficient.[2] Thyroid peroxidase (TPO) is an iron-containing enzyme that is involved in the first two steps in thyroid hormone synthesis.[3] Anemic women in one study had lower body temperatures and lower triiodothyronine (T3) and thyroxine (T4) levels than controls. Iron supplementation corrected the anemia, raised body temperature, and raised thyroid levels.[4] In this case, lack of iron caused the limited thyroid hormone production.

Low ferritin can cause negative reactions like palpitations, nervousness, and anxiety in someone starting thyroid hormone replacement. Someone described the sensation as similar to being shot out of a cannon. It is therefore imperative that ferritin not be at the bottom of the reference range before starting thyroid hormone medication.[5] But what causes low ferritin?

- Poor gut health from celiac or Crohn's disease (autoimmune diseases), or the use of antacids will prevent iron from being absorbed.[6] Ferritin levels rose in iron deficient celiac patients after they adopted a gluten-free diet.[7]
- Inadequate meat consumption or being vegetarian will keep ferritin low. Young women tend to be iron deficient because they don't consume enough iron in their diet, even when they're not vegetarian.[8]

- The hypothyroid condition and autoimmune thyroid disease are associated with chronic, unexplained anemia.[9]
- Excessive blood loss from heavy menstrual periods will keep iron levels low, and heavy periods are a hypothyroid symptom in women.[10]
- Donating blood too frequently (more than three times a year) can induce iron deficiency.[11]
- Intestinal bleeding due to high aspirin intake, an ulcer, or colon cancer can also keep iron levels low.[12]

Hereditary hemochromatosis (HH) is a genetic disorder which causes excess iron to be retained in the body. This can damage organs like the pituitary gland, heart, thyroid, liver, testes, etc. It is possible to have low ferritin with this disease, so a full iron panel should be run to make an accurate diagnosis. Iron supplementation would obviously be contraindicated with hemochromatosis.

If one does not have hemochromatosis, consumption of high iron foods such as red meat, the elimination of gluten from one's diet for a trial period, or probiotics/yogurt to restore gut health may help raise ferritin levels. A non-constipating iron supplement, ferrous bisglycinate, is highly recommended on several thyroid forums and has successfully raised iron and ferritin levels in patients. Sometimes iron/ferritin levels will not increase unless thyroid hormone is also prescribed. In one study, the addition of 75 mcg levothyroxine daily to iron supplementation raised hemoglobin, hematocrit, red blood cell count, iron, transferrin saturation, ferritin, and Free T4 significantly more than just iron supplementation.[13] Liver pills are another option for raising iron levels. Iron infusions should be a last resort because they have some serious drawbacks, including fatal allergic reactions.[14]

Iron Deficiency Anemia (IDA) vs. Anemia of Chronic Disease (ACD)

Iron deficiency anemia should be verified with blood tests before anyone supplements iron. Because iron is used by bacteria and cancer cells for their growth, it is imperative that patients have a full iron panel to rule out something called anemia of chronic disease, which can also cause a low serum iron reading, low transferrin saturation percent, and low hemoglobin.[15] Supplementing iron in this case amounts to feeding the pathogens, which is not a good idea. It also defeats the body's protective mechanism of limiting available iron when pathogens are present. The body is purposely shunting available iron to ferritin to get it out of circulation and out of the pathogens' reach.[16]

Iron deficient patients will have low hemoglobin/hematocrit, low ferritin, low iron, low transferrin iron saturation percent, low MCH,[17] and high total iron binding capacity (TIBC).[18] A good chart that compares Iron Deficiency Anemia (IDA) with Anemia of Chronic Disease (ACD) is available at irondisorders.org.

Ferritin levels can rise when infection, inflammation, or cancer is present, appearing normal or high in a state of iron deficiency. Because someone can have both Iron Deficiency Anemia and Anemia of Chronic Disease simultaneously, multiple tests are looked at to confirm a diagnosis. An elevated C-Reactive Protein (CRP) blood test is a marker of chronic inflammation,[17] and would be another diagnostic for Anemia of

Chronic Disease. In Anemia of Chronic Disease, there will be a slight drop in hemoglobin to low normal levels, along with a normal or high ferritin. Serum iron and transferrin saturation percent will also be low. Total iron binding capacity (TIBC) is low in Anemia of Chronic Disease because even though there are ample iron stores, they are not easily mobilized.[15]

Iron Deficiency Anemia, once confirmed, should be treated by supplementing iron. On the other hand, iron should not be supplemented in Anemia of Chronic Disease, but the underlying condition should be addressed. This can be as benign as a urinary tract infection, a head or chest cold, mononucleosis, tonsillitis or strep, stomach or intestinal flu, and bacterial infections such as *H. pylori*. But Anemia of Chronic Disease can also indicate something more serious such as kidney disease, hepatitis, tumors, or cancer, so it should be investigated.[15] Autoimmune conditions associated with Anemia of Chronic Disease include rheumatoid arthritis, lupus, and inflammatory bowel disease.[19]

If iron lab results don't point to Iron Deficiency Anemia or Anemia of Chronic Disease but still seem unusual, further research into unusual iron disorders might be warranted. Apparently iron overload or anemia is a consequence of certain disease states, and managing the disease state can positively impact the iron dysfunction. Some are mentioned at http://www.irondisorders.org/rare, and a visit with a hematologist for further testing might not be out of order.

Cortisol

Cortisol levels must be sufficient for someone to tolerate thyroid hormone. Cortisol levels that remain at the bottom of the reference range all day (found in Addison's disease) require supplemental hydrocortisone before thyroid hormone can be taken, or symptoms as severe as vomiting can occur.[20] [21] This is because thyroid hormone increases cortisol clearance from the body. A true adrenal crisis (when cortisol levels fall to zero) can be fatal.[22] For others who are low, but not flat-lined, supporting the adrenals and raising thyroid hormone *very* slowly has often worked. Thyroid and corticosteroid binding globulin (CBG) have an inverse relationship, so as thyroid is raised, CBG goes down, leaving more cortisol free. Thyroid and cortisol levels usually rise and fall in tandem.[23]

Other cofactors

Iodine, iron, selenium, Vitamin A, and zinc are all essential for normal thyroid hormone metabolism, and can be obtained from diet or daily multi-vitamins. Iron works in conjunction with iodine and has reduced goiters in those who were anemic, when iodine alone did not work.[3] Selenium is a component of the deiodinase enzymes that convert T4 to T3.[24] It also protects the thyroid gland from damage by excessive iodide exposure. Vitamin A works in conjunction with iodine and lowers Thyroid Stimulating Hormone (TSH) stimulation and the risk of goiter.[25] Zinc appears to be involved in thyroid conversion, because T3 levels rise on zinc supplementation,[26] and a deficiency correlates with reverse T3 production.[27] A comparison of zinc and selenium levels between hypothyroid and normal patients showed that serum zinc and selenium levels were significantly lower in the hypothyroid patients.[28]   However, zinc should never be supplemented without proper testing, because a balance needs to be maintained between zinc and copper. People in the autistic spectrum tend to be low in zinc and high in copper.[29] But for those who are not autistic, supplementing zinc without copper can create a copper deficiency, and cause serious unintended side effects such as anemia and neuropathy.[30] Bariatric surgery patients with copper deficiencies may present with anemia, leukopenia (low white blood cell count) and myeloneuropathy, which iron supplementation and B12 does not correct, but copper does.[31] Long-term treatment with high doses of zinc can negatively affect the immune system or result in zinc poisoning.[32] Diarrhea, nausea, vomiting, and dizziness are signs of zinc toxicity.[33] In fact, all of these cofactors are *trace* elements, and are toxic at high levels.

Why do so many people today seem to have autoimmune problems? One hypothesis is that the standard western diet (high in sugar and refined carbohydrates and low in protein) contributes to a deficiency of essential nutrients such as zinc, selenium and vitamins A, B, C and E, which results in disturbed immune function and autoimmunity. These nutrients, along with methionine, cysteine, and arginine (amino acids obtained from protein in the diet), are needed to produce the enzymes and other cofactors which help regulate immune responses to antigens. Lack of these essential nutrients can lead to a shift in the balance of the immune system's T-helper cells, known as TH1 or TH2. TH2 dominance is associated with chronic (viral) infections, obesity, atherosclerosis, auto-immunity, allergies and cancer.[34] Ongoing research confirms that lack of adequate protein, fats, Vitamins A, C, D, E, selenium, copper, and zinc affects immune activity and the development of allergies.[35]

Conclusion

Iron problems are common topics of discussion on nearly every thyroid forum. Many thyroid patients suffer from true iron deficiency and low ferritin, and safely take iron supplements to raise their levels. Others, however, have Anemia of Chronic Disease, which is much more difficult to treat. Because iron can feed pathogens, it is imperative that a full iron panel be run before iron is ever supplemented. Perplexing iron labs may need the interpretation of a hematologist.

If iron and hemoglobin levels don't rise even with iron supplementation, copper levels should also be tested and supplemented, if necessary. Zinc is another metal that should not be supplemented without proper testing, because zinc toxicity can induce more problems.

Key points

- Several cofactors are essential for normal thyroid metabolism; in fact, iodine, iron, selenium, zinc, and vitamin A are all found in most daily multi-vitamins and may be enough for some patients.
- Iodine is a component of thyroid hormone.

- Iron is a component of the enzymes that produce thyroid hormone; correcting iron deficiencies has normalized thyroid levels for some people.
- Selenium is a component of the enzymes that convert T4 to T3.
- Zinc is involved with thyroid conversion and a healthy immune system.
- Vitamin A works with iodine and lowers TSH stimulation and goiter risk.
- Adequate ferritin levels are essential to tolerate supplemental thyroid hormone; low levels can cause anxiety and palpitations when thyroid hormone is started.
- Possible causes of low iron levels are poor gut health (celiac, Crohn's disease, or antacid use), a diet low in protein (vegetarian), heavy menstrual periods (a hypothyroid sign), too frequent blood donations, and intestinal bleeding (aspirin use, ulcers, or colon cancer).
- Iron or liver supplements are one way to raise iron levels, provided that the person does not have Anemia of Chronic Disease, which resembles an iron deficiency, but is much more serious. Full iron labs should always be run to differentiate between Anemia of Chronic Disease and Iron Deficiency Anemia before iron is supplemented.
- Adequate cortisol levels are essential when thyroid hormone is started. Starting at too high a dose of prescription thyroid hormone without sufficient cortisol can trigger an adrenal crisis.
- Poor diet can lead to autoimmunity and allergies; the importance of nutrition is often overlooked.
- Unnecessary zinc supplementation can create a copper deficiency, which can lead to anemia and neuropathy.
- Copper deficiencies can present as anemia, leukopenia (low white blood cell count) and myeloneuropathy in bariatric surgery patients.

---

[1] Takamatsu, Junta, et al. "Serum ferritin as a marker of thyroid hormone action on peripheral tissues." *Journal of Clinical Endocrinology & Metabolism* 61.4 (1985): 672-676.

[2] DellaValle, Diane M., and Jere D. Haas. "Impact of iron depletion without anemia on performance in trained endurance athletes at the beginning of a training season: a study of female collegiate rowers." *International Journal of Sport Nutrition andExercise Metabolism* 21.6 (2011): 501.

[3] Zimmermann, Michael B., and Josef Köhrle. "The impact of iron and selenium deficiencies on iodine and thyroid metabolism: biochemistry and relevance to public health." *Thyroid* 12.10 (2002): 867-878.

[4] Beard, John L., M. J. Borel, and Janice Derr. "Impaired thermoregulation and thyroid function in iron-deficiency anemia." *The American journal of clinical nutrition* 52.5 (1990): 813-819.

[5] Shakir, K. M., et al. "Anemia: a cause of intolerance to thyroxine sodium." *Mayo Clinic Proceedings*. Vol. 75. No. 2. Elsevier, 2000.

[6] Al-Quaiz, Joharah M. "Iron deficiency anemia." *Saudi Med J* 22.6 (2001): 490-496.

[7] Harper, Jason W., et al. "Anemia in celiac disease is multifactorial in etiology." *American journal of hematology* 82.11 (2007): 996-1000.

[8] Hawk, Susan N., Kimberly Grage Englehardt, and Cindi Small. "Risks of iron deficiency among vegetarian college women." *Health* 4 (2012): 113-119.

[9] Sibilla, Rosanna, et al. "Chronic unexplained anaemia in isolated autoimmune thyroid disease or associated with autoimmune related disorders." *Clinical endocrinology* 68.4 (2008): 640-645.

[10] Moragianni, Vasiliki A., and Stephen G. Somkuti. "Profound hypothyroidism-induced acute menorrhagia resulting in life-threatening anemia." *Obstetrics & Gynecology* 110.2, Part 2 (2007): 515.

[11] Brittenham, Gary M. "Iron deficiency in whole blood donors." *Transfusion* 51.3 (2011): 458-461.

[12] Rockey, Don C., and John P. Cello. "Evaluation of the gastrointestinal tract in patients with iron-deficiency anemia." *New England Journal of Medicine* 329.23 (1993): 1691-1695.

[13] Cinemre, Hakan, et al. "Hematologic effects of levothyroxine in iron-deficient subclinical hypothyroid patients: a randomized, double-blind, controlled study." *Journal of Clinical Endocrinology & Metabolism* 94.1 (2009): 151-156.

[14] Fishbane, Steven. "Safety in iron management." *American journal of kidney diseases* 41 (2003): 18-26.

[15] Iron Disorders Institute, Anemia of Chronic Disease, http://www.irondisorders.org/anemia-of-chronic-disease Accessed 9/18/2013.

[16] Pieracci, Fredric M., and Philip S. Barie. "Iron and the risk of infection." *Surgical Infections* 6.S1 (2005): s41-s46.

[17] Muñoz, Manuel, José Antonio García-Erce, and Ángel Francisco Remacha. "Disorders of iron metabolism. Part II: iron deficiency and iron overload." *Journal of clinical pathology* 64.4 (2011): 287-296.

[18] Iron Disorders Institute, "How do I know if I am anemic?" http://www.irondisorders.org/Websites/idi/files/Content/854256/FActsAnemia.pdf

[19] Weiss, Guenter, and Lawrence T. Goodnough. "Anemia of chronic disease." *New England Journal of Medicine* 352.10 (2005): 1011-1023.

[20] Murray, Jonathan Stephen, Rubaraj Jayarajasingh, and Petros Perros. "Lesson of the week: Deterioration of symptoms after start of thyroid hormone replacement." *BMJ: British Medical Journal* 323.7308 (2001): 332.

[21] Arlt, Wiebke, and Bruno Allolio. "Adrenal insufficiency." *The Lancet* 361.9372 (2003): 1881-1893.

[22] Choudhary, Nidhi, et al. "Thyroxine replacement precipitating adrenal crisis." Endocrine Abstracts 19 (2009): 64.

[23] Dumoulin, Sonia C., et al. "Opposite effects of thyroid hormones on binding proteins for steroid hormones (sex hormone-binding globulin and corticosteroid-binding globulin) in humans." *European journal of endocrinology* 132.5 (1995): 594-598.

[24] Triggiani, Vincenzo, et al. "Role of iodine, selenium and other micronutrients in thyroid function and disorders." Endocrine, Metabolic & Immune Disorders-Drug Targets (Formerly Current Drug Targets-Immune, Endocrine & Metabolic Disorders) 9.3 (2009): 277-294.

[25] Zimmermann, Michael B., et al. "Vitamin A supplementation in iodine-deficient African children decreases thyrotropin stimulation of the thyroid and reduces the goiter rate." *The American journal of clinical nutrition* 86.4 (2007): 1040-1044.

[26] Maxwell, Christy, and Stella Lucia Volpe. "Effect of zinc supplementation on thyroid hormone function." *Annals of Nutrition and Metabolism* 51.2 (2007): 188-194.

[27] Nishiyama, S., et al. "Zinc supplementation alters thyroid hormone metabolism in disabled patients with zinc deficiency." *Journal of the American College of Nutrition* 13 (1994).

[28] Al-Juboori, Iham Amir, Rafi Al-Rawi, and Hussein Kadhem A-Hakeim. "Estimation of Serum Copper, Manganese, Selenium, and Zinc in Hypothyroidism Patients." *IUFS Journal of Biology* 68.2 (2010): 121-126.

[29] Bjørklund, Geir. "The role of zinc and copper in autism spectrum disorders." *Acta Neurobiol Exp* 73 (2013): 225-236.

[30] Sharma, Vivek R. "Copper Deficiency: Clinical Review of an Obscure Imitator." *J Med Sci* 32.1 (2012): 001-007.

[31] Pereira, Andrea Z., et al. "Copper deficiency anemia: A complication after bariatric surgery." *IJNutrology* 6.2 (2013).

[32] Chasapis, Christos T., et al. "Zinc and human health: an update." *Archives of toxicology* 86.4 (2012): 521-534.

[33] Driscoll, Marcia S., et al. "Nutrition and the deleterious side effects of nutritional supplements." *Clinics in dermatology* 28.4 (2010): 371-379.

[34] Sprietsma, J. E. "Modern diets and diseases: NO–zinc balance." *Medical hypotheses* 53.1 (1999): 6-16.

[35] Faria, Ana Maria Caetano, et al. "Food components and the immune system: from tonic agents to allergens." *Frontiers in immunology* 4 (2013).

11

Graves' Hyperthyroidism: Modified Block and Replace Treatment with Antithyroid Drugs + Levothyroxine

Radioactive iodine (RAI) cures Graves' disease.

—what some endocrinologists say

Graves' disease is an autoimmune disease where Thyroid Stimulating Hormone (TSH) Receptor antibodies provide constant stimulation to the TSH Receptor, which causes thyroid hormone to be produced non-stop. The antibodies mimic the function of TSH. In normal people, the TSH is part of a negative feedback loop, where the production and presence of thyroid hormone lowers TSH, so that production slows down. With Graves' disease, the antibodies override the feedback loop and production never stops. TSH levels are typically close to zero, which means the body *can* sense that thyroid hormone is available and more does not need to be produced, but it continues to be produced anyway, due to stimulation from the antibodies. The hyperthyroid state is a serious one, and can be fatal if left untreated. For this reason, Graves' patients today are offered the same three options that have been around for decades: antithyroid drugs, a thyroidectomy to surgically remove the thyroid, or a radioactive iodine (RAI) pill which destroys the thyroid. Each option has pros and cons.

Antithyroid drugs (ATDs) to lower Graves' antibodies

The difference between Graves' and Hashimoto's patients is not simply that Graves' patients are hyperthyroid and Hashimoto's patients are hypothyroid. Graves' patients have specific antibodies that can disfigure the eyes (thyroid eye disease or TED), the skin (pretibial myxedema, acropachy), and affect other organs in addition to causing goiters, so the antibodies need to be controlled. There are antithyroid drugs (ATD) available today that can do this, such as methimazole, carbimazole, tapazole, or propylthiouracil. But they not only reduce the antibodies, they also reduce the synthesis of any thyroid hormones.[1] So long-term, they induce hypothyroidism. Patients have achieved remission, or the reduction of their antibodies to a point where they are no longer problematic, by using antithyroid drugs, usually for several years. Because antithyroid drugs induce a hypothyroid state, the patient is then dealing with hypothyroid, instead of hyperthyroid symptoms. To keep thyroid levels close to normal, a block and replace regimen can be used. *Block* refers to the blocking effect the antithyroid drugs have on both thyroid hormones *and* antibodies, and *replace* refers to the replacement of thyroid hormone (usually levothyroxine or T4) that keeps a Graves' patient's free thyroxine (FT4) levels close to mid-range.

If antithyroid drugs lower thyroid levels, making the patient hypothyroid, shouldn't they just lower the antithyroid drug dose and let thyroid levels return to normal?

Antithyroid drugs lower the antibodies, which is one of the reasons they are prescribed, because of the damage antibodies can do to the body. If the Graves' antibodies, TSI (Thyroid Stimulating Immunoglobulin) and TRab (TSH Receptor antibodies, also known as Thyroid Binding Inhibitory Immunoglobulins or TBII) are still high, it seems unwise to reduce the antithyroid drug dose, even if thyroxine (T4) and triiodothyronine (T3) levels have already come down. The antithyroid drug dose should be based on the level of both Graves' antibodies, TSI and TRab. TSI antibodies mimic the action of TSH, causing excess secretion of both T4 and T3, making patients hyperthyroid. There are also antibodies that block the action of TSH, called blocking TRab, which instead make patients hypothyroid.[2] The thyroid gland itself is not the problem; it's the antibodies that are controlling it.

Antibody and thyroid levels rapidly drop once antithyroid drugs are started, and frequent monitoring (every 4-6 weeks or less) of these antibodies and thyroid levels (TSH, Free T3, Free T4) is imperative when this protocol is first started. Some have had to lower their dose within the first week, so the patient needs to be very aware of hypothyroid symptoms (feeling cold, constipated, etc.). Antithyroid drugs are powerful medications. The initial antithyroid drug dose is lowered after 4-12 weeks (or sooner) if antibody levels have come down, and many maintain a dose of only 5 mg methimazole for years.[1] The antibody levels are what should determine the antithyroid drug dose, *not* TSH levels. TSH can remain suppressed for years in someone with Graves' because of *TSH* Receptor antibodies, even when actual T3 and T4 levels have fallen below the reference range.[3] These are not the same antibodies found in Hashimoto's patients; those are the TPO (thyroid peroxidase) and Tg (thyroglobulin) antibodies (although Graves' patients can also have these antibodies). A person with Hashimoto's usually does not have a suppressed TSH, while a Graves' patient usually does.

Antithyroid drugs can have serious side effects, and the risk increases if the dose is kept too high for too long.[4] The dose will most likely be kept too high if a doctor tries to dose a Graves' patient by their TSH. A Graves' patient can be either hyperthyroid *or* hypothyroid while on ATDs, with a TSH near zero, even with T4 and T3 levels *below* the reference range, because the antibodies are artificially stimulating the TSH Receptors. The TSH is no longer an indication of whether a Graves' patient has an excess or deficiency of thyroid hormone (T4 and T3) when high levels of TRab are present. If the patient is now suffering from hypothyroid symptoms, thyroid hormone such as levothyroxine can be prescribed to bring levels up to mid-range, while maintaining the antithyroid drug dose. If thyroid levels are allowed to drop too low, the patient can again experience hyperthyroid symptoms, from being *hypo*thyroid. Norepinephrine rises to compensate for the lack of thyroid hormone[5] and causes an increase in heart rate, blood pressure, and terrible anxiety. It is possible to lead a somewhat normal life with the antithyroid drugs controlling the antibodies, and the supplemental thyroid medication keeping the patient euthyroid or normal.

Why should patients *replace* or add thyroid hormone, instead of coping with the hypothyroid state?

One theory is that being in a hypothyroid state will stimulate the antibodies, as the body may try to increase thyroid levels through that route. Graves' has developed in patients who were first diagnosed with Hashimoto's thyroiditis.[6] These people went from a hypo-thyroid state to a hyperthyroid state, simply by creating additional antibodies. Plus, being hypothyroid has its own set of risks and health problems, so healthy thyroid levels should be restored by taking thyroid hormone in addition to antithyroid drugs. Free T3 and Free T4 should be close to mid-range or higher, not bottom-of-range. Healthy people have levels that *start* just below mid-range [see Chapter 21, Reference Ranges, for further explanation on why reference ranges start too low].

To get Free T3 and Free T4 levels to mid-range often means supplementing T4 *and* T3, but some doctors are reluctant to do this because Graves' patients already have a sup-pressed TSH. Normally, a suppressed TSH means the patient is hyperthyroid, but a measurement of the actual thyroid hormones, Free T3 and Free T4, will show the patient's true state. A patient cannot be hyperthyroid with thyroid levels at the bottom of the reference range. TSH is a pituitary hormone, not a thyroid hormone, and with TSH Receptor antibodies, the TSH cannot be used as a diagnostic at all. Doctors are reluctant to prescribe any T3 because of the possibility of pituitary atrophy, since T3 is known to suppress TSH. But a study that examined Graves' patients on block and replace therapy found that after three months of methimazole (when free T4 and total T3 were normal), 22 out of 45 patients (almost 50%) still had detectable TSI Graves' antibodies. Patients who still showed TSI had significantly lower TSH values than those who no longer had TSI. This suggests that it is the TSI antibodies affecting the TSH, not the level of free T4 or total T3, because those were comparable between the two groups. The suppressed TSH is therefore not from pituitary atrophy or a breakdown of the pituitary-thyroid axis, but the continued presence of TSI antibodies. A TSH-Receptor was found in the pitui-tary, which means the antibodies could exert an effect there.[7]

The pituitary atrophy hypothesis is further discredited by the fact that TSH levels increase within weeks after discontinuation of T4 therapy (in patients treated with TSH suppressive doses of T4 for thyroid cancer),[8] suggesting that the pituitary-thyroid axis can revive quickly. Secondly, not all patients treated for Graves' hyperthyroidism exhibit long-term TSH suppression. And thirdly, a decreased level of TSH after a one year course of antithyroid drugs may simply mean the antibodies are still active, not that the pituitary has atrophied. It may be premature to discontinue the antithyroid drugs if TSH is still suppressed after a year. Continued TSH suppression in Graves' disease is only found in a subset of Graves' patients--those likely to relapse after antithyroid drug therapy, or those with persistent TSI.[7]

A block and replace study successfully used 100 μg of thyroxine in conjunction with 10 mg of methimazole as a maintenance dose.[9] Another study contradicted this one, saying that replacement with T3 or placebo was better than replacement with T4.[10] This might be because T3 is the active hormone that relieves symptoms, and the T4 did not convert to enough T3, leaving the patient hypothyroid. Antithyroid drugs may impede conversion of T4 to T3. Insufficient conversion is the main problem most hypothyroid patients (non-Graves') have with T4 medications. It should be noted that a normal thyroid produces both T4 *and* T3.

Graves' orbitopathy (eye disease) patients in one study showed that long-term (80 months), low-dose block (5 mg methimazole/day or 200 mg propylthiouracil/day) and replace (100 mcg/day levothyroxine) kept 90% of the patients stable, with antibodies within range, and a normal TSH.[11]

Are antithyroid drugs for everyone?

Antithyroid drugs don't work for everyone; for some the dose is too high, then too low, as their thyroid continues to act erratically from the antibody stimulation. Antithyroid drugs can affect the liver if the dose is kept too high for too long. A significant decrease in white blood cells (agranulocytosis) can be a serious problem. Vasculitis (blood vessel inflammation that decreases blood supply to the organs) and kidney failure are also potential side effects. Some of these side effects can be fatal, but do seem to be dose-related.[3] In one hospital, agranulocytosis was significantly higher in patients taking 30 mg methimazole daily compared to those taking only 15 mg daily. This hospital now recommends a starting dose of 15 mg daily.[12] Another study found no difference in remission rates after one year of therapy between 10 or 40 mg of methimazole. As expected, adverse reactions were higher on 40 mg.[13] Antithyroid drugs continue to be used because they have worked for some patients. They have successfully lowered antibodies to the point where a patient can be said to be in a state of remission, and no longer needs medication. Their own thyroid works properly again. Others get their antibodies under control with the antithyroid drugs and are able to wean off them, but must still take supplemental thyroid hormone, because their own thyroid gland doesn't produce enough thyroid hormone.

If radioactive iodine (RAI) or thyroidectomy could immediately fix the hyperthyroid condition, why should patients even consider antithyroid drugs?

Thyroid removal (thyroidectomy) or destruction (RAI) does not eliminate the antibodies, because those are actually made in the white blood cells, not in the thyroid. In some patients, the antibodies rise after RAI, and their condition worsens.[3] The thyroid gland is not the cause of the hyperthyroid condition; it is actually the TSH Receptor antibodies that are the problem, by causing overstimulation of the thyroid.

Radioactive iodine and thyroidectomy each have their own risks. If there is any evidence of thyroid eye disease (TED), RAI is contraindicated, for it can exacerbate the condition to the point of disfigurement. Smokers are at greater risk for TED complications. There is also the risk of damage to other surrounding tissues, since they will also be subject to radiation. It is also contraindicated in pregnancy.[3]

Thyroidectomy risks are surgical—parathyroids could be damaged since they are embedded in the thyroid gland, and they are essential for bone health. Vocal cords are also close to the gland and at risk of damage.[3] So are other nerves to the shoulder. Then there is the usual risk of any surgery with anesthesia.

Some RAI or thyroidectomy patients are happy with their results, and glad to no longer be dealing with hyperthyroid symptoms. Some people with Graves' do not develop TED, but there is no way to tell who is at risk for this complication. It is possible that another factor, in addition to the Graves' antibodies, is responsible for TED.[14] [15] [16] While it is assumed that TED is simply from TRab attacking the eyes, it doesn't explain how up to 5% of Hashimoto's Thyroiditis patients have TED who do not possess any TRab.[17] In fact, there is a case study of a woman who had normal (mid-range) T3, T4, and TSH levels, with no detectable TRab (0%), who had Grave's ophthalmopathy. Her TPO and Tgab were also negative. But further testing showed TSI to be over range.[18] Other drugs such as thiazolidinediones (TZD), used to control blood sugar, have induced TED in those with pre-existing Graves' or autoimmune thyroid disease and Type 2 diabetes mellitus. TED symptoms appeared within six months of starting TZD.[19]

Are there any other options besides antithyroid meds, thyroidectomy, and radioactive iodine to control the Graves' antibodies?

LDN (low dose naltrexone) is a prescription substance which has helped some Graves' patients significantly reduce their antibodies. Positive first person testimonies can be found on Graves' and LDN forums throughout the internet, and there are a few medical journal studies on LDN[20] that reported positive results in other autoimmune conditions like Crohn's,[21] multiple sclerosis,[22] and fibromyalgia.[23] LowDoseNaltrexone.org and LDNScience.org are two websites with a great deal of information that patients can share with their doctors.

I personally have never taken LDN or an anti-thyroid medication, nor did I have a thyroidectomy (I had RAI), but enough Graves' patients have had positive results with LDN that I felt it should be mentioned [see Lucy's story in Chapter 5]. Graves' patients should certainly investigate LDN before resorting to irreversible options like RAI or a thyroidectomy, which do not always decrease, and may even increase the antibodies. If Graves' antibody levels are high, they must be addressed because of the damage they can do. This is especially critical if the woman is of child-bearing age and may become pregnant, because high antibodies can affect an unborn child with a condition called neonatal Graves. In fact, any woman who has ever had Graves should have her antibodies tested if she becomes pregnant, so the antibodies can be treated.[3] Dangerous levels of antibodies may still be present even after RAI or a thyroidectomy, because, as stated earlier, the antibodies are not actually made in the thyroid, but in the white blood cells.

Aspartame, a sugar substitute, has also been implicated in some cases of Graves'; symptoms resolved when aspartame was eliminated from the diet.[24]

European diagnosis and treatment of Graves' disease[25]

In Europe, ultrasound is the primary imaging procedure for determining the cause of thyrotoxicosis (Graves' is not the only cause). Ultrasound is considered highly sensitive, reliable, convenient, and non-invasive. In the U.S., however, a radioactive iodine uptake is most often performed, even though iodine is really the last thing that should be given to a Graves' patient, because iodine can be used to manufacture more thyroid hormone. An abnormal ultrasound can predict autoimmune thyroid dysfunction before the patient displays positive antibodies. Ultrasounds can also detect increased vascularity (blood flow) that is associated with Graves' disease.

Radioactive iodine uptake (or scintigraphy) reveals less about the thyroid gland than ultrasound, so is not used as often in Europe. A physical examination may point to Graves' disease, and a simple blood test will confirm the presence of Graves' antibodies, which completes the diagnosis. Radioactive imaging is costly and exposes the patient to radioactivity, so is difficult to justify over ultrasound and blood testing. Ultrasound is also far superior in identifying thyroid nodules or thyroid cancer when compared to scintigraphy.

Anti-thyroid drugs are the first choice for treating autoimmune hyperthyroidism in European countries, and TRab are monitored to determine the effectiveness of treatment. Radioactive iodine is not the first treatment choice because of its known risk for developing or worsening Graves' orbitopathy, 20% after RAI vs. 5% after ATDs.

European medical centers rarely perform thyroidectomies unless thyroid cancer is present. Laser therapy for hyperfunctioning nodules is also more common in Europe, and is a good choice for solitary nodules; it can reduce hyperfunctioning nodules while not affecting nearby tissue.

Japanese and Korean diagnosis and treatment of Graves' disease[26]

Graves' disease is managed differently in different parts of the world. Surveys from the American Thyroid Association, the European Thyroid Association, and the Japan Thyroid Association show that American endocrinologists use fewer diagnostic tests than their counterparts in other countries. RAI was the first choice of treatment for 69% of American respondents, but only 22% of European, and 11% of Japanese respondents.

The reason fewer Japanese are given RAI may be due to radiophobia in the culture, due to the 1945 atomic bombings of Hiroshima and Nagasaki. The Japanese are aware that childhood thyroid cancers developed after the 1986 Chernobyl nuclear power plant accident in Russia, and these fears have been renewed with the Fukushima nuclear power plant accident in 2011.

In Japan, antithyroid drugs like methimazole (MMI) are the first choice of treatment, and levothyroxine is sometimes administered at the same time to keep thyroid levels up. The Graves' antibodies (TRab) are measured more frequently, first for diagnosis, and later to determine when antithyroid drug therapy can be decreased or even halted. In Asian countries, the protocol is considered a long-term therapy that continues for years, whereas the American protocol only lasts for 12-18 months, after which RAI is adminis- tered if the patient relapses. Long-term remission rates approach 67% in those who have followed the protocol for years; in contrast, only 20% reach remission in shorter treat- ment periods. Patients are tested every 2-3 weeks for at least 2-3 months after first starting antithyroid drugs, so that side effects can be quickly detected. MMI at 15 mg/day is used for mild and moderate cases of Graves', while 30 mg/day is used for severe cases. Propylthiouracil, another antithyroid drug, is not recommended initially because of a high frequency of side effects.

Antibody measurements are used to differentiate between Graves' disease and gesta- tional thyrotoxicosis and postpartum thyrotoxicosis. Ultrasound further clarifies whether the condition is from Graves' disease or destructive thyroiditis.

Conclusion

In the U.S., if antithyroid drugs are ineffective, RAI is recommended, whereas in Euro- pean and Asian countries, thyroidectomies are usually performed if antithyroid drugs are ineffective. Recurrence rates are actually lower with thyroidectomies than RAI, and RAI is contraindicated with any sign of TED.[27]

The treatment a Graves' patient chooses is a very personal decision, and patients should realize that all therapies have pros and cons. Therefore, patients should thoroughly research any protocols and discuss them with their doctor; gut instincts should not be ignored when making a decision.

Key points

- Graves' is more than just being hyperthyroid. The antibodies associated with Graves' disease can cause serious damage to the eyes, skin, and other organs.
- Antithyroid drugs are usually the first line of treatment, but they induce hypothy- roidism. Therefore, supplemental thyroid hormone should be prescribed in addition to antithyroid drugs to keep the patient's thyroid levels close to mid- range, or wherever they feel best.
- Antithyroid drugs are powerful and some patients may need to lower their dose after only one week, or they may become severely hypothyroid and/or suffer from side effects of the medication.
- Antithyroid drugs should not be stopped until the *antibodies* have decreased to a more normal level. That is the goal, because the antibodies are responsible for the hyperthyroid state. If the antibodies normalize, then thyroid levels may nor- malize. Antibody levels must be monitored.
- Higher antithyroid doses (greater than 15 mg methimazole, for example) usually result in more side effects without any improvement over a lower dose of 10 mg. ATDs should be viewed as a long-term therapy (years) and prescribed at the low- est effective possible dose (5-10 mg).

- Methimazole can be taken in a maintenance dose of 5 mg for years, combined with added levothyroxine.
- TSH cannot be used to determine a Graves' patient's thyroid levels, because the antibody is to the TSH Receptor; TSH is usually close to zero whether the patient has low or high thyroid levels.
- Antithyroid drugs don't work for all patients because of side effects, and thyroidectomy and RAI are the usual second choices offered.
- Anyone with even a hint of TED should not have RAI. RAI can induce TED in unsuspecting patients who show no signs prior to the RAI.[28]
- Depending on the severity of Graves', other options such as LDN or diet modifications may be helpful. Some have successfully combined them with low doses of antithyroid drugs. Severe cases may not have that luxury—some sort of treatment must be chosen, because the body cannot withstand a constant high heart rate forever.

---

[1] RSK Sinha, Antithyroid Drugs. Clinical Medicine: a Practical Manual for Students & practitioners by Agarwal. Vol. 1. Jaypee Brothers Publishers, 2007.

[2] Furmaniak, Jadwiga, Jane Sanders, and Bernard Rees Smith. "Blocking type TSH receptor antibodies." Autoimmunity Highlights (2013): 1-16.

[3] Chung, Yun Jae, et al. "Continued suppression of serum TSH level may be attributed to TSH receptor antibody activity as well as the severity of thyrotoxicosis and the time to recovery of thyroid hormone in treated euthyroid Graves' patients." Thyroid 16.12 (2006): 1251-1257.

[4] Abraham, Prakash, and Shamasunder Acharya. "Current and emerging treatment options for Graves' hyperthyroidism." Therapeutics and clinical risk management 6 (2010): 29.

[5] Coulombe, Pierre, Jean H. Dussault, and Peter Walker. "Catecholamine metabolism in thyroid disease. II. Norepinephrine secretion rate in hyperthyroidism and hypothyroidism." Journal of Clinical Endocrinology & Metabolism 44.6 (1977): 1185-1189.

[6] Wasniewska, Malgorzata, et al. "Frequency of Hashimoto's thyroiditis antecedents in the history of children and adolescents with Graves' disease." Hormone research in paediatrics 73.6 (2010): 473-476.

[7] Mark F. Prummel, Leon JS Brokken. "The physiological and clinical relevance of the TSH Receptor in the anterior pituitary." Hot Thyroidology (www.hotthyroidology.com). October , No 1 , 2003. http://www.hotthyroidology.com/ausgabe.php?ID=121

[8] Valle, Laticia A., et al. "In Thyroidectomized Patients with Thyroid Cancer, a Serum Thyrotropin of 30 μ U/mL After Thyroxine Withdrawal Is Not Always Adequate for Detecting an Elevated Stimulated Serum Thyroglobulin." Thyroid 23.2 (2013): 185-193.

[9] Hashizume, Kiyoshi, et al. "Administration of thyroxine in treated Graves' disease: effects on the level of antibodies to thyroid-stimulating hormone receptors and on the risk of recurrence of hyperthyroidism." New England Journal of Medicine 324.14 (1991): 947-953.

[10] Mastorakos, G., et al. "T4 but not T3 administration is associated with increased recurrence of Graves' disease after successful medical therapy." Journal of endocrinological investigation 26.10 (2003): 979-984.

[11]Laurberg, Peter, et al. "Sustained control of Graves' hyperthyroidism during long-term low-dose antithyroid drug therapy of patients with severe Graves' orbitopathy." Thyroid 21.9 (2011): 951-956.

[12] Takata, Kazuna, et al. "Methimazole-induced agranulocytosis in patients with Graves' disease is more frequent with an initial dose of 30 mg daily than with 15 mg daily." Thyroid 19.6 (2009): 559-563.

[13] Reinwein, D., et al. "A prospective randomized trial of antithyroid drug dose in Graves' disease therapy. European Multicenter Study Group on Antithyroid Drug Treatment." Journal of Clinical Endocrinology & Metabolism 76.6 (1993): 1516-1521.

[14] Lahooti, Hooshang, Kishan R. Parmar, and Jack R. Wall. "Pathogenesis of thyroid-associated ophthalmopathy: does autoimmunity against calsequestrin and collagen XIII play a role?." Clinical Ophthalmology (Auckland, NZ) 4 (2010): 417.

[15] Stan, Marius N., and Rebecca S. Bahn. "Risk factors for development or deterioration of Graves' ophthalmopathy." Thyroid 20.7 (2010): 777-783.

[16] Tjiang, Hilman, et al. "Eye and eyelid abnormalities are common in patients with Hashimoto's thyroiditis." Thyroid 20.3 (2010): 287-290.

[17] Tani, Junichi, and Yuji Hiromatsu. "Genetic Susceptibility to Graves' Ophthalmopathy." Edited by Spaska Angelova Stanilova (2013): 1.

[18] Yanai, Hidekatsu, and Hiroko Yamazaki. "Grave's Ophthalmopathy in the Absence of Abnormal Thyroid Hormone and Thyrotropin Levels and Thyrotropin Receptor Antibody." Thyroid 6.1 (2010): 1-3.

[19] Menaka, R., et al. "Thiazolidinedione precipitated thyroid associated ophthalmopathy." JAPI 58 (2010): 243.

[20] Meng, Jingjuan, et al. "Low dose naltrexone (LDN) enhances maturation of bone marrow dendritic cells (BMDCs)." International Immunopharmacology 17.4 (2013): 1084-1089.

[21] Zagon, Ian S., and Patricia J. McLaughlin. "Targeting opioid signaling in Crohn's disease: new therapeutic pathways." Expert Review of Gastroenterology & Hepatology 5.5 (2011): 555-558.

[22] McLaughlin, P. J., and I. S. Zagon. "A New Biotherapeutic Approach for the Treatment of Multiple Sclerosis." Transl Med 3 (2013): e119.

[23] Younger, Jarred, et al. "Low-dose naltrexone for the treatment of fibromyalgia: Findings of a small, randomized, double-blind, placebo-controlled, counterbalanced, crossover trial assessing daily pain levels." Arthritis & Rheumatism 65.2 (2013): 529-538.

[24] Roberts, H. J. "Aspartame disease: A possible cause for concomitant Graves' disease and Pulmonary hypertension." Texas Heart Institute Journal 31.1 (2004): 105.

[25] Kahaly, George J., Luigi Bartalena, and Laszlo Hegedüs. "The American Thyroid Association/American Association of Clinical Endocrinologists guidelines for hyperthyroidism and other causes of thyrotoxicosis: a European perspective." Thyroid 21.6 (2011): 585-591.

[26] Yamashita, Shunichi, Nobuyuki Amino, and Young Kee Shong. "The American Thyroid Association and American Association of Clinical Endocrinologists hyperthyroidism and other causes of thyrotoxicosis guidelines: viewpoints from Japan and Korea." Thyroid 21.6 (2011): 577-580.

[27] Liu, Jing, et al. "Total thyroidectomy: a safe and effective treatment for Graves' disease." Journal of Surgical Research 168.1 (2011): 1-4.

[28] Vannucchi, G., et al. "Graves' orbitopathy activation after radioactive iodine therapy with and without steroid prophylaxis." Journal of Clinical Endocrinology & Metabolism 94.9 (2009): 3381-3386.

12

High Altitude Sickness:
a Hypothyroid Condition?

You have a headache too?

—often heard around high altitude ski resorts

High altitude sickness or Acute Mountain Sickness (AMS) is a cluster of symptoms that affect people who ascend too rapidly to higher elevations, usually above 8,000 feet (2,500 meters). Many who plan a vacation to high altitude ski areas like Colorado are hit with the typical symptoms of headache, insomnia, a faster heart rate, and occasionally nausea, fatigue, dizziness, and loss of appetite. Hypoxia, or lack of oxygen, is said to cause all of these symptoms, but what exactly happens that causes hypoxia?

Adrenal dysfunction: low thyroid levels and low cortisol levels exacerbate high altitude sickness

Low oxygen triggers an increase in the thyroid deiodinase enzyme (D3) that inactivates the thyroid hormones: thyroxine (T4) converts to reverse triiodothyronine (rT3), and triiodothyronine (T3) is converted to diiodothyronine (T2). This reduces cell metabolism and reduces oxygen consumption.[1][2] A normal person becomes hypothyroid, and if they are already hypothyroid or undermedicated, they become worse. According to an article in *5280*, a Denver, Colorado magazine, more than 20% of the visiting tourists are hit with high altitude sickness.[3] Maybe this reflects the number of undiagnosed or undermedicated hypothyroid patients? I certainly have an extremely difficult time at high altitudes: I get a throbbing headache, my heart rate increases, I feel the need to drink water constantly, and I end up tossing and turning all night, when I'm usually a deep sleeper.

Glucocorticoids such as prednisolone, prednisone, or dexamethasone are used to treat altitude sickness. One study showed that after someone from sea level arrived by air to an altitude of 11,350 feet (3,450 meters), both adrenocorticotropic hormone (ACTH) and plasma cortisol levels rose until day eight. The body responds to higher altitude by increasing cortisol. Glucocorticoid treatment from day one on test subjects significantly lowered the severity of symptoms.[4] Hypothyroid patients frequently suffer from relative adrenal insufficiency, where their cortisol levels have downregulated to match their lower thyroid levels. An inability of their adrenals to provide adequate cortisol would certainly result in a more severe state of high altitude sickness. The high altitude sickness symptoms of nausea, dizziness, and fatigue are also signs of low cortisol.

In a study of men who ascended to 14,270 feet (4,350 meters), both thyroid hormones (T3 and T4), norepinephrine, and cortisol became elevated, while Thyroid Stimulating Hormone (TSH) did not change.[5] Interestingly, norepinephrine tends to be elevated in hypothyroid patients.[6] Thyroid and cortisol levels came up naturally in these men in response to the higher altitude. Anyone who is manually dosing their thyroid hormone may not have this natural response. In hindsight, the last time I was at high altitude, I did not sleep well at all and had a rapid heart rate. My Free T4 was at the very bottom of the reference range on desiccated thyroid, though my Free T3 was close to mid-range. I have since changed to a combination dose of desiccated plus T4, to balance both my T3 *and* T4 levels.

A low T3 syndrome was found in a similar study on men who climbed Mt. Everest and spent seven weeks at high altitude. They acclimatized at a base camp of 17,000 feet (5,200 meters) for two months, before ascending to elevations between 24,600 feet (7,500 meters) and 29,000 feet (8,850 meters). None of them developed high altitude sickness. Blood work after returning to base camp showed increased Free T4 levels, but decreased Free T3 levels. Their Free T3 levels dropped below the reference range, yet there was an average weight loss of 11 pounds (5 kg). There was no change in their TSH, dehydroepiandrosterone sulfate (DHEA-S), cortisol, or ACTH from their levels seven weeks earlier at sea level, although prolactin and progesterone were both higher.[7] Elevated prolactin is associated with hypothyroidism,[8] and progesterone is known to stimulate respiration.[9] Since none of these men developed severe high altitude sickness, the seven weeks at base camp may have given their bodies time to fully acclimate to the higher altitude. Their results also imply that the low T3 syndrome is the body's way of handling lower oxygen levels, because lower T3 levels lower cellular oxygen requirements.

Reverse T3 was measured in another high altitude expedition; reverse T3 levels rose during the trek, along with T4 levels and thyroxine binding globulin (TBG). Reverse T3 levels may have risen in response to physical exertion.[10]

Sleep quality was studied in two men shortly after they arrived at the South Pole (9,300 feet or 2,900 meters). There was complete loss of stage 3 and 4 sleep for all nights recorded; those are the deeper stages of sleep. In addition, one man suffered from Acute Mountain Sickness and had a 100% increase in stage 1 and 50% decrease in rapid eye movement (REM) sleep.[11] Interestingly, hypothyroid patients also have significantly less stage 3 and 4 sleep.[12]

At high altitudes with lower oxygen levels, normal breathing and respiration rates are essential. Slow respiration is a hypothyroid symptom, and may contribute to hypothyroid patients getting even less oxygen at higher altitudes, which would compound their symptoms. One study of hypothyroid patients found respiratory muscle weakness in both the inhalation and exhalation muscles and the weakness positively correlated with thyroid levels. In other words, the lower the thyroid levels, the weaker the respiratory muscles.[13] This muscle weakness is reversible if thyroid hormone is prescribed and thyroid levels are brought up.

High altitude will certainly be a problem for someone who is hypothyroid and possibly undermedicated or undiagnosed. But knowing this, are there any measures that can be taken to reduce high altitude sickness symptoms, or must hypothyroid patients always choose low elevations to live, work, and vacation?

High altitude sickness treatments

Anyone who still feels hypothyroid even though they are taking prescription thyroid hormone should have their thyroid hormone levels (Free T3 and Free T4) checked. Unfortunately, many are only given a TSH test, which often does not reflect thyroid levels.

Sleeping at an elevation below 6,500 feet or 2,000 meters helps, because a lower sleeping altitude is one of the most important factors, along with rate of ascent, which determines whether someone develops high altitude sickness. *Climb high, sleep low*, is a rule that mountain climbers follow.[14]

Drinking lots of water to keep the body hydrated is important at high altitudes because of the dry air. Dehydration is a known cause of headaches, and for me, just drinking a lot of water keeps the headache away. Hypothyroid patients tend to be dehydrated even at sea level, because insufficient thyroid hormone often results in low aldosterone, a hormone involved in sodium, potassium and fluid balance.[15]

Limiting physical activity in the first few days allows the body to acclimate to the higher altitude. If vacationing in a mountainous area, consider buying a half-day ski pass, or doing half-day hikes for the first few days. Check the elevation of any destination before booking the trip, and remember that 8,000 feet (2,500 meters) is when those who are susceptible usually become symptomatic. I had a coworker book a dream trip to the Alps with her daughter for her high school graduation gift. She (the mother) had no idea she could not tolerate the altitude until she was already there and had to return to the base city, while her daughter went ahead without her.

Sleeping at a lower elevation the first night before heading to the final, higher destination also helps the body acclimate. Denver, Colorado is already over 5,000 feet in elevation, but that is still less than the 8,000-13,000 feet found at the ski resorts. Look for other nearby towns with lower elevations for lodging. Remember, one of the best ways to acclimate is to *sleep low*. Or pick a lower elevation ski resort altogether. A list of ski resorts in the western U.S., by elevation, can be found at wherewevacation.com.

Alcohol and any drug that suppresses respiration (large doses of narcotic pain medications or sedatives like sleeping pills) should be avoided. Respiration normally slows when asleep, is naturally slower in someone who is hypothyroid, and the addition of alcohol or drugs could result in dangerously low levels of oxygen while asleep.[16] People on thyroid internet forums have reported waking at night gasping for air when staying at high altitudes. Actually, when my thyroid levels were too low, I would also awake in the middle of the night gasping for air, and this was at sea level. This is called periodic breathing, where breathing slows and even stops for short periods.[17] It's possible this is just another form of sleep apnea.[18] I would dream that I was underwater and running out of air, deep in a lake or the ocean, and would be swimming to the surface. I would awake with a huge gasp, right when my head would surface in the dream. My heart would be rapidly pounding when I woke, and a rapid heartbeat is one way the body compensates for low oxygen levels. I would also wake up in a sweat, and this could be from noradrenaline that was pumped out to compensate for low cortisol levels, to keep blood sugar levels stable. I am happy to say that I have not had these dreams for a while, now that I'm on a higher dose of thyroid medication, when I used to have them every few days just a few years ago.

Diamox or acetazolamide is a drug that is sometimes prescribed to help high altitude sickness.[16] This is a sulfa drug, so caution is advised. More than one thyroid patient has reported extreme reactions to sulfa drugs. This may be due to a genetic inability to metabolize certain drugs.[19] I personally ended up in the emergency room (ER) in what seemed like anaphylactic shock when I was once prescribed a sulfa antibiotic.

Headache is usually the first symptom of high altitude sickness that most people experience and should not be ignored, because it can progress to high altitude pulmonary edema (HAPE) or high altitude cerebral edema (HACE) and left untreated, can be fatal. Swelling of the lungs and brain are the problem. Someone with high altitude pulmonary edema will have difficulty breathing and walking uphill. A dry cough and audible chest congestion are not good signs, nor are white lips and blue fingernails. Someone with high altitude cerebral edema will display loss of coordination (ataxia) and confusion. This can progress into a coma, and then death. With any of these symptoms, medical help should be sought and immediate descent to a lower altitude may be required.[16]

Conclusion

There are many beautiful cities, parks, and ski resorts at high altitudes that are worth living, working, and/or vacationing in. It would be a shame to exclude visiting these areas because of a medical condition that is mostly correctable. Since high altitudes are more difficult to tolerate if someone is hypothyroid, patients should certainly explore the possibility that they are undermedicated if they suffer from high altitude sickness, especially if they are being dosed by TSH. Skiers may want to look into ski resorts with peak elevations below 8,000 feet. Reviews of some lower elevation ski resorts can be found at wherewevacation.com.

Key points

- Headache, insomnia, a faster heart rate, and occasionally nausea, fatigue, dizziness, and loss of appetite are all symptoms of high altitude sickness, caused by a lack of oxygen.
- To accommodate to lower oxygen levels at higher altitudes, the body lowers available thyroid hormone to decrease oxygen consumption at the cellular level. Someone who is already hypothyroid may feel worse at altitude.
- Cortisol levels normally rise when someone moves to a high altitude. Hypothyroid patients with low cortisol may have a difficult time at altitude and may benefit from glucocorticoids.
- In several studies, T4 levels increased at altitude. The rise in T4 may compensate for the simultaneous rise in TBG, which binds thyroid hormone.

- Sleep is fitful at altitude, and a complete loss of the deeper stages of sleep has been documented. Hypothyroid patients don't reach the deeper stages of sleep either and the combination often results in insomnia.
- Slowly climbing in altitude (over days) and sleeping at lower elevations helps the body acclimate.
- It is important to drink lots of liquids because hypothyroid patients tend to be somewhat dehydrated, and the dry air at altitude only compounds the problem, resulting in headaches.
- Most people become symptomatic around 8,000 feet or 2,500 meters.
- Alcohol, narcotic pain medications, and sedatives like sleeping pills should be avoided because they can depress respiration, resulting in dangerously low oxygen levels while asleep.
- Signs that medical help should be sought: difficulty breathing while walking uphill, a dry cough and audible chest congestion, white lips and blue fingernails. Someone with high altitude cerebral edema will display loss of coordination (ataxia) and confusion.

---

[1] Diano, Sabrina, and Tamas L. Horvath. "Type 3 deiodinase in hypoxia: to cool or to kill?" *Cell metabolism* 7.5 (2008): 363-364.

[2] Ma, Yaluan, et al. "Thyroid hormone induces erythropoietin gene expression through augmented accumulation of hypoxia-inducible factor-1." *American Journal of Physiology-Regulatory, Integrative and Comparative Physiology* 287.3 (2004): R600-R607.

[3] Lindsey B. Koehler and Natasha Gardner. Low On 02 - The ultimate guide to living at altitude: Slope Sick. 5280, The Denver Magazine. Oct 2009.

[4] Basu, M., et al. "Glucocorticoids as prophylaxis against acute mountain sickness." *Clinical endocrinology* 57.6 (2002): 761-767.

[5] Richalet, Jean-Paul, Murielle Letournel, and Jean-Claude Souberbielle. "Effects of high-altitude hypoxia on the hormonal response to hypothalamic factors." *American Journal of Physiology-Regulatory, Integrative and Comparative Physiology* 299.6 (2010): R1685-R1692.

[6] Christensen, Niels Juel. "Increased levels of plasma noradrenaline in hypothyroidism." *Journal of Clinical Endocrinology & Metabolism* 35.3 (1972): 359-363.

[7] Benso, Andrea, et al. "Endocrine and metabolic responses to extreme altitude and physical exercise in climbers." *European Journal of Endocrinology* 157.6 (2007): 733-740.

[8] Honbo, Ken S., Andre J. Van Herle, and Katherine A. Kellett. "Serum prolactin levels in untreated primary hypothyroidism." *The American journal of medicine* 64.5 (1978): 782-787.

[9] Saaresranta, Tarja, and Olli Polo. "Hormones and breathing." *CHEST Journal* 122.6 (2002): 2165-2182.

[10] Wright, A. D. "Birmingham Medical Research Expeditionary Society 1977 Expedition: thyroid function and acute mountain sickness." *Postgraduate medical journal* 55.645 (1979): 483-486.

[11] Joern, Albert T., et al. "Short-term changes in sleep patterns on arrival at the South Polar Plateau." *Archives of Internal Medicine* 125.4 (1970): 649.

[12] Kales, Anthony, et al. "All night sleep studies in hypothyroid patients, before and after treatment." *Journal of Clinical Endocrinology & Metabolism* 27.11 (1967): 1593-1599.

[13] Siafakas, N. M., et al. "Respiratory muscle strength in hypothyroidism." *CHEST Journal* 102.1 (1992): 189-194.

[14] Peacock, Andrew J. "ABC of oxygen: Oxygen at high altitude." *BMJ: British Medical Journal* 317.7165 (1998): 1063.

[15] Saruta, T., et al. "Renin and aldosterone in hypothyroidism: relation to excretion of sodium and potassium." *Clinical endocrinology* 12.5 (1980): 483-489.

[16] Altitude Hypoxia Explained, Altitude Research Center, Anschutz Medical Campus, University of Colorado Denver. http://www.altituderesearch.org/hypoxia/altitude-hypoxia-explained

[17] Nussbaumer-Ochsner, Yvonne, et al. "Effect of short-term acclimatization to high altitude on sleep and nocturnal breathing." *Sleep* 35.3 (2012): 419.

[18] Taylor, A. "High-altitude illnesses: Physiology, risk factors, prevention and treatment." *RMMJ* 2.1 (2011): e0022.

[19] Kumari, Rashmi, Dependra K. Timshina, and Devinder Mohan Thappa. "Drug hypersensitivity syndrome." *Indian Journal of Dermatology, Venereology, and Leprology* 77.1 (2011): 7.

13

Hormone Replacement for Men
(Testosterone Replacement Therapy)

Of course you're tired . . . you're old!

—what older people are told

Andropause (male menopause) seems to hit men around age 50, when their declining testosterone levels ("low T") begin to affect their health. Osteoporosis, sexual dysfunction, fatigue, gynecomastia (male breasts), and metabolic syndrome are just a few of the symptoms.[1] Should they start hormone replacement? This is a bigger decision than it is for women, because if a woman starts hormone replacement and doesn't like it, she can just stop, and she returns to her previous state. But testosterone replacement therapy (TRT) in men shuts down natural testicular function, which causes the testicles to shrink. The hypothalamus (a gland located in the brain) normally releases gonadotropin-releasing hormone (GnRH) when testosterone levels are low, which stimulates the release of luteinizing hormone (LH) and follicle-stimulating hormone (FSH) by the anterior pituitary (also located in the brain). LH stimulates the production of testosterone, but once the testosterone reaches a certain blood concentration, it inhibits the release of GnRH by the hypothalamus, which in turn, limits the release of LH by the anterior pituitary, thus reducing testosterone production. Because it interferes with this feedback loop, TRT can shut down natural testosterone production. This is similar to taking any thyroid medication with triiodothyronine (T3) in it, which suppresses Thyroid Stimulating Hormone (TSH) and any natural thyroid production. There are also potential side effects of TRT that patients should be aware of before committing to this protocol: high estradiol, erythrocytosis or thick blood, fluid retention, benign prostatic hyperplasia, gynecomastia, and testicular atrophy or infertility, to name just a few.[2] Some of these side effects can be controlled by taking smaller doses of testosterone more often (more than once a week), or by managing the estradiol levels with supplements or drugs.

Causes of low testosterone

Aging and any head injury that could damage the hypothalamus or pituitary gland may result in low testosterone levels. It can also be caused by other hormone deficiencies, diet, and drugs. Sometimes, just bringing thyroid hormone levels up will raise testosterone.[3] In other cases, the elimination of soy products, which are estrogenic, has brought levels back up.[4] Statins will also lower testosterone, because testosterone is made from cholesterol, and statins lower cholesterol.[5] High cholesterol can be a sign of low thyroid levels.[6]

Testosterone levels can also decrease from excessive exercise like long-distance running, cycling, or rowing. This is similar to the reduced hormone levels found in women long-distance runners, whose menstrual periods stop.[7] Exercise is stressful to the body, and strenuous exercise and overtraining can negatively impact the hypothalamic-pituitary-gonadal (HPG) axis that regulates hormones. Cortisol levels rise in response to strenuous exercise, and this can indirectly inhibit LH and testosterone production. Some studies indicate that overtraining may induce hypogonadotropic hypogonadism (low sex hormones due to a pituitary or hypothalamus problem).[8]

Testosterone replacement therapy (TRT)

Because natural testicular function shuts down on TRT, it is imperative that the cause of low testosterone be determined *before* starting any TRT protocol. Tests should be performed to determine whether the patient has primary dysfunction (the testicles have stopped functioning), or secondary dysfunction (the testicles work, but the pituitary is not sending the LH signal). If the patient is secondary, injectable Human Chorionic Gonadotropin[9] (HCG) or Human Menopausal Gonadotropin[10] (HMG) will stimulate the testicles to produce testosterone and help maintain testicle size. If the patient has primary dysfunction, then there are basically three options: transdermal patches or gels such as Androgel or Testim, injectable testosterone ester formulations such as testosterone cypionate, or subcutaneous testosterone pellet implants. Some insurance companies cover the shots but not the gels or pellets, while others cover some or none of the options. Shots are much less expensive than gels. Creams or gels can also be made by compounding pharmacies for far less than the cost of the name-brand gels. Anecdotally, some men do very well on the pellets, but it does require a minor surgical procedure and tends to be very expensive. Insurance may or may not cover the procedure.

Pellets that are implanted under the skin (subcutaneous) in a surgical procedure appear to be the most physiological testosterone replacement therapy; they cause an initial increase in testosterone levels, which then level out and produce stable levels for months.[11] Estradiol levels remain stable too.[12] This is in contrast to intramuscular injections, which were originally given by doctors once a month, at 400 mg/shot. Both testosterone and estradiol levels peaked way above the normal range (in roughly 2-3 days), and then eventually dropped below the man's original levels.[13] These men would feel great shortly after the shots, but horrible in the last couple of weeks before their next shot. In addition, estrogen levels would skyrocket as the body tried to lower the excess testosterone.[14]

Over time, they figured out that a lower dose more often, like 100 mg/week, resulted in more physiological levels, because testosterone levels did not rise and fall so drastically. Some men administer their testosterone shots every three days. Weekly shots are a good starting point, but symptoms such as low energy by day 7 suggest that shorter intervals (every 3-6 days) at lower doses might work even better. Note that just like thyroid doses range from ½ grain – 5+ grains, testosterone shots can range from 25 mg to over 100 mg per shot. It is all very individual, and patients should work with a doctor and get frequent lab tests when starting out. If thyroid levels are low, it will usually limit testosterone's life in the body and patients will have to dose more frequently. This is because sex hormone binding globulin (SHBG) levels affect the life of testosterone, and low thyroid levels are one cause of low SHBG.[15] Insulin resistance or diabetes is another cause, although low thyroid levels may also be the cause of insulin resistance.[16] It is imperative that thyroid levels be monitored along with testosterone levels when on TRT, because they are interrelated, with the replacement of one hormone affecting the other.[17] Occasionally, TRT unmasks a thyroid deficiency which then requires treatment.[18] Most doctors will run a TSH test to check thyroid health, but unfortunately, TSH levels are not specific enough to detect thyroid hormone deficiencies, and more specialized thyroid tests must be requested [see Blood Tests, Chapter 9].

Testosterone cypionate is prescribed as an intramuscular injection, but some men are now successfully using it subcutaneously, or injected into fat just under the skin.[19] They are reaping the benefits of subcutaneous testosterone pellets, but without the expense and hassle of a surgical procedure and related complications, and the added ability to easily adjust the dose. They inject smaller amounts (as low as 25 mg) of testosterone cypionate into their belly fat at more frequent intervals (usually twice a week). Some men who experienced problems with estradiol on the higher dose intramuscular injections no longer have them when injecting subcutaneously.

Side effects of TRT

Estrogen in men is a common side effect of testosterone replacement therapy because of the aromatization (conversion) of testosterone to estrogen. Diindolylmethane (DIM) is an over-the-counter (OTC) supplement that helps some (not all) men keep their estrogen levels down.[20] It alters estrogen metabolism pathways. Sometimes, if thyroid and liver health can be optimized, estrogen levels will normalize without medication. This is because thyroid energy powers the liver, which is responsible for processing out all the hormones.[21] If thyroid levels are low, liver function will be suboptimal, and estrogen can build up. There are also genetic mutations in liver detoxification enzymes that may affect estrogen metabolism. DIM is not effective for all men, and there are prescription aromatase inhibitor medications like Arimidex or Aromasin that can help control estrogen levels. It is often difficult to get the dosage correct, however, and sometimes estrogen is too high, then too low. This can negatively affect a man's ability to have and maintain erections.

Hereditary hemochromatosis (HH) is a genetic, inherited disease where the body loads too much iron. Total iron levels, percent saturation, and ferritin will be high. One does not "get" this condition from testosterone replacement therapy. Too much iron in the blood can damage organs, so periodic bloodletting is standard practice for anyone with hemochromatosis or high iron levels. Over time, high iron levels can damage the testicles and cause hypogonadism (low testosterone).

Thick blood or erythrocytosis can result from testosterone replacement therapy. Red blood cells (RBC), hematocrit, and hemoglobin will all be high and over the reference range.[22] This is not the same as having too much iron and is an unrelated condition. A CBC or Complete Blood Count should be run when testosterone is tested to monitor this condition. Donating blood is the standard treatment for either hereditary hemochromatosis or thick blood, but if done too often in someone without hemochromatosis (more than twice a year), it may deplete stored iron (ferritin) and lead to iron deficiency.[23] [24] This can lead to other problems like anemia and fatigue and will lower thyroid function, since thyroid needs adequate ferritin to work.[25] Multiple enzymes have iron as a component, so multiple biochemical processes will be negatively affected if ferritin drops too low.[26]

Testosterone, hydrocortisone,[27] and thyroid[28] are all known to affect RBC levels. Any one of these hormones in excess can cause erythrocytosis or thick blood. Lower the excessive hormone, and the blood returns to normal. If thyroid levels are low, bringing them up may allow the testosterone dose to be reduced, and the erythrocytosis will resolve. If testosterone, cortisol, and thyroid levels are optimal (neither too high nor low), blood should return to normal and there would be no need to donate blood all the time. Sometimes just taking a smaller testosterone dose more often does the trick. For example, a 100 mg shot given every 10 days is theoretically equivalent to a 50 mg shot given every 5 days. In reality, some patients report that they are able to use less testosterone when splitting a dose, because less is aromatized to estradiol. The smaller dose creates less of a spike in testosterone (and estradiol), creating a more physiological (natural) level, and possibly, no thick blood.

For some hypothyroid men, the amount of T3 in natural desiccated thyroid may be too much, and they might do better combining T4 (levothyroxine) with a lower dose of desiccated thyroid split throughout the day. If they are taking T3-only to combat reverse T3, this will raise both SHBG and estradiol to unnatural levels,[29] and result in more imbalance. High SHBG is correlated with osteoporosis and fracture risk in men.[30] In one study, T3 doses of 50-75 mcg daily resulted in accelerated bone turnover that resulted in bone loss.[31]

Conclusion

In spite of what people may be led to believe from television advertisements, testosterone replacement for men is not as simple as swallowing a daily vitamin pill. Testosterone is just one hormone amongst many that are used in the human body (cortisol, estradiol, thyroid, etc.), and their levels are all intertwined through multiple feedback mechanisms. When one hormone is added, others are affected. Sometimes they are affected negatively, in which case those other hormones must now be brought into balance. TRT is a constant balancing act. For younger men who would otherwise have the testosterone levels of a 90-year-old man, TRT can restore their testosterone levels and return some of the energy they had when they were younger. For that reason, many hypogonadal men consider the balancing act a small price to pay for the health benefits they receive.

Key points

- TRT shuts down natural testicular function and is a lifetime protocol.
- Testing should be performed before starting TRT to determine the cause of low testosterone: does the patient suffer from primary or secondary hypogonadism?
- Low testosterone can be from aging, hypothalamus or pituitary damage, low thyroid levels, poor diet, statins, overtraining, and iron overload.
- High estradiol is a side effect of TRT and may be controlled with DIM or pharmaceutical anti-estrogens.
- Thyroid levels should be monitored when on TRT, because the two hormones are interrelated.
- Thick blood can be caused by too much testosterone, hydrocortisone, or thyroid
- Erythrocytosis is a side effect of TRT, but blood should not be donated more than twice a year, because it depletes iron levels, inducing another set of problems.
- Lower doses of testosterone administered at shorter intervals may give a more physiologic response and resolve erythrocytosis.
- Subcutaneous injections may reduce estradiol and result in more even levels of testosterone
- Too much T3 raises estradiol and SHBG in men, and may lead to osteoporosis.

[1] Dohle, G. R., et al. "Guidelines on male hypogonadism." Eur Ass Urol (2012).

[2] Rhoden, Ernani Luis, and Abraham Morgentaler. "Risks of testosterone-replacement therapy and recommendations for monitoring." New England Journal of Medicine 350.5 (2004): 482-492.

[3] Pantalone, Kevin M., and Charles Faiman. "Male hypogonadism: More than just a low testosterone." Cleveland Clinic Journal of Medicine 79.10 (2012): 717-725.

[4] Kraemer, William J., et al. "The Effects of Soy and Whey Protein Supplementation on Acute Hormonal Reponses to Resistance Exercise in Men." Journal of the American College of Nutrition 32.1 (2013): 66-74.

[5] Schooling, C. Mary, et al. "The effect of statins on testosterone in men and women, a systematic review and meta-analysis of randomized controlled trials." BMC medicine 11.1 (2013): 1-9.

[6] Shashi, A., and N. Sharma. "Lipid Profile Abnormalities In Hypothyroidism." International Journal of Science & Nature 3.2 (2012).

[7] Wheeler, Garry D., et al. "Reduced serum testosterone and prolactin levels in male distance runners." JAMA: the journal of the American Medical Association 252.4 (1984): 514-516.

[8] Du Plessis, S., et al. "Is there a link between exercise and male factor infertility." Open Reprod Sci J 3 (2011): 105-13.

[9] Roth, M. Y., et al. "Dose-dependent increase in intratesticular testosterone by very low-dose human chorionic gonadotropin in normal men with experimental gonadotropin deficiency." Journal of Clinical Endocrinology & Metabolism 95.8 (2010): 3806-3813.

[10] Ho, Christopher Chee Kong, and Hui Meng Tan. "Treatment of the Hypogonadal Infertile Male—A Review." Sexual Medicine Reviews 1.1 (2013): 42-49.

[11] Kelleher, S., et al. "Testosterone release rate and duration of action of testosterone pellet implants." Clinical endocrinology 60.4 (2004): 420-428.

[12] Cantrill, Judith Anne, et al. "Which testosterone replacement therapy?." Clinical endocrinology 21.2 (1984): 97-107.

[13] Behre, H. M., et al. "Pharmacology of testosterone preparations." Testosterone, Action, Deficiency, Substitution (2004): 405-444.

[14] Tenover, J. Lisa. "The androgen-deficient aging male: current treatment options." Reviews in Urology 5.Suppl 1 (2003): S22.

[15] Cavaliere, Humberto, Neusa Abelin, and Geraldo Medeiros-Neto. "Serum Levels of Total Testosterone and Sex Hormone Binding Globulin in Hypothyroid Patients and Normal Subjects Treated with Incremental Doses of L-T4 or L-T3." Journal of andrology 9.3 (1988): 215-219.

[16] Maratou, Eirini, et al. "Studies of insulin resistance in patients with clinical and subclinical hypothyroidism." European Journal of Endocrinology 160.5 (2009): 785-790.

[17] Meikle, A. Wayne. "The interrelationships between thyroid dysfunction and hypogonadism in men and boys." Thyroid 14.3, Supplement 1 (2004): 17-25.

[18] Tahboub, Rundsarah, and Baha M. Arafah. "Sex steroids and the thyroid." Best Practice & Research Clinical Endocrinology & Metabolism 23.6 (2009): 769-780.

[19] Al-Futaisi, Abdullah M., et al. "Subcutaneous administration of testosterone." Saudi Med J 27.12 (2006): 1843-1846.

[20] Smith, Sunyata, et al. "3, 3′-Diindolylmethane and genistein decrease the adverse effects of estrogen in LNCaP and PC-3 prostate cancer cells." The Journal of Nutrition 138.12 (2008): 2379-2385.

[21] Amar, Dotan, et al. "The transition of human estrogen sulfotransferase from generalist to specialist using directed enzyme evolution." Journal of molecular biology 416.1 (2012): 21-32.

[22] Fernández-Balsells, M. Mercè, et al. "Adverse effects of testosterone therapy in adult men: a systematic review and meta-analysis." Journal of Clinical Endocrinology & Metabolism 95.6 (2010): 2560-2575.

[23] Yousefinejad, Vahid, et al. "The evaluation of iron deficiency and anemia in male blood donors with other related factors." Asian journal of transfusion science 4.2 (2010): 123.

[24] Simon, Toby L., Philip J. Garry, and Elizabeth M. Hooper. "Iron stores in blood donors." JAMA: the journal of the American Medical Association 245.20 (1981): 2038-2043.

[25] Akhter, S., et al. "Thyroid Status in Patients with Low Serum Ferritin Level." Bangladesh Journal of Medical Biochemistry 5.1 (2013): 5-11.

[26] Beard, John L. "Iron biology in immune function, muscle metabolism and neuronal functioning." The Journal of Nutrition 131.2 (2001): 568S-580S.

[27] Fisher, James W. "Increase in circulating red cell volume of normal rats after treatment with hydrocortisone or corticosterone." Proceedings of the Society for Experimental Biology and Medicine. Society for Experimental Biology and Medicine (New York, NY). Vol. 97. No. 3. Royal Society of Medicine, 1958.

[28] Das, K. C., et al. "Erythropoiesis and erythropoietin in hypo-and hyperthyroidism." Journal of Clinical Endocrinology & Metabolism 40.2 (1975): 211-220.

[29] Southren, A. Louis, et al. "The conversion of androgens to estrogens in hyperthyroidism." Journal of Clinical Endocrinology & Metabolism 38.2 (1974): 207-214.

[30] Lormeau, C., et al. "Sex hormone-binding globulin, estradiol, and bone turnover markers in male osteoporosis." Bone 34.6 (2004): 933-939.

[31] Smith, Steven R., et al. "The effects of triiodothyronine on bone metabolism in healthy ambulatory men." Thyroid 13.4 (2003): 357-364.

14

Hormone Replacement for Women (Estrogen & Progesterone)

You use a tri-est gel topically?

—an incredulous ob-gyn, who only prescribes oral, pharmaceutical estrogen

Insomnia, incontinence, and vaginal dryness and itching can often be relieved with bioidentical hormone replacement therapy (BHRT) in post-menopausal or even peri-menopausal women. There are a number of different thoughts and protocols on how to best implement this from different doctors, books, websites, etc., so I will just tell you what I chose, and why.

Oral, sublingual, vaginal, or transdermal delivery was the first decision I had to make, and I chose transdermal (applied to the skin), because it is absorbed without first passing through the liver, and the dosage can be easily adjusted. Oral estrogen first passes through the liver, which raises thyroid binding globulin (TBG), which binds to and reduces thyroid hormone (free thyroxine or FT4), so is not the best choice for someone like me who is also taking thyroid hormone.[1] There's also no way to tell how much is lost when it passes through the liver, and it's difficult to adjust fixed oral doses without getting another prescription. Sublingual and vaginal delivery may also work well; in fact, vaginal delivery may be the most natural since the hormones would enter in the uterine area, instead of through the intestinal tract (how natural is that?). But transdermal seemed like it would be the easiest method to adjust, for me.

There are three different forms of prescription estrogen: estrone (E1), estradiol (E2), and estriol (E3). Estradiol and estrone are considered "parent" estrogens, because over a dozen estrogen metabolites derive from them, including estriol. Estradiol is considered the most potent type, and is primarily from the ovaries. It is thought to play a role in the development of breast cancer. Estriol appears to have mixed effects on breast cancer cells, depending on the type of receptor.[2] The three different estrogens can be prescribed in various combinations, and the number of estrogens in the formula determines the name of the formula: estradiol (E2), bi-est (E2+E3), or tri-est (E1+E2+E3). I chose tri-est, because it seemed more complete and more closely replicates a female body's natural output, in the same way that desiccated thyroid replicates normal thyroid function by containing all the hormones in the thyroid gland, and not just T4. I take about 0.8 mg of topical estrogen on days 1-25 and follow a formula by Dr. Jonathan Wright called Esnatri that I have compounded. This formula is 90% estriol (E3), 7% estradiol (E2), and 3% estrone (E1). My dose equates to 0.72 mg estriol, 0.056 mg estradiol and 0.024 mg estrone. The estradiol component of my dose is miniscule next to others who are only prescribed estradiol.

The large estriol component in my tri-est formula is based on three findings:[3]

1. Circulating estriol *significantly* exceeds the sum of circulating estrone and estradiol at any point in the menstrual cycle in healthy, pre-menopausal women.

2. Japanese women have the lowest rates of breast cancer in the world and the highest serum estriol levels worldwide. This appears to be the effect of a relatively high iodine diet (when compared to the standard U.S. diet).

3. Estrone and estradiol are considered slightly pro-carcinogenic, while estriol is considered neutral or anti-carcinogenic. Iodine encourages conversion of both estrone and estradiol to estriol.

Premarin is another form of estrogen that doctors prescribe and is called an equine estrogen because it is made from horse urine. It does not contain the human estrogens. While it would not be my first choice for estrogen, some find it very effective. Unfortunately, it can raise sex hormone binding globulin (SHBG), lower free testosterone, lower Free T4, and raise free cortisol levels.[4] It may also increase the risk of breast cancer in women who have a polymorphism in their Catechol O-methyl transferase (COMT) detoxification enzyme, because they would already have suboptimal detoxification, and one of the equine estrogen metabolites further inhibits COMT.[5]

The Women's Health Initiative study analyzed the effects of Premarin and a progestin, medroxyprogesterone acetate (MPA), on women's health. Because Premarin is made from horse urine, it contains metabolites that are foreign to the human body. MPA is a synthetic progesterone, also foreign to the human body. The study was halted before completion in 2002 because results indicated that the progestin had negative effects on the heart (increased the risk of coronary heart disease) and breasts (increased the risk of breast cancer).[6] This is not the same bioidentical estrogen and progesterone obtained from compounding pharmacies. Some progestins increase the proliferation of specific progesterone receptors that are overexpressed on breast cancer cells, which means they may encourage breast cancer. This progesterone receptor membrane component-1 (PGRMC1) was also found in serum samples of lung cancer patients and may be a cancer marker.[7] Other studies also implicate synthetic progestin in breast cancer cell proliferation through different mechanisms.[8]

When I first researched BHRT several years ago, everything I read said that estrogen should always be balanced with progesterone. It did not matter whether one had a uterus or not, and progesterone was somewhat protective against cancer. Studies showed a lower incidence of cancer if estrogen replacement was combined with bioidentical progesterone replacement. The relative risks for breast cancer were higher for estrogen therapy alone, and even higher for estrogen plus synthetic progestins.[9] Dr. John Lee's books on transdermal progesterone made a lot of sense, and following his guidelines, I w take about 12 mg of topical progesterone for two weeks out of the month. The actual proportion of estrogen to progesterone that a woman needs is very individual and is often found through trial and error. I found that if I took more than 12 mg of progesterone, it made my breasts ache in the second half of the cycle. Everything I read suggested I needed *more* progesterone if they ached, not less, but my experience was the opposite. Today, I'm finding studies that confirm what my body was telling me; cell proliferation of the breast during the luteal phase (second half) may be when cancer starts.[10] Progesterone peaks during the luteal phase. Recent studies present conflicting results: progesterone is a risk factor for breast cancer, but loss of progesterone receptors is associated with more invasive breast cancer.[11] In other words, the presence of progesterone may limit later stages of tumor progression. The bottom line is that progesterone has multiple effects, and normal breast cells and cancerous breast cells may respond differently. Different microenvironments may also play a role in the different responses.[12] Levels of iodine, thyroid hormones (specifically triiodothyronine or T3), Vitamin D, and other hormones and antioxidants may all play a role in the response to progesterone.

One thing I learned from experience is that progesterone is a natural antagonist of aldosterone. Aldosterone is a hormone involved in the control of water and electrolyte balance and helps to retain sodium, so someone doesn't have to go to the bathroom all the time. If aldosterone is low, the person will have to urinate multiple times throughout the day. Progesterone has a high affinity for the mineralocorticoid receptor, which means it competes with aldosterone.[13] Anyone's who's been pregnant should remember the effect of their high progesterone levels at the time (frequent bathroom trips). When my progesterone dose is too high, I become very thirsty and go to the bathroom multiple times throughout the night, I'm guessing because my aldosterone is blocked from the mineralocorticoid receptor by progesterone. Decreasing my dose gave me the benefit of deeper sleep without the frequent bathroom trips.

Testosterone at only 0.1 mg gave me acne, but I found pregnenolone in pill form to be a good substitute. I used to take 2.5 mg twice a week, or 5 mg/week, until I decided that was also turning into testosterone too. Pregnenolone may be a good alternative for someone who is looking to increase their testosterone and/or dehydroepiandrosterone (DHEA) indirectly. I could not tolerate DHEA either and only 1.25 mg gave me acne.

Breast cancer has many causes, but we still don't know exactly what triggers cancer development or we would know how to prevent it, instead of treat it after the fact. What we do know is that estrogen and/or progesterone are somehow involved, because an oophorectomy (removal of the ovaries), which eliminates the primary source of both hormones, lowers the risk of both breast and ovarian cancer in those who are genetically susceptible.[14] Detoxification enzymes process estrogen and progesterone for elimination through urine or feces, and there are numerous detoxification enzyme mutations and deficiencies that may play a role in cancer. COMT was mentioned earlier, but sulfotransferase (SULT), UDP-glucuronosyltransferase (UGT), and glutathione S-transferases (GST) are other enzymes that may also play a role.[15] Environmental toxins like cigarette smoking are also implicated.[16] My personal opinion is that our genetic detoxification enzyme makeup is what makes some of us more susceptible to cancer. How else is it possible for some people to smoke for years and not develop cancer, while others are diagnosed at an early age? They are exposed to the same toxin, so the difference must be in the individual's susceptibility. And that would be the ability to detoxify any toxin.

Thyroid levels may play a role because metabolism speeds up or slows down depending on the amount of thyroid hormone available. A slow metabolism implies slower detoxification with longer exposure to toxins. Therefore, if thyroid is not optimized, it might be wise not to start estrogen replacement until that is corrected. Breast tenderness during the second half of the cycle suggests that thyroid, estrogen, and/or progesterone levels need adjusting because one or more of these are either too high or too low. Hyperthyroidism will raise SHBG and decrease the rate that estradiol clears from the body.[17] This may explain why some women on the T3-only protocol report painful breasts. In fact, high T3 levels are positively associated with breast cancer, but not other cancers.[18] Some studies show that thyroid hormone stimulates tumor growth and metastasis, and that hypothyroidism actually prolongs survival.[19]

There are doctors and internet groups who say that saliva labs are better than serum for monitoring sex hormones, yet there are other doctors and groups who say just the opposite, that serum is better. Out of curiosity, I did saliva and serum labs one day apart to see if the labs would show a great disparity, and the surprise was that for estrogen and progesterone, they didn't. Both were within the normal range. I was absolutely meticulous about not applying the hormones to my face/neck area, and not getting the topical hormones on my fingertips for a few days prior to the saliva testing, to ensure that I would not contaminate/skew the saliva results. The other result that surprised me was the dehydroepiandrosterone-sulfate (DHEA-S), which was almost at the top-of-range in serum, but rock bottom in saliva. One study found that salivary DHEA-S is influenced by saliva flow rate and is only present at 1% of the unbound concentration in serum.[20] In other words, the DHEA-S serum level will always be higher than the saliva result.

Should estradiol be high or low or in the middle of the range when supplementing? That depends on the woman's natural levels before menopause. High estrogen women are very busty and curvaceous; they have naturally high levels. Low estrogen women are tall, lean, and fairly flat-chested, with boyish figures. If you look at families, most of the women in a family will have a similar build. This is normal and healthy for them, because they were obviously able to reproduce. A naturally low estrogen woman would only need a small dose of hormone to restore estrogen levels to what is normal *for her*. Some women may also need less hormone to achieve the same results because they process hormones out at a slower rate than others. The sex hormones are better dosed by symptoms rather than lab results, though lab results can be used as rough guidelines to determine when a dose is too high or too low.

Conclusion

Thanks to bioidentical hormone replacement therapy, I now fall asleep easier and sleep deeper, I look younger because of the tri-est, the vaginal dryness and itching is gone, the incontinence from laughing or sneezing is gone, and I have great muscle tone for someone my age. You will note that I am taking extremely low doses next to what others are prescribed. More is not always better.

However, hormone replacement is not without risk, and anyone considering it should research the topic thoroughly, especially if there is any history of cancer in their family. It's a very personal decision. Women who have never taken supplemental estrogen

/or progesterone have been diagnosed with breast cancer, so post-menopausal /rmone supplementation cannot be blamed in those cases. There is ample evidence that /ral pharmaceutical replacement options are not in women's best interests, because they create foreign metabolites. I prefer topical bioidentical hormones. Estriol is the estrogen found in abundance in the female body, so it makes no sense to supplement only estradiol, even though estradiol is considered more potent. To me, that is analogous to taking only T3—it's an incomplete form of replacement that will cause an imbalance.

Not every doctor will prescribe the topical bioidentical hormones, and in fact, my insurance will not cover estriol, because it is not FDA approved in any form. My insurance does cover Premarin, oral or cream estradiol, and oral progesterone. When the doctor who originally prescribed my BHRT stopped taking my insurance, I went to another ob-gyn for my annual check-up. When I mentioned I took estrogen, he said, "Premarin?" And when I told him no, that I was taking a tri-est gel topically, he looked incredulous. At the next open season, I will switch to an insurance plan that my previous ob-gyn takes, or I will consider paying for her visits "out-of-network." While it will cost me more, it will be more than worth it to consult with someone who listens to patients and is actually familiar with bioidentical female hormones. In fact, she told me that while she initially prescribed Premarin (because that's what she was taught to prescribe), she now prescribes bioidentical hormones because that's what her patients have requested.

Key points

- Hormones can be administered four different ways: orally, sublingually, vaginally, or transdermally. Oral estrogen is not the best choice for someone also on thyroid hormone, because it lowers Free T4.

- There are three types of prescription estrogen: estrone (E1), estradiol (E2), and estriol (E3). Estradiol can be prescribed individually or in combination with estriol as bi-est or tri-est. Premarin (horse urine) is another prescription choice that some women are happy with.

- Estriol is the most abundant form of estrogen found in healthy, pre-menopausal women. Japanese women, who have the lowest rates of breast cancer, have the highest levels of estriol in the world.

- The Women's Health Initiative study in 2002 reported increased risks of coronary heart disease and breast cancer and scared women away from hormone supplementation. The hormones studied were Premarin and a synthetic progestin, not bioidentical hormones. Because these create foreign metabolites in the body, the results are not interchangeable with bioidentical supplementation.

- Cell proliferation in the breast occurs during the luteal phase, when progesterone peaks. Progesterone, like the estrogens, is considered a risk factor in breast cancer.

- Pregnenolone may be a good substitute for testosterone or DHEA in women who cannot tolerate either directly.

- Genetic detoxification enzyme mutations or deficiencies may play a role in cancer development.

- High T3 levels are associated with breast cancer, but not other cancers. High T3 levels raise SHBG and lower estradiol clearance from the body.
- There shouldn't be much difference between saliva and serum labs, except for DHEA-S. The serum level is more accurate for DHEA-S.
- Women have widely different natural estrogen levels, as seen in the range of body types. Some women may only need to supplement small amounts of hormone to relieve menopausal symptoms.

---

[1] Mazer, Norman A. "Interaction of estrogen therapy and thyroid hormone replacement in postmenopausal women." *Thyroid* 14.3, Supplement 1 (2004): 27-34.

[2] Lappano, Rosamaria, et al. "Estriol acts as a GPR30 antagonist in estrogen receptor-negative breast cancer cells." *Molecular and cellular endocrinology* 320.1 (2010): 162-170.

[3] Wright, Jonathan V. "Bio-Identical Steroid Hormone Replacement: Selected Observations from 23 Years of Clinical and Laboratory Practice." *Annals of the New York Academy of Sciences* 1057.1 (2005): 506-524.

[4] Shifren, Jan L., et al. "A randomized, open-label, crossover study comparing the effects of oral versus transdermal estrogen therapy on serum androgens, thyroid hormones, and adrenal hormones in naturally menopausal women." *Menopause* 14.6 (2007): 985-994.

[5] Chang, Minsun. "Dual roles of estrogen metabolism in mammary carcinogenesis." *BMB Rep* 44.7 (2011): 423-434.

[6] Manson, JoAnn E., et al. "Estrogen plus progestin and the risk of coronary heart disease." *New England Journal of Medicine* 349.6 (2003): 523-534.

[7] Neubauer, H., et al. "Possible role of PGRMC1 in breast cancer development." *Climacteric* 0 (2013): 1-5.

[8] Diaz Flaqué, María C., et al. "Progestin drives breast cancer growth by inducing p21^{CIP1} expression through the assembly of a transcriptional complex among Stat3, progesterone receptor and ErbB-2." *Steroids* (2012).

[9] Fournier, Agnès, Franco Berrino, and Françoise Clavel-Chapelon. "Unequal risks for breast cancer associated with different hormone replacement therapies: results from the E3N cohort study." *Breast cancer research and treatment* 107.1 (2008): 103-111.

[10] Brisken, Cathrin. "Progesterone signalling in breast cancer: a neglected hormone coming into the limelight." *Nature Reviews Cancer* 13.6 (2013): 385-396.

[11] Obr, Alison E., and Dean P. Edwards. "The biology of progesterone receptor in the normal mammary gland and in breast cancer." *Molecular and cellular endocrinology* 357.1 (2012): 4-17.

[12] Kim, I Julie, Takeshi Kurita, and Serdar E. Bulun. "Progesterone action in endometrial cancer, endometriosis, uterine fibroids, and breast cancer." *Endocrine reviews* 34.1 (2013): 130-162.

[13] Caprio, M., et al. "Potential role of progestogens in the control of adipose tissue and salt sensitivity via interaction with the mineralocorticoid receptor." *Climacteric* 11.3 (2008): 258-264.

[14] Eisen, Andrea, et al. "Breast cancer risk following bilateral oophorectomy in BRCA1 and BRCA2 mutation carriers: an international case-control study." *Journal of Clinical Oncology* 23.30 (2005): 7491-7496.

[15] Hevir, N., et al. "Expression of estrogen and progesterone receptors and estrogen metabolizing enzymes in different breast cancer cell lines." *Chemico-Biological Interactions* 191.1 (2011): 206-216.

[16] Reynolds, Peggy. "Smoking and breast cancer." *Journal of mammary gland biology and neoplasia* (2013): 1-9.

[17] Olivo, Jaime, et al. "Estrogen metabolism in hyperthyroidism and in cirrhosis of the liver." *Steroids* 26.1 (1975): 47-56.

[18] Tosovic, Ada, et al. "Triiodothyronine levels in relation to mortality from breast cancer and all causes: a population-based prospective cohort study." *European Journal of Endocrinology* 168.4 (2013): 483-490.

[19] Moeller, Lars C., and Dagmar Führer. "Thyroid hormone, thyroid hormone receptors, and cancer: a clinical perspective." *Endocrine-related cancer* 20.2 (2013): R19-R29.

[20] Gatti, R., and E. F. De Palo. "An update: salivary hormones and physical exercise." *Scandinavian Journal of Medicine & Science in Sports* 21.2 (2011): 157-169.

15

Hormone Supplements for Men:
Saw Palmetto, Stinging Nettle, & Hair Loss Drugs

Does anyone really want to get old?

Dihydrotestosterone (DHT) is believed to be the cause of male pattern baldness and prostate problems. Therefore, men seeking to address these two problems often take DHT inhibitors. Saw Palmetto is an over-the-counter (OTC) men's supplement that is considered a DHT inhibitor. It inhibits the hormone pathway of testosterone to DHT. However, the alternative pathway is to estradiol (a form of estrogen). This is not what most men want, because estrogen is the female hormone! There are also prescription DHT inhibitors or 5-alpha reductase inhibitor drugs called finasteride (Proscar, Propecia) and dutasteride (Avodart). Men take these drugs hoping to grow more hair, but some have also developed erectile dysfunction, ejaculation disorders, low libido and gynecomastia (male breasts).[1] These side effects appear to be permanent in some men, for they persist even after stopping the medication.[2] Low thyroid levels may be a contributing factor, because low thyroid levels also cause hair loss.[3] In one case study, a hypothyroid man (taking levothyroxine) given 1 mg/day of finasteride developed enlarged breasts four months after starting treatment.[4]

DHT metabolites play an essential role in mental health, therefore, inhibiting DHT may not be wise. One of these DHT metabolites, 3α-diol (or 5α-androstane, 3α, 17α-diol), has been shown to reduce anxiety, depression, and cognitive decline in older rats. When the rats were given indomethacin, which blocks the conversion of DHT to 3α-diol, they showed decreased cognitive performance and increased anxiety. Reduced gamma-aminobutyric acid (GABA) receptor function is associated with anxiety and depression,[5] and 3α-diol has actions at the GABA receptors in the hippocampus in the brain.[6] When DHT is inhibited, then the DHT metabolite 3α-diol will decrease, which would lead to lower GABA function, which is associated with anxiety and depression. In short, DHT inhibitors could induce anxiety and depression. Studies confirm that finasteride, even in low doses, may cause depression in some men. A decrease in several other important hormones, including DHEA and pregnenolone, has also occurred during finasteride treatment.[7] Hormones are essential to good health, so any decrease (from normal) is not good.

Some men have high Sex Hormone Binding Globulin (SHBG) levels, which may interfere with their testosterone levels. The T3-only protocol, or even high levels of T3 from desiccated thyroid, will raise SHBG.[8] Stinging nettle, an OTC supplement, is believed to reduce SHBG, and has been taken for this effect. However, stinging nettle has caused gynecomastia in a male, and galactorrhoea (breast milk) in a woman who was not breastfeeding at the time. Both subjects had been drinking nettle tea for about a month before the onset of their symptoms, which decreased once they stopped taking the herb.[9]

Testosterone raising supplements ordered online may have undesirable side effects as well. One medical journal report profiled a 19-year-old male who developed "fluid retention," lack of libido, and erectile dysfunction after taking an online supplement to increase his libido. He was found to have high serum testosterone and raised Luteinising Hormone (LH), the pituitary hormone that stimulates testosterone production.[10]

Aggressive prostate cancer developed in two men within months of their starting daily consumption of an unnamed herbal/hormonal dietary supplement. An analysis of the product showed it contained both testosterone and estradiol. A warning letter from the Food & Drug Administration (FDA) to the manufacturer led to the product being removed from the market.[11]

In the U.S., testosterone is a controlled substance regulated by the Drug Enforcement Administration (DEA). This means it can only be obtained with a valid prescription from a physician. Anything sold online (without a prescription) may not really be testosterone. Buyer beware.

Conclusion

Hormones and their pathways are extremely complicated. Attempting to lower or raise just one hormone usually affects an entire cascade with undesirable side effects. Research is highly recommended before any supplement is taken; many have experienced results they did not anticipate!

Key points

- Even OTC supplements can negatively affect hormones.
- Some hair loss drugs have serious side effects.
- DHT, considered to be the cause of hair loss, creates beneficial metabolites. If DHT is inhibited, these metabolites are decreased, and anxiety and depression can result.

---

[1] Marihart, Sibylle, Mike Harik, and Bob Djavan. "Dutasteride: a review of current data on a novel dual inhibitor of 5α reductase." *Reviews in urology* 7.4 (2005): 203.

[2] Irwig, Michael S. "Persistent Sexual Side Effects of Finasteride: Could They Be Permanent?" *Journal of Sexual Medicine* 9.11 (2012): 2927-2932.

[3] Harrison, Shannon, and Wilma Bergfeld. "Diffuse hair loss: its triggers and management." *Cleveland Clinic journal of medicine* 76.6 (2009): 361-367.

[4] Ramot, Yuval, Tali Czarnowicki, and Abraham Zlotogorski. "Finasteride induced Gynecomastia: Case report and Review of the Literature." *International journal of trichology* 1.1 (2009): 27.

[5] Earnheart, John C., et al. "GABAergic control of adult hippocampal neurogenesis in relation to behavior indicative of trait anxiety and depression states." *The Journal of neuroscience* 27.14 (2007): 3845-3854.

[6] Frye, Cheryl A., et al. "3α-androstanediol, but not testosterone, attenuates age-related decrements in cognitive, anxiety, and depressive behavior of male rats." *Frontiers in aging neuroscience* 2 (2010).

[7] Dušková, Michaela, Martin Hill, and Luboslav Stárka. "The influence of low dose finasteride, a type II 5α-reductase inhibitor, on circulating neuroactive steroids." *Hormone Molecular Biology and Clinical Investigation* 1.2 (2010): 95-102.

[8] Carani, Cesare, et al. "Multicenter study on the prevalence of sexual symptoms in male hypo-and hyperthyroid patients." *Journal of Clinical Endocrinology & Metabolism* 90.12 (2005): 6472-6479.

[9] Sahin, Mustafa, et al. "Gynaecomastia in a man and hyperoestrogenism in a woman due to ingestion of nettle (Urtica dioica)." *NZ Med J* 120.1265 (2007): U2803.

[10] McDonald, Tim J., et al. "A novel case of a raised testosterone and LH in a young man." *Clinica Chimica Acta* 412.21 (2011): 1999-2001.

[11] Shariat, Shahrokh F., et al. "Herbal/hormonal dietary supplement possibly associated with prostate cancer progression." *Clinical Cancer Research* 14.2 (2008): 607-611.

16

Hyperthyroid Symptoms
(Anxiety, Tachycardia)
with Hypothyroid Labs

You can't possibly be hypothyroid—you're too thin!

—common misconception

Anxiety, high blood pressure, panic attacks, a fast heart rate, and hypoglycemia can actually be symptoms of low thyroid levels. Unfortunately, because of the misleading Thyroid Stimulating Hormone (TSH) test, which for most comes back "normal," the correct diagnosis of hypothyroidism is seldom made. Patients complaining of these symptoms may be prescribed blood pressure medications (such as beta blockers) and/or anti-anxiety medications (such as benzodiazepines). Neither of these pharmaceutical prescriptions corrects the low thyroid condition that caused the symptoms in the first place, and both have side effects. These people may feel hungry all the time and may either gain or lose weight, depending on their cortisol levels. Someone who is severely hypothyroid may actually be quite thin because they have very little cortisol; they resemble patients with Addison's disease, whose adrenal glands produce little to no cortisol. Thyroid lab results will show low levels of the thyroid hormones triiodothyronine (T3), thyroxine (T4), or both. Sometimes the T3 and T4 will *barely* be within the reference range, but statistically, anything within the reference range is considered "normal."

The anxiety, tachycardia (fast heart rate), and high blood pressure these people experience is not from being hyperthyroid, but from noradrenaline that the adrenals are secreting for energy to compensate for the lack of thyroid hormone. Without thyroid hormone, the heart can beat too slowly; noradrenaline quickly raises it. Blood pressure can also drop when hypothyroid; noradrenaline will raise it. In one study, noradrenaline was three times higher in hypothyroid subjects than normal controls when lying down.[1] This may explain why my heart always felt like it was racing whenever I laid down (when I was undermedicated), and why I couldn't fall asleep. I had radioactive iodine treatment to destroy my thyroid when I was hyperthyroid, so I cannot possibly be hyperthyroid now unless I take an overdose of thyroid medication. When I was only taking ½ grain of desiccated thyroid and obviously undermedicated, my pulse was 100 beats per minute and my blood pressure (BP) was 170/100 mmHg. Raising my dose to 2 grains brought the pulse back into the 80s and BP down to about 130/80 mmHg. This is completely counterintuitive, which is why it's so difficult to understand. Thyroid and noradrenaline (norepinephrine) have an inverse relationship.[2] [3] [4] [5] An inverse relationship simply means that two variables move in opposite directions from each other. In this particular case, as thyroid levels decrease, norepinephrine increases. Conversely, as thyroid levels rise, norepinephrine decreases. Norepinephrine is one of the hormones involved in the "fight or flight response" that causes hyperarousal.

A few of these people will actually have a TSH that is high enough for them to be diagnosed as hypothyroid, but when they start taking prescription thyroid hormone in any form, they feel worse. When they try to raise their thyroid dose by the lowest increment available, ¼ grain of desiccated thyroid or 25 mcg of T4, they get hyperthyroid symptoms, so they return to their previous dose, which keeps them hypothyroid. Their intolerance may be due to low cortisol[6] and/or low iron/ferritin. If ferritin is low (usually less than 50 ng/mL,[7] but keep in mind that everyone's threshold is different), taking thyroid hormone, especially anything with T3, will cause palpitations, nervousness, and feelings of restlessness.[8] They should return to their previous dose or temporarily stop treatment, and address the low cortisol and low iron problems with supplements, if lab tests confirm that they are truly low in iron or cortisol. A full iron panel and ferritin test should be performed to determine whether the person is truly anemic (low iron) or dealing with Anemia of Chronic Disease (low iron caused by a disease state). In some cases, like hereditary hemochromatosis (iron loading), iron should not be supplemented. Patients taking supplemental iron need to have their levels monitored regularly, because too much iron can be toxic.

If someone is never properly diagnosed as hypothyroid, they will continue to suffer from their symptoms. Hyperthyroidism causes many negative psychiatric symptoms, but so does hypothyroidism: depression, panic attacks,[9] auditory and visual hallucinations, distortions of taste and smell,[10] and paranoid delusions[11] have been reported. Normal brain function is *highly* dependent on adequate thyroid levels and a quick Google Scholar search for "psychiatry hypothyroid" brings up journal articles published in 2013 with the phrases: acute psychosis, acute mania, dementia, major depressive disorder, and delusions, all on the first page!

An insatiable appetite can be either a hyperthyroid or hypothyroid symptom. In the hyperthyroid state, high T3 levels raise the metabolism, and increased food intake is required to meet that demand. In the hypothyroid state, extremely low cortisol can result from extremely low thyroid levels. Thyroid and cortisol usually rise and fall in tandem.[12] One of cortisol's functions is to keep blood sugar stable; without cortisol, blood sugar will drop and the person becomes hypoglycemic. This person has to eat all the time to keep blood glucose up. I had to eat every 1.5 - 2 hours when I was in this state (even in the middle of the night), lest I have another hypoglycemic attack, which was like a panic attack: my heart would suddenly race, I'd get very hot and break out in a sweat, my whole body would shake, I would lose control of my hands (computer mouse would be released), and then it would all just stop. This is called a hypoglycemic seizure. I no longer have them now that I'm on a higher dose of thyroid medication. I lost a considerable amount of weight while taking only 1/2 grain, and I looked gaunt. Now that I'm taking significantly more thyroid medication, I actually eat less and have regained 20 pounds, but it's a much healthier look.

Low cortisol as a cause of hypoglycemia is illustrated in a case study of a 7-year-old girl with zero cortisol. She had a genetic adrenocorticotropic hormone (ACTH) deficiency, and her plasma ACTH was undetectable (ACTH signals the body to release cortisol). She had severe hypoglycemia, was admitted to the hospital unconscious, and regained consciousness after treatment with intravenous glucose. Her daily treatment now consists of oral hydrocortisone in three divided doses; this has resolved her symptoms and normalized her blood glucose.[13]

Hyperpigmentation, or the darkening of the skin in certain areas (armpits, anogenital area, gums) is another symptom of low cortisol and the resulting high ACTH that tells the adrenals to produce more cortisol. Hyperpigmentation is a common feature of Addison's disease or chronic primary adrenal insufficiency, where melanocyte-stimulating hormone (MSH) and ACTH are high.[14] Hyperpigmentation is also found in hyperthyroid patients, or anyone taking more thyroid hormone than their adrenals can handle. Hyperthyroid patients displayed high ACTH levels that reduced once their thyroid levels were brought down with anti-thyroid drugs.[15] Someone can also be very low in cortisol but have normal looking skin if their problem is with the hypothalamus (low corticotropic-releasing hormone or CRH) or pituitary (low ACTH) hormones that signal cortisol production. My darkened skin areas have lightened considerably since switching from 100% desiccated to mostly T4 with a little desiccated. I can only guess that lowering the T3 resulted in the need for less cortisol and therefore, my ACTH decreased.

Conclusion

The TSH test that is used to diagnose hypothyroidism is not accurate enough to catch all cases, and many people suffer from a myriad of physical and mental symptoms because they cannot get diagnosed or treated. Psychiatry has recognized the importance of thyroid function for mental health, but unfortunately, this knowledge has not been passed on to mainstream medicine. I have had two panic attacks in my life, and now understand how frightening they can be. I realized that they were just hypoglycemic attacks and if I ate often enough, I could prevent them. Of course, the actual cause was that I was too low in thyroid hormone at the time, and sure enough, as I raised my dose, they stopped completely. Some people live with chronic anxiety and repeated panic attacks, and my heart goes out to them.

Key points

- Anxiety, high blood pressure, panic attacks, a fast heart rate, and hypoglycemia can actually be symptoms of low thyroid levels
- The TSH test is not sensitive enough to catch all cases of hypothyroidism. Most with symptoms of high blood pressure and anxiety will be prescribed blood pressure medications and anti-anxiety medications, which can sometimes have severe side effects.
- A hypothyroid person can be quite thin if they also have low cortisol levels.

- Noradrenaline compensates for lack of thyroid hormone by raising both heart rate and blood pressure, which can drop when hypothyroid.
- Low cortisol and low iron levels may cause an intolerance to thyroid hormone.
- Normal brain function is highly dependent on thyroid hormone; low levels may cause acute psychosis, acute mania, dementia, major depressive disorder, panic attacks, auditory, olfactory and visual hallucinations, and paranoid delusions.
- An insatiable appetite can be a hyperthyroid or hypothyroid symptom. In severe hypothyroidism, cortisol levels drop, and the person becomes hypoglycemic and hungry all the time.
- Hyperpigmentation is another low cortisol sign. It can also be a sign that a patient is taking too much thyroid hormone.

[1] Christensen, Niels Juel. "Increased levels of plasma noradrenaline in hypothyroidism." Journal of Clinical Endocrinology & Metabolism 35.3 (1972): 359-363.

[2] Faber, J., et al. "Hemodynamic changes after levothyroxine treatment in subclinical hypothyroidism." Thyroid 12.4 (2002): 319-324.

[3] Fommei, Enza, and Giorgio Iervasi. "The role of thyroid hormone in blood pressure homeostasis: evidence from short-term hypothyroidism in humans." Journal of Clinical Endocrinology & Metabolism 87.5 (2002): 1996-2000.

[4] Manhem, P., B. Hallengren, and B-G. Hansson. "Plasma noradrenaline and blood pressure in hypothyroid patients: effect of gradual thyroxine treatment." Clinical endocrinology 20.6 (1984): 701-707.

[5] Levey, Gerald S., and Irwin Klein. "Catecholamine-thyroid hormone interactions and the cardiovascular manifestations of hyperthyroidism." The American journal of medicine 88.6 (1990): 642-646.

[6] Murray, Jonathan Stephen, Rubaraj Jayarajasingh, and Petros Perros. "Lesson of the week: Deterioration of symptoms after start of thyroid hormone replacement." BMJ: British Medical Journal 323.7308 (2001): 332.

[7] Vaucher, Paul, et al. "Effect of iron supplementation on fatigue in nonanemic menstruating women with low ferritin: a randomized controlled trial." Canadian Medical Association Journal 184.11 (2012): 1247-1254.

[8] Shakir, K. M., et al. "Anemia: a cause of intolerance to thyroxine sodium." Mayo Clinic Proceedings. Vol. 75. No. 2. Elsevier, 2000.

[9] Kikuchi, Mitsuru, et al. "Relationship between anxiety and thyroid function in patients with panic disorder." Progress in Neuro-Psychopharmacology and Biological Psychiatry 29.1 (2005): 77-81.

[10] McConnell, Robert J., et al. "Defects of taste and smell in patients with hypothyroidism." The American journal of medicine 59.3 (1975): 354-364.

[11] Heinrich, Thomas W., and Garth Grahm. "Hypothyroidism presenting as psychosis: myxedema madness revisited." Primary care companion to the Journal of Clinical Psychiatry 5.6 (2003): 260.

[12] Dumoulin, Sonia C., et al. "Opposite effects of thyroid hormones on binding proteins for steroid hormones (sex hormone-binding globulin and corticosteroid-binding globulin) in humans." European journal of endocrinology 132.5 (1995): 594-598.

[13] Torchinsky, Michael Y., Robert Wineman, and George W. Moll. "Severe Hypoglycemia due to Isolated ACTH Deficiency in Children: A New Case Report and Review of the Literature." International journal of pediatrics 2011 (2011).

[14] Ten, Svetlana, Maria New, and Noel Maclaren. "Addison's disease 2001." *Journal of Clinical Endocrinology & Metabolism* 86.7 (2001): 2909-2922.

[15] Mishra, Sunil Kumar, Nandita Gupta, and Ravinder Goswami. "Plasma adrenocorticotropin (ACTH) values and cortisol response to 250 and 1 μg ACTH stimulation in patients with hyperthyroidism before and after carbimazole therapy: case-control comparative study." *Journal of Clinical Endocrinology & Metabolism* 92.5 (2007): 1693-1696.

17

Insulin Resistance and T3 Levels

T3 doesn't raise blood sugar.

—a diabetic following the T3-only protocol

High blood sugar, insulin resistance, and high fasting blood glucose may all be caused by high triiodothyronine (T3) levels. Many on the T3-only protocol or high doses of desiccated thyroid notice their blood sugar levels rising, because thyroid levels, either too high *or* too low, have a direct impact on blood glucose.

Hypothyroidism may cause high blood sugar and insulin resistance

Glycated hemoglobin (A1C), a measure of average blood glucose levels over several months, is generally higher than normal in hypothyroid patients. In one study, replacement with thyroid hormone brought the A1C down, but it did not lower fasting blood glucose.[1] This study shows that the hypothyroid condition causes an average blood glucose that is higher than normal.

Insulin resistance appears when thyroid levels are too low *or* too high.[2] Correcting the hypothyroid condition is beneficial, but replacement with too much thyroid hormone may result in continued insulin resistance.

Pre-diabetics who had both high insulin levels and insulin resistance had lower T3 levels and higher thyroxine (T4) levels than normal, glucose-tolerant subjects. This resulted in a low T3/T4 ratio. This study confirms that a certain level of T3 is essential for normal glucose metabolism.[3]

Sex Hormone Binding Globulin (SHBG) is secreted by the liver and is positively correlated with thyroid levels—it rises when hyperthyroid and falls when hypothyroid. Low levels therefore suggest a hypothyroid condition. Low SHBG is also a biomarker of insulin resistance, metabolic syndrome, and a risk factor for developing high blood sugar and type 2 diabetes, especially in women.[4]

High T3 & high T4 may cause high blood sugar and insulin resistance

Blood sugar problems may be caused by either low or high thyroid levels. The following are some studies that show the direct correlation of rising T3 and T4 levels with high fasting blood glucose and insulin resistance.

Type 2 diabetics with metabolic syndrome showed a positive correlation between their Free T3 levels and fasting blood glucose. In other words, the higher their Free T3, the higher the fasting blood glucose.[5]

Insulin sensitivity (which is desirable, as opposed to insulin insensitivity), measured with an insulin sensitivity index (ISI), was negatively correlated with both Free T3 (FT3) and Free T4 (FT4). In other words, the higher the FT3 and FT4 levels, the lower the insulin sensitivity. Likewise, Homeostasis Model Assessment (HOMA), a measure of insulin resistance (which is undesirable), was positively correlated with both FT3 and FT4. In other words, as FT3 and FT4 increased, so did insulin resistance. This correlation was apparent even when FT3 and FT4 were within the normal reference range. Insulin allows glucose to enter the body's cells, which provides them with energy. In insulin resistance, cells don't respond, even to normal amounts of insulin. Insulin resistance is a feature of type 2 diabetes.[6]

Insulin resistance was measured in Graves' hyperthyroid patients before and after treatment with antithyroid drugs that brought their thyroid levels down into the normal range. Insulin resistance, measured by HOMA, decreased once their thyroid levels decreased to a more normal level.[7] Serum glucose and insulin levels did not significantly change before and after treatment of the hyperthyroidism. However, Body Mass Index (BMI)-adjusted insulin levels fell as both FT3 and FT4 also fell.

Thyroid hormone stimulates glucose production from the liver and at high levels, induces liver insulin resistance. In a comparison of hyperthyroid vs. normal patients, hepatic glucose production (HGP) or glucose produced by the liver was 20% higher in hyperthyroid patients. After an intravenous infusion of glucose, insulin levels increased 66% in the hyperthyroid patients vs. 37% in normal patients. The excess insulin showed a diminished inhibitory effect on glucose production, suggesting liver insulin resistance.[8] In other words, even though more insulin was released, it did not inhibit glucose production as much as it should have.

Since insulin resistance is affected by thyroid hormone levels, a comparison was made between a ratio of T3/reverse T3 (rT3) of insulin resistant and insulin sensitive subjects. The T3/rT3 ratio was significantly higher in insulin resistant subjects, who had a higher proportion of T3 to rT3.[9] Since a high ratio is actually the goal of the T3-only protocol, and quite a few on the protocol notice their blood glucose rising, the safety of this protocol should be questioned. The protocol itself may be inducing insulin resistance.

A suppressed Thyroid Stimulating Hormone (TSH) that is below the reference range or close to zero, is also correlated with higher insulin levels, insulin resistance, and lower insulin sensitivity when compared to control subjects, even though Free T4 and T3 may be within the reference range. Insulin resistance, as measured by HOMA-IR, showed a positive relationship with T3 levels throughout the whole sample population of both controls and those on thyroid replacement. In other words, as T3 rose, so did insulin resistance.[10]

Conclusion

Blood sugar problems are a common topic of discussion on many thyroid forums. Some patients keep their Free T3 levels at the top or even above the reference ranges, and many are now starting to report elevated fasting blood glucose levels. Low-carb diets are the common recommendation, although it seems, from the research shown in this chapter, that many are just taking too much T3.

If thyroid levels were graphed with blood sugar problems, it would form a u-shaped curve, like most hormones. There is a small range of thyroid hormone which keeps blood sugar and insulin at healthy levels, but either too much or too little thyroid hormone will cause blood sugar problems. Apparently thyroid reference ranges are too broad, because symptoms of both too much and too little thyroid hormone are appearing in subjects whose Free T3 and Free T4 values are within the reference ranges.

Key points

- Blood sugar is affected by thyroid hormone levels that are either too high or too low.
- A higher than normal A1C is found in hypothyroid patients.
- Insulin resistance appears when thyroid levels are too high or too low.
- A low T3/T4 ratio is found in pre-diabetics who have both high insulin levels and insulin resistance.
- Low SHBG, which correlates with low thyroid levels, is a biomarker of insulin resistance, metabolic syndrome, and a risk factor for developing high blood sugar and type 2 diabetes, especially in women
- High Free T3 levels correlate with high fasting blood glucose.
- High Free T3 and Free T4 levels correlate with lower insulin sensitivity.
- High Free T3 and Free T4 levels correlate with insulin resistance, which is a feature of type 2 diabetes
- Too much thyroid hormone causes liver insulin resistance; more insulin is released in response to glucose but has a decreased effect.
- The T3/rT3 ratio was significantly higher in insulin resistant subjects, who had a higher proportion of T3 to rT3.
- A suppressed TSH is also correlated with higher insulin levels, insulin resistance, and lower insulin sensitivity when compared to control subjects, even though Free T4 and T3 may be within the reference range.

---

[1] Kim, Mee Kyoung, et al. "Effects of thyroid hormone on A1C and glycated albumin levels in nondiabetic subjects with overt hypothyroidism." *Diabetes Care* 33.12 (2010): 2546-2548.

[2] Kapadia, Kunal B., Parloop A. Bhatt, and Jigna S. Shah. "Association between altered thyroid state and insulin resistance." *Journal of pharmacology & pharmacotherapeutics* 3.2 (2012): 156.

[3] Farasat, Tasnim, Abdul Majeed Cheema, and Muhammad Naeem Khan. "Hyperinsulinemia and insulin resistance is associated with low T3/T4 ratio in pre diabetic euthyroid pakistani subjects." *Journal of Diabetes and its Complications* (2012).

[4] Pugeat, Michel, et al. "Sex hormone-binding globulin gene expression in the liver: drugs and the metabolic syndrome." *Molecular and cellular endocrinology* 316.1 (2010): 53-59.

[5] Taneichi, Haruhito, et al. "Higher serum free triiodothyronine levels within the normal range are associated with metabolic syndrome components in type 2 diabetic subjects with euthyroidism." *Tohoku Journal of Experimental Medicine* 224.3 (2011): 173.

[6] Lambadiari, Vaia, et al. "Thyroid hormones are positively associated with insulin resistance early in the development of type 2 diabetes." *Endocrine* 39.1 (2011): 28-32.

[7] Chu, Chih-Hsun, et al. "Hyperthyroidism-associated insulin resistance is not mediated by adiponectin levels." *Journal of thyroid research* 2011 (2011).

[8] Wennlund, Anders, et al. "Hepatic glucose production and splanchnic glucose exchange in hyperthyroidism." *Journal of Clinical Endocrinology & Metabolism* 62.1 (1986): 174-180.

[9] Ruhla, S., et al. "T3/rT3-ratio is associated with insulin resistance independent of TSH." *Hormone and metabolic research* 43.2 (2011): 130.

[10] Rezzonico, Jorge, et al. "The association of insulin resistance with subclinical thyrotoxicosis." *Thyroid* 21.9 (2011): 945-949.

18

Iodine – Cure or Curse?

There's no such thing as iodine toxicity; you're experiencing bromide detox.

—Explanation given for the acne, runny nose, metallic taste, headaches, coughing, etc. experienced by some people on the high dose iodine protocol (these are symptoms of iodine poisoning)

Iodine evokes polar opposite reactions amongst thyroid patients. Some patients rave about iodine's benefits and claim it cured their cancer. Others blame the high dose iodine protocol for all their current thyroid problems and say it induced the hyper or hypothyroidism they must now live with. Like most thyroid topics, this story has two sides, and I wanted to know what the "real facts" were (as opposed to made up "facts"). I spent months reading countless medical journal articles, and had to brush up on my knowledge of chemistry and biochemistry to analyze what I read. This chapter becomes quite technical in places, because readers need to understand how iodine works in the body to see the fallacy of the arguments the high-dose iodine proponents make. For those of you who do not wish to wade through the technical arguments, I would direct you to the *Conclusion* and *Key Points* sections at the end, where the research is summarized. For the other scientific types out there like me, read on and I will do my best to explain this highly complex topic.

Iodine terminology

Iodine is one of five non-metallic elements (fluorine, chlorine, bromine, iodine, astatine) referred to as *halogens*. For those who took chemistry and remember the periodic table, they are all in the same column on the far right of the table and considered a *group* because of their similar properties. Their ions have a negative charge and form compounds called *salts* with positive ions. *Sodium chloride* (NaCl) is the halogen compound most people are familiar with; it is the chemical name for table salt. Potassium is in the same chemical group as sodium and thus has similar properties. Sodium and potassium are both alkali metals, found in the leftmost column in the periodic table. Their ions have positive charges and thus combine well with the negatively charged halogens to make salts. *Potassium iodide* (KI) is another halogen compound that has been used as a medication for various ailments for over a century.

The words *iodide* and *iodine* are often used interchangeably, although they are not the same chemically. *Iodide* refers to the single, negatively charged iodine atom, represented as I⁻. When two of these atoms join together, they form a molecule of iodine, chemically represented as I_2 and referred to as *molecular* or *elemental iodine*. Because the body appears to use iodide in some organs (thyroid) and iodine in others (breasts), both forms were combined in a formula called *Lugol's solution*, created in 1829 by French physician Jean Guillaume Auguste Lugol. Iodoral, a pill form of Lugol's, was created in 1997 by Guy Abraham, M.D., and is sold by his company Optimox Corporation. There are other iodine products available as well.

The U.S. Government's daily Recommended Dietary Allowance (RDA) for iodine is 150 micrograms (mcg). Both Lugol's and Iodoral provide iodine in milligram (mg) amounts, which is 1000 times more than a microgram. Lugol's comes in 2%, 5%, and other concentrations. One drop of 2% Lugol's has 1 mg iodine + 1.5 mg iodide. The lowest dose of Iodoral has 5 mg iodine + 7.5 mg iodide, or the equivalent of 5 drops of 2% Lugol's. Iodoral is available in a 12.5, 25, or 50 mg tablet.

Both Lugol's and Iodoral are referred to as *inorganic iodine* because the chemical definition of *organic* means the molecule has a carbon atom, and their formula does not contain carbon. The formula is a solution of I_2 (iodine) + KI (potassium iodide). Amiodarone is a high iodine pharmaceutical drug prescribed for heart rhythm problems. It contains about 75 mg iodine in a 200 mg tablet. It is considered an organic form of iodine because it contains carbon (C). The molecular formula for amiodarone is $C_{25}H_{29}I_2NO_3$. Amiodarone has triggered both hyper and hypothyroidism in patients,[1] but the high-dose iodine proponents claim that is because it is a form of organic iodine. However, both Lugol's and Iodoral, which are both inorganic, have triggered the same reactions.

The Iodine Project

Based upon his personal belief that high doses of iodine are beneficial, Guy Abraham, M.D., started the Iodine Project[2] to focus on iodine research around 1998. Through his company, Optimox Corporation, he designed, monitored, and funded studies of patients on Iodoral through Jorge D. Flechas, MD. According to Abraham, high doses of iodine in liquid form had an unpleasant taste, would be difficult to measure accurately, and could cause gastric irritation and stain clothing, so a precisely quantified tablet form of Lugol's was created, which was later named Iodoral. Hakala Apothecaries compounded the tablets. Tablets ranged in strength from 1 to 12.5 mg and the 12.5 mg dose was tested in 10 female subjects, 7 of whom had fibrocystic breast symptoms. Measurement of various blood and thyroid parameters pre and post-testing led them to conclude, by their standards, that 12.5 mg was a safe dose, and the results of this study were published[3] in 2002 in an alternative health journal, *The Original Internist* (not peer-reviewed). Many of Abraham's papers, which were originally published in *The Original Internist*, can be read on his website, optimox.com.

Much of this chapter addresses statements made in three of Dr. Abraham's papers published in *The Original Internist* titled:

- *The Wolff-Chaikoff Effect: Crying Wolf?*[4] published in 2005

- *The history of iodine in medicine Part III: thyroid fixation and medical iodophobia*[5] published in 2006, and

- the Epilogue from *Orthoiodosupplementation: Iodine sufficiency of the whole human body*[6] published in 2002.

Abraham's articles are regularly cited on iodine forums when the Wolff-Chaikoff effect is being challenged. This effect occurs when excess iodine is ingested and thyroid hormone synthesis and release stops. Dr. Abraham does not believe in the Wolff-Chaikoff effect, otherwise known as iodine induced hypothyroidism, even though it has been observed in numerous individuals over the years. Anyone considering a high-dose iodine protocol should read the above papers for themselves.

Iodine's role in the body

The sodium-iodide symporter (NIS) is the name of the cell membrane protein that transports iodide into cells. It is highly expressed in the thyroid, as expected. But it is also expressed in the stomach, salivary glands, and *lactating* mammary gland. It should not be active in a woman who is not pregnant or breastfeeding. Lower levels of NIS have been detected in the small intestine, colon, rectum, pancreas, kidney, bile duct, lung, lacrimal (tear) glands, heart, placenta, testes, ovaries, prostate gland, adrenal gland, thymus, and pituitary gland,[7] but NIS is *not* found in every cell in the body. NIS is a transporter, not a receptor, as some iodine proponents incorrectly state. A transporter is like a truck, and merely moves things from point A to point B. A receptor is similar to the lock in the lock and key analogy. Once the correct key is inserted into a lock, a door opens. Thyroid and other hormones are the keys that activate cellular receptors (the locks) and initiate a chemical reaction. Thyroid receptors are found in every cell of the body, and that is confirmed by numerous studies. However, a search for the phrase "iodine receptor" in PubMed (the U.S. National Library of Medicine database with over 22 million citations) returns zero results for that phrase. After all, iodine is not a hormone; it is an element. Only when iodine is coupled with the amino acid tyrosine does it "become" thyroid hormone. Many of the beneficial effects of iodine are from the higher levels of thyroid hormone that are produced. Iodine is also found in the extracellular fluid, like all of the halogens, and this fluid runs throughout the entire body.

NIS's main function is to concentrate iodide in the thyroid gland to produce the two thyroid hormones, triiodothyronine (T3) and thyroxine (T4). Thyroid Stimulating Hormone (TSH) increases NIS expression, which results in enhanced iodide uptake and thyroid hormone synthesis.[8] This is an important point, because many with thyroid problems have almost non-existent TSH, even though they are extremely hypothyroid, not hyperthyroid, as conventional medicine assumes (a low TSH normally indicates high thyroid levels, while a high TSH indicates low thyroid levels). Without TSH, NIS won't function properly. It is important to note that NIS stands for sodium-iodide symporter, which means sodium is an essential component. A sodium (salt) restricted diet may limit the sodium available to NIS.

When iodine intake is deficient, the thyroid compensates by activating angiofollicular units (AFUs) outside the thyrocytes (the follicles that absorb iodine). These AFUs consist of adjacent capillaries (blood vessels) and, combined with the thyrocytes, act as a functional unit. The thyroid gland microvasculature (blood supply) expands rapidly, which brings in additional nutrients and oxygen while optimizing the iodine supply. If this autoregulation fails, a goiter may form as another means of adaptation. In the early stages of iodine deficiency, most AFUs are inactive. But with TSH stimulation, the AFUs are activated and after repeated periods of high, low, and moderate cell activity, multinodular goiters (enlarged thyroid glands) can result.[9]

In pregnant or breastfeeding women, the hormones prolactin and oxytocin induce NIS expression in the mammary gland; breast milk contains enough iodide to fulfill the newborn's iodine requirements. There should be no NIS in non-lactating women, yet NIS has been found in breast cancer tumor samples. In fact, studies show that some estrogen receptor positive breast cancer tumors show high intensity NIS staining equivalent to thyroid tissue.[10] In other words, these breast cancer tumors can transport as much iodide as a thyroid gland.

Apparently there's a synergy between prolactin (primarily a pituitary hormone) and estradiol (E2, an estrogen) in the regulation and proliferation of breast cancer cells. Prolactin alone induced little to no response in some breast cancer cells, but cell proliferation was greatly enhanced in cultures with estradiol.[11] Prolactin stimulates milk production in women who are breastfeeding. Levels *should* be high after childbirth. But prolactin can also rise when a woman is not breastfeeding, but is hypothyroid. Some other causes of high prolactin include pituitary tumors and kidney failure. When non-breastfeeding women with a high TSH and high prolactin levels were treated with thyroid hormone, their prolactin returned to normal levels.[12] These women were infertile and treatment with thyroxine resulted in pregnancy for three out of four women within the following year.

Higher E2 levels are associated with the BRCA1 (Breast Cancer susceptibility gene 1) gene mutation, which is a known risk factor for breast cancer.[13] E2 levels in the breast also tend to be higher in obese, post-menopausal women.[14] In one study, both E2 and prolactin were higher in hypothyroid women compared to normal women, and both levels decreased after thyroxine replacement was started to treat their hypothyroidism.[15] These women also had enlarged ovaries and/or cysts, also known as PCOS (polycystic ovary syndrome), which also resolved once thyroid hormone levels improved.

Men are not immune from high prolactin levels, and there's a case study of a man who became unconscious from myxedema coma, which is the severest, most hypothyroid state before death. He had initially sought help at an infertility clinic, where he was found to have low serum testosterone, decreased semen volume, decreased sperm motility, and elevated serum prolactin. He was actually diagnosed as hypothyroid at another clinic when he presented with insomnia, lethargy, and general malaise. After several months on thyroid hormone replacement, his sperm count, total testosterone and prolactin levels normalized.[16]

Prolactin appears to be associated with tumor growth throughout the body—in the breast, prostate, colon, rectum, and the central nervous system (brain).[17] Serum prolactin is also elevated in ovarian and endometrial cancers.[18] Since low thyroid levels may cause high prolactin, and high prolactin is associated with tumors, it seems that low thyroid levels are associated with tumor growth. Prolactin has a positive correlation with TSH; in other words, as TSH rises (indicating hypothyroidism), prolactin also rises.[19]

Antipsychotic drugs can also elevate prolactin. High prolactin (hyperprolactinemia) occurs in almost 42% of men and 75% of women with schizophrenia who are treated with prolactin-raising antipsychotics, such as risperidone.[20] Hyperprolactinemia clinical symptoms include gynecomastia (male breasts), galactorrhea (lactating when not breast-feeding), menstrual irregularities, infertility, sexual dysfunction, acne and hirsutism (excess hair growth in women). Some studies suggest an association between hyperprolactinemia and bone mineral density loss and breast cancer. Other side effects are sedation, hypotension, constipation, cognitive impairment, weight gain, blood sugar problems, and high triglycerides.[21] All of these symptoms can also be found in hypothyroid patients, which raises the question: do antipsychotics induce hypothyroidism, and the high prolactin is just a reflection of that state? Or were these people hypothyroid to start with, but because their TSH was "normal," they were prescribed antipsychotic medications instead? Both low and high thyroid levels have been associated with psychosis and depression.[22]

About 6% of non-lactating women show radioiodine uptake in their breasts, which means that their breasts are absorbing iodine, which is not normal. Radioiodine uptake should only be present in lactating breasts, when a mother's breasts are absorbing iodine to be incorporated into breast milk for the infant. Uptake can be a sign of cancer. Moderately elevated prolactin levels were found in 24% of these cases, and galactorrhea in 48%.[23]

Earlier in this section, hypothyroidism was listed as a cause of elevated prolactin. Prolactin activates NIS, and this would then cause iodine absorption in breasts, which is not normal for a non-lactating woman. Because prolactin is associated with tumors, non-lactating breasts should not absorb iodine, and some breast cancer tumors display high levels of NIS, it can be hypothesized that whole body scans that display iodine uptake in the breasts may be showing the early stages of breast cancer. If this is true, it would be prudent for prolactin to be tested in those who display hypothyroid symptoms, but whose TSH appears "normal," since studies show there is sometimes no relationship of TSH to thyroid levels. In fact, a normal TSH does not guarantee good health; people with the metabolic syndrome often have a normal TSH.[24] Theoretically, elevated prolactin could be used as a diagnostic marker for hypothyroidism and/or cancer risk, since several studies have shown an inverse relationship of prolactin to thyroid levels.

Iodine fights cancer

NIS is found in tumors, where it would not normally be expected. There is also some indication that iodine (I_2) uptake does not require NIS or pendrin (another iodide transporter), but diffuses into cells and binds to proteins or lipids that then inhibit cell proliferation.[25] In other words, iodine may enter some cells without a specific transporter.

Molecular iodine (not iodide or I-) induces apoptosis, or cell death, and this feature gives iodine its anti-tumor effects. Iodine's anti-tumor effects have been observed in different types of tumors, not just breast cancer.[26] Medical studies show these effects only occur when iodine is taken in milligram doses, which puts the high-dose iodine protocol at odds with what is considered a safe dose for thyroid function (microgram doses).

Iodine has documented beneficial effects: it has induced tumor regression and is often used to normalize fibrocystic breasts.[27] One hypothesis is that iodine inhibits or modulates the estrogen pathways, which are implicated in some breast cancers.[28] Dr. David Derry believes that the thyroid gland reaches iodine saturation at only 2-3 mg iodine daily, and that iodine doses above this amount will prevent breast cancer, because any remaining iodine will then flood the extracellular fluids in the body, which triggers the death of any abnormal or atypical cells (apoptosis). He has found that in the very *early* stages, iodine can reverse abnormalities in fibrocystic breasts. When thyroid hormone is taken along with iodine, it makes the patient stronger, both physically and psychologically, and also strengthens their connective tissue, so the cancer cannot metastasize to other organs. Dr. Derry's hypothesis is that tight connective tissue will contain the cancer where it is.[29]

In one study, women with breast pain were given a placebo, 1.5 mg, 3 mg, or 6 mg of molecular iodine daily for six months. The iodine treated groups reported an improvement in pain compared to the placebo group. Physicians used three criteria to assess improvement: breast pain, tenderness, and nodularity per cycle. Reductions in *all* three criteria were reported by some in the 3 mg/day (25%) and 6 mg/day (18.5%) groups, but none in the placebo or 1.5 mg/day groups. The higher the iodine dose, the more women in the group that reported less breast pain.[30] The report states that this is consistent with prior observations that 3-6 mg/day is the effective dose for treating pain and fibrocystic breasts.

Another study on rats treated to induce cancer showed that continuous iodine treatment reduced the incidence of mammary cancer to 30% vs. 72.7% in the controls. Discontinuation of the iodine treatment resulted in an increase in mammary cancer incidence. The first tumor also developed later in the iodine treated rats: 12 weeks instead of 10 weeks compared to the controls. Iodide did not have the same positive effect as iodine.[31]

The thyroid gland uses iodine to manufacture other iodocompounds besides thyroid hormone. One compound synthesized by the thyroid is an iodinated arachidonic acid (AA) derivative, IL-δ, also known as δ-iodolactone or *delta iodolactone*. It regulates thyroid cell proliferation and goiter growth, but also inhibits cell growth and induces apoptosis (cell death) in other non-thyroid cell lines, such as colon cancer cells. Mice implanted with colon cancer cells and then given IL-δ had a 70% tumor growth delay compared to controls.[32]

One study hypothesizes that δ-iodolactone is the iodine compound that inhibits cell proliferation and induces apoptosis in differentiated thyroid carcinoma cells and breast cancer cells; it could be a key player in the fight against thyroid or breast cancer.[33]

The prostate also benefits from iodine and δ-iodolactone; both cancerous and normal prostate cells take up iodine and iodide (independent of NIS) and benefit from its anti-proliferative and apoptotic effects. Some of the cancerous cell lines were more sensitive to iodine than iodide. Iodine impaired tumor growth in mice implanted with human prostate cancer cells.[34]

Iodine and hyperthyroidism

Hyperthyroid patients are most at risk when using iodine because iodine can exacerbate the hyperthyroid state. Iodine provides the raw material to produce more thyroid hormone, which is the last thing a hyperthyroid patient needs. Known as "thyroid storm," this uncontrolled hyperthyroid state can be deadly. Hyperthyroidism can produce a non-stop, rapid heartbeat which wears out the heart and can lead to congestive heart failure and pulmonary edema (fluid in the lungs), which is considered an emergency (life-threatening) situation. High doses of Lugol's iodine solution (elemental iodine and potassium iodide in water) were used in the past to treat hyperthyroidism and Graves' disease before the pharmaceutical anti-thyroid medications (methimazole, propylthiouracil, etc.) were produced. Therefore, proponents of the high-dose iodine protocol advise people suffering from Graves' to take iodine, not avoid it, because they believe iodine deficiency causes hyperthyroidism. That is potentially dangerous advice because not all Graves' patients respond the same way to iodine supplementation.

The problems associated with Graves' disease are not solely from the effect of high thyroid levels. Graves' antibodies cause specific issues that are not seen in someone who is simply taking too much thyroid hormone. Since specific genes associated with both Graves' and Hashimoto's autoimmune thyroid disease have been identified,[35] iodine deficiency cannot be said to be the only cause, though it could certainly be a contributing factor. Graves' disease even affects some Japanese,[36] who generally eat an iodine sufficient diet. Protruding eyes are a problem for some Graves' patients, and the Graves' antibodies can also affect the skin of the shins and hands, as well as various other organs. The antibodies are diagnostic for Graves', and a patient can have very high antibodies and very little thyroid hormone if they've had radioactive iodine treatment in the past. The hyperthyroid state of Graves' is often preceded by a hypothyroid phase; this is called *hypothyroid Graves'* in medical literature.[37] A patient may exhibit hypo or hyperthyroid symptoms, but the level of Graves' antibodies determines the severity of the disease.

Thyroid hormone is produced when the thyroid gland is stimulated by the appropriately named Thyroid Stimulating Hormone (TSH) produced in the pituitary gland. A high TSH is a signal to the thyroid to produce more hormone; likewise, a low TSH is a signal that less thyroid hormone needs to be produced. For those with Graves' disease, there is another signal that can lead to thyroid hormone production: TSH Receptor antibodies (TRab) or Thyrotrophin Binding Inhibiting Immunoglobulins (TBII) in the stimulating mode. (Some laboratories call the test for these antibodies TRab, others TBII.) TSH Receptor antibodies stimulate the TSH Receptor in the same way that a high TSH does—with the end result of more thyroid hormone production. Thyroid Stimulating Immunoglobulin (TSI) measures how strong this stimulation signal is, and is reported as a percentage. When both the TSH Receptor antibodies and TSI are high, it is analogous to a car's gas pedal being pressed to the floor, resulting in full acceleration. TSH has already dropped to zero, so there's no stimulation coming from TSH at all; the normal feedback loop is working. The only reason thyroid hormone continues to be produced in excessive amounts is because of the high levels of TSI and TRab (or TBII) antibodies. Thyroid hormone will continue to be produced non-stop until those antibodies decrease (the gas pedal is released). If more iodine (gas) is added (while the gas pedal is still stuck), the car would be expected to accelerate, and this effect has been observed in some Graves' patients who started on the high-dose iodine protocol. They report intolerable, rapid heart rates, exhaustion, and extremely elevated Free T3 (FT3) and/or Free T4 (FT4) levels.

On an iodine forum, one person with Graves' taking 50 mg a day of Lugol's for a couple of months reported a FT3 nearly four times higher than the top of the reference range, and a FT4 nearly three times higher than the top of the reference range. She was taking all the required supplements recommended for the protocol. When she asked whether or not she should continue on iodine, she was asked if she had taken her thyroid medication that morning before testing, because that could cause the high levels she reported. She replied that she was not taking any thyroid hormone. There's a lesson to be learned here: internet advice can be dangerous. Another Graves' patient was taking 50 mg of Iodoral and all the required supplements. In only one month, her FT3 rose from 180% of the reference range to 260%, and her FT4 rose from 130% to 180%. The iodine had worsened her condition, not improved it, as she had hoped. Her cholesterol had also dropped to 134 mg/dL (normal is less than 200). Cholesterol has an inverse relationship to thyroid hormone, and her low cholesterol confirms that she is making too much thyroid hormone. In another case, a 20-year-old male taking 37.5 mg Iodoral for chronic fatigue was hospitalized for tachycardia and shortness of breath. His heart rate was 120-150 beats per minute, he'd lost 56 pounds over the last two years, and his thyroid gland was tender and mildly enlarged. He was placed on four pharmaceuticals (propylthiouracil, propranolol, potassium perchlorate, and prednisolone) to bring his thyroid levels down into the normal range.[38]

Since iodine is the raw material from which thyroid hormone is produced, providing additional iodine to Graves' patients may exacerbate the hyperthyroid state, unless the Wolff-Chaikoff effect halts thyroid hormone production. Ironically, high-dose iodine proponents dismiss the Wolff-Chaikoff effect because they believe it is only a temporary condition. But if iodine only causes a temporary shutdown of thyroid hormone production, when production resumes it can be at an even higher level than before, since more iodine is now available to produce thyroid hormone. This can be an extremely dangerous situation for a Graves' patient. Lugol's is used by surgeons to induce this temporary halt in thyroid hormone production to stabilize the patient before a thyroidectomy. They are fully aware that the effect wears off and that they only have a small window of time in which to perform a successful operation.

In one study, the window only lasted for 21 days. Hyperthyroid patients given 150 mg potassium iodide daily had a decrease in thyroid hormones (T4, T3, and reverse T3), although T3 did not fall into the normal range in all cases. After 21 days, some patients' T4 and T3 levels started rising, while others remained in the normal range even after 6 weeks. The study's authors concluded that iodide treatment for hyperthyroidism is variable and unpredictable.[39]

Radioactive iodine has been a treatment option for hyperthyroidism since the 1940s. Propylthiouracil, a prescription anti-thyroid drug, blocks the formation of thyroid hormone and also blocks T4 to T3 conversion, thus resulting in very little T3, the active hormone. It was approved by the United States Food and Drug Administration (FDA) in 1947. Methimazole, another anti-thyroid drug, was approved in 1950 and also blocks thyroid hormone production. According to the high-dose iodine proponents, who believe that iodine *cures* Graves', the benefit of Lugol's was forgotten when these pharmaceuticals appeared. A review of older articles on Graves' treatment shows that Lugol's was indeed used to induce the Wolff-Chaikoff effect, to stop thyroid hormone synthesis and release and make the patient less hyperthyroid. However, Lugol's was being used to stabilize Graves' patients before thyroidectomy. It was not considered a cure at all.

Preexisting nodules or *any* underlying thyroid abnormality may cause some of the negative reactions people report from iodine, possibly because these nodules absorb iodine and then overproduce. Yet Lugol's in high doses has been used to halt Graves' hyperthyroid attacks, while others swear that the iodine protocol induced their Graves' or Hashimoto's (autoimmune hypothyroid condition).[40] Apparently, high doses of iodine can correct *mild* cases of diffuse toxic goiter, but in severe cases of Graves', the decrease in thyroid hormone release is transient and only lasts a month or two. In 1960, a surgeon in Great Britain, Oliver Garrod, noted that a high dose of Lugol's solution before surgery reduced vascularity (blood supply to the thyroid gland) and increased the firmness of the thyroid gland, which was beneficial in surgery.[41] Surgery would be scheduled 14-21 days after Lugol's treatment was started, when its positive effects were greatest. In severe cases, carbimazole (an anti-thyroid pharmaceutical) was often used before Lugol's, to minimize the risk of a post-operative thyroid crisis.

A Canadian surgeon, Gordon S. Fahrni, noted in 1929 that a certain amount of iodine is essential to keep the thyroid gland healthy, and when levels fall below that threshold, goiter develops. He noted that the prolonged use of iodine in hyperthyroid patients seems to lose its effectiveness over time, with an initial improvement followed by a severe worsening of symptoms. Some patients relapsed into thyroid storm (uncontrolled hyperthyroidism), which was often fatal at that time. After thyroidectomy, some of his patients grew new goiters. If this happened, he gave them 60-120 mg of Lugol's daily, but only until their symptoms subsided, at which point they would be weaned off of the iodine. Each time symptoms returned, they would be put back on Lugol's, but only until symptoms diminished. Dr. Fahrni did this because he had observed that prolonged use of iodine diminished its effectiveness for these patients. He believed iodine starvation was the cause of regrowth of these thyroid stumps. Based on this theory, he prescribed Lugol's to all his patients for two to three months post-thyroidectomy, in gradually decreasing doses. Patients who complied with this protocol had no recurrence. Those who did not take the Lugol's for the prescribed time sometimes grew new goiters.[42]

A British surgeon, J. Douglas Robertson, noted in a 1948 study that 180 mg of iodine taken daily generated four different responses in thyrotoxic patients: 1) a decrease in metabolism to normal, 2) a decrease in metabolism (but still above normal), 3) a rapid decrease followed by a rapid increase in metabolism back to previous high levels or even higher, and 4) an increase in metabolism. He also noted that these responses were only for those with thyrotoxicosis; it did not apply to normal people. While 180 mg daily was used in these cases, the study's author stated that any dose over 6 mg would produce the maximum effect. In the last two types of cases, iodine actually made the thyrotoxicosis worse.[43]

Correct and Incorrect Use of Iodine in the Treatment of Goiter was published by Emil Goetsch in an American surgical journal in 1934. Doctors noticed that iodine had different effects on different types of goiters. Simple colloid (inactive) goiter is the only type of goiter that can safely be corrected or prevented with small amounts of iodine combined with small amounts of thyroid extract. Even then, prolonged iodine supplementation can occasionally result in hyperthyroidism. Non-toxic as well as toxic goiters can be activated and exacerbated with iodine. Graves' thyroid glands change the first time iodine is given; the enlarged gland reverts to a normal state and initially, the patient improves and experiences remission. However, if a surgical thyroidectomy is not performed, the patient often relapses into an exacerbated hyperthyroid state within 1-3 months. Even small doses of iodine over a prolonged period can induce an uncontrollable hyperthyroid state in these patients. Unfortunately, the positive effects of iodine on a Graves' gland may only work the first time; it becomes relatively insensitive to iodine after that. If the patient later becomes thyrotoxic again, additional iodine can fuel a thyroid storm instead of halting it, and can be fatal.[44]

A paper written in 1927 by an American surgeon, Joseph DeCourcy, provided detailed descriptions of how Graves' thyroid glands differed from others. He observed that glands treated with iodine before surgery were firm and fluid-filled (edematous). When the gland was cut open, a watery fluid would exude. This effect was not seen in ordinary colloid goiters or other enlarged glands not previously treated with iodine. He believed iodine pre-treatment led to rapid formation of colloid material in an iodine-famished gland, resulting in back pressure or distention, which caused edema (water retention). The edema would render the gland temporarily inactive and unable to function, but with time, new blood vessels grew, the gland accommodated to the increased pressure, and the patient became toxic again.[45]

In 1930, another American doctor, David Marine, observed that large doses of iodine given to dogs with goiters resulted in similar thyroid changes, from soft and spongy to firm, about 4 days after treatment was started. An examination of their thyroid glands showed this was due to an accumulation of colloid material. Human patients experience the same effect, complaining that their gland is painful, larger, and firmer, about 7 days after the start of iodine treatment.[46]

A surgeon in Montreal made an interesting observation in 1944 which still holds true today, 70 years later: "the proponents of iodine medication have all been physicians; the warnings against misuse have all come from surgeons." As a surgeon, he observed over 4,800 cases in 22 years, and believes that iodine thyrotoxicosis does exist, because many patients came to the clinic in a thyrotoxic state after using iodine for long periods. The biggest problem is that once a patient becomes thyrotoxic, it usually continues for a long time even after the iodine is withdrawn.[47] At that point, a thyroidectomy would be extremely risky; patients have died shortly after these surgeries from thyroid storm. Keep in mind this was back in the 1940s—Graves' patients have more options today and experience much better results.

An examination of over one hundred years of iodine case studies concluded that *some* individuals can tolerate very high levels of iodine with no apparent side effects and that iodine doses of less than or equal to 1 mg/day are probably safe for the majority of the population. However, even this low dose may cause adverse effects in *some* individuals. Exposure to excessive iodine through foods, dietary supplements, topical medications, or iodinated contrast media (used for visualization in medical procedures) has resulted in thyroiditis, goiter, hypothyroidism, hyperthyroidism, sensitivity reactions, or acute responses in some individuals. Adverse effects are more likely in those who have been iodine deficient for a while, have underlying thyroid disorders, or who are sensitive to iodine.[48]

Japanese iodine intake

One drop of 2% Lugol's has approximately 2.5 mg of iodine, while the lowest dose of Iodoral is 12.5 mg, or five times stronger. This higher dose is based on the assumption that Japanese people consume that amount of iodine daily from their diet and they're considered to be "the healthiest people in the world" with the highest life expectancy.[49] But other studies suggest the Japanese don't really consume that much iodine. Three different studies that incorporated daily food surveys in their calculations determined that daily iodine intake of the Japanese was less than 5 mg. The first study calculated daily iodine intake to be 1-3 mg/day,[50] the second 471 mcg,[51] and the third up to 1.9 mg, or up to 4.7 mg at university hospitals.[52] The Korean diet is also high in fish and seaweed, and a Korean study calculated daily iodine intake ranging from 0.06 to 4.09 mg.[53]

Even studies in Japan are concluding that high iodine intake may be responsible for some cases of hypothyroidism. When iodine intake was restricted in Japanese hypothyroid subjects for 6-8 weeks, their elevated TSH (indicating hypothyroidism) decreased, and their low Free T4 (the main hormone produced by the thyroid) increased, which means there was an inverse relationship—thyroid levels increased when iodine intake decreased. These subjects did not have thyroid antibodies,[54] which means their low thyroid levels resulted from too much iodine, not an autoimmune condition. Another study performed in the coastal areas of Japan where kelp is produced found that 1) hypothyroidism may be associated with the amount of iodine ingested; 2) hypothyroidism is more prevalent and marked in subjects consuming excessive amounts of iodine; and 3) excessive intake of iodine should be considered a cause of hypothyroidism and chronic thyroiditis in these areas.[55]

A portion of the Japanese population tests positive for autoimmune antibodies: anti-thyroglobulin antibodies (TGAb) and anti-thyroid peroxidase antibodies (TPOAb) were present in over 13% of the population in four different areas in Japan. Urinary iodine excretion was 1.5 mg/day in Nishihara.[56] If we assume these people are iodine sufficient, then based on current iodine loading test interpretation they should excrete 90% of the iodine they consumed the previous day. This calculates to a daily iodine consumption rate of approximately 1.7 mg (1.5 mg/90% excretion rate).

An analysis of urinary iodine excretion in male Japanese university students resulted in much lower levels than expected. On days when seaweed was not part of their diet, they excreted, on average, 153 mcg of iodine. On those days when seaweed was included, urinary iodine increased to 1.1 mg.[57] Another study based on urinary iodide excretion of Japanese concluded that daily dietary intake was approximately 470 mcg.[58] None of these studies that examined Japanese iodine intake, whether through diet or urinary excretion, approach the 12.5 mg in the smallest dose of Iodoral.

Iodine and hypothyroidism

Can iodine worsen or induce hypothyroidism? Unfortunately, the answer appears to be yes. The high-dose iodine proponents are adamant that this does not happen, but there are enough different biochemistries that it can and does happen to some people. When high levels of iodine are ingested, the thyroid gland stops synthesizing and releasing hormone. Although it is dismissed by some, the Wolff-Chaikoff effect has been observed in countless people for over a century. The sudden decrease in thyroid levels is the intended effect when treating a hyperthyroid person. But the same effect would make a normal person hypothyroid. In normal people, this shutdown is temporary and normal production and release of thyroid hormone resumes within a few weeks after the iodine is stopped. For a few, however, the shutdown becomes permanent, and the person will need prescription thyroid hormone to replace what they've lost. Those most likely to experience this effect are newborns and fetuses, patients with chronic systemic diseases, euthyroid (normal thyroid level) patients with autoimmune thyroiditis, patients treated with recombinant interferon-α who developed transient thyroid dysfunction, and Graves' disease patients previously treated with radioactive iodine (RAI), surgery or antithyroid drugs.[59] Iodide given in large doses for asthma and pulmonary conditions has induced goiters, hypothyroidism, and myxedema in some patients.[60] In two patients with underlying Hashimoto's autoimmune thyroiditis, supplementation with Iodoral resulted in severe symptomatic hypothyroidism.[61]

Japanese patients with primary hypothyroidism (blood tests revealing a TSH > 40) were studied while on a typical high iodine diet, and then for 3-15 weeks after they avoided high iodine foods. After iodine in their diet was restricted, 52% had serum T3, T4, and TSH return to normal levels. After only two weeks, both T3 and T4 rose, while TSH dropped dramatically. Excess iodine intake in these cases had induced a reversible form of hypothyroidism. The remaining subjects showed no change in their lab values and were considered to have irreversible hypothyroidism. All the reversible cases had goiters, while less than half of the irreversible group did. Those who had a normal or high 24-hour iodine uptake test had reversible cases; those with a low uptake were irreversible. A normal thyroid should take up iodine; this suggests the thyroid glands in the irreversible cases with low uptake were not functioning properly.[62]

Thyroid biopsies from iodine-induced hypothyroid patients were found to have common abnormalities. Electron microscope examinations revealed severe interference with thyroid hormone biosynthesis in the follicular cells, where thyroid hormone is produced. In some patients, thyroid function reverted back to normal after iodine restriction.[63]

Thyroid gland enlargement is another effect of high iodine intake. After healthy male volunteers were given 27 mg iodine daily for a month, measurements showed their thyroid glands had grown significantly, TSH and thyroglobulin rose, and free T4 decreased. One month after discontinuation of the iodine, thyroid gland volume and function returned to baseline levels.[64] This echoes the previous study, where excess iodine induced a reversible form of hypothyroidism.

High iodine intake (one 12.5 mg Iodoral per day) when pregnant can result in congenital hypothyroidism in newborns.[65] Either too much or too little iodine may harm the fetus because iodine crosses the placenta. If too much iodine induces the Wolff-Chaikoff effect, the fetus will have less thyroid hormone than it should, which can lead to fetal hypothyroidism. Such infants are born with T4 levels below the reference range and are placed on levothyroxine shortly after birth. In some the condition is temporary; in others it may be permanent. In one case, a fetus developed a goiter while still in the womb of a mother taking potassium iodide.[66] Congenital goiter and hypothyroidism of the newborn are the most common results of excess iodide intake while pregnant, but mental retardation and death have also been reported.[67]

The same effect was seen in Japanese infants whose mothers ate a moderately high iodine diet consisting of kombu soups and seaweed while pregnant (up to 3.2 mg iodine daily). In one study, 34 infants tested positive for congenital hypothyroidism, and 12 required levothyroxine because of persistent low T4 and/or high TSH levels.[68]

The negative effects of a high iodine diet are seen in animals too. Foals (baby horses) were born with goiters on farms where the mares (mother horses) were fed a high iodine diet. On three farms, the percentage of goitrous foals correlated to the level of iodine in the diet. In other words, the higher the iodine level in the diet, the more foals were born with goiters. The maximum safe daily iodine intake for horses has been calculated as 50 mg/day. At one farm where daily iodine consumption amounted to 288-432 mg/day, 50% of the foals were born with goiters.[69] Iodine is concentrated across the placenta and breast milk so a fetus or nursing foal receives a much higher concentration of iodine for their body weight than the mother. This explains why the newborn foal may have a goiter while the mother may not. Note also that if 50% of the foals had goiters, 50% did not. What is an excess for one is not for another. Biochemistry is extremely individual.

A human mother who had eight children illustrates the same concept. The mother took 600 mg potassium iodide daily for over 10 years for chronic asthma. Three pregnancies occurred while on the medication; those children were normal and did not have goiters at birth. The mother's thyroid gland was also normal in size and she did not display any hypothyroid symptoms. Her 8th child was born with an enlarged thyroid, many clinical symptoms of hypothyroidism, and blood work confirmed low thyroid levels. The infant was prescribed desiccated thyroid and the goiter disappeared by the time he was a year old.[70]

Iodine or bromine toxicity?

High-dose iodine proponents claim that iodine is used by every single cell in the body and is an essential element, therefore it is impossible for someone to react negatively to it. When people report negative reactions, they are told they are experiencing bromine toxicity, not iodine toxicity, even though it was iodine they ingested. Our environment today is toxic and full of bromine, they say, even though bromine was measurable in human blood a century ago, in the 1920s.[71] They are told that iodide is pushing out bromide from their cells, which is causing a detox reaction. They further insist that there is no such thing as iodism, or iodine poisoning/toxicity, or even an allergy to iodine. Rather, people who experience side effects are probably not taking enough of the required supplements ("companion nutrients") of sea salt, magnesium, Vitamin C, and selenium, in spite of the fact that the patients say they *are*. So whom do we believe? Can iodine be toxic? Or is it really bromide release that's causing the reactions?

Bromine concentration in the ocean is over 1000 times that of iodine.[72] Fish,[73] shell-fish,[74] seaweed,[75] and sea vegetables[76] all contain bromine. Anyone who consumes a lot of seafood ingests a lot of bromine. A study that compared urinary bromine levels between coastal Japanese and inland Chinese confirmed that the Japanese had significantly higher bromine levels.[77] In fact, bromine in the teeth and bones of archaeological samples can identify those from coastal versus inland regions, and is indicative of a marine diet.[78] The Japanese label of "healthiest people in the world" doesn't make sense if bromine is really that toxic. Bromine is even found in trace levels in newborns, and in adults at a 20 to 1 ratio to iodine by weight.[79] Both iodine and bromine are found in the plasma and urine of healthy individuals; bromine concentration is about 70 times higher than iodine in plasma, and 38 times higher in a 24-hour urine collection.[80]

The Dead Sea has a higher level of bromine than any other ocean water, yet Dead Sea salt baths are renowned for their healing properties. When patients with psoriasis bathe in the Dead Sea for four weeks, their serum bromine levels increase 2-3 fold, and their physical and mental state improves.[81] The major elements in the Dead Sea, in decreasing order of concentration, are magnesium, sodium, calcium, and potassium. Chlorine is the halide in highest concentration (212 gm/liter), followed by bromine (5 gm/liter). Iodine isn't even mentioned in this analysis, probably because it is only found in trace amounts.

There are many pairs of opposing elements in nature where an imbalance either way causes problems; sodium-potassium and calcium-magnesium are two such examples. It would be reasonable to hypothesize that iodine-bromine is another one of those pairs. Iodine is a component of thyroid hormone, which increases metabolism and alertness, while bromine has the opposite effect, and has been used as a sedative.[82] The Japanese consume a lot of seaweed, which is high in both iodine *and* bromine, but it doesn't seem to negatively affect their health. Perhaps seaweed's high iodine content is balanced by its high bromine content. The Japanese don't follow a "protocol"—they just naturally consume a high iodine (and bromine) diet. Iodine supplements do not have the bromine balance that nature intended.

It appears that when any one halide is taken in excess, another halide is displaced to maintain equilibrium, and that may be the cause of toxic symptoms. In rat studies, bromide replaces chloride in body tissues and fluids, but it replaces iodide in the thyroid gland.[83] This action is reversible, and taking a large amount of chloride (salt is sodium chloride) will flush out both bromide and iodide.[84] Salt water is the standard treatment for either iodine or bromine toxicity. The salt loading protocol (drinking large quantities of sea salt water to trigger urination) may work not just because it flushes out bromine, but because it flushes out the excess iodine that was ingested. In one case, a woman who had taken bromides for ten years was admitted to a hospital with bromoderma (skin lesions from excess bromide). Upon admittance, her urine contained no bromide and was declared normal. However, when she was given intravenous saline, she had a severe reaction. Her urine became strongly positive for bromide and her kidneys showed signs of severe stress (large amounts of albumin in her urine).[85] The woman was not taking iodide, and bromide only appeared in high quantities after she was flushed with another halide, sodium chloride (salt water). This suggests that bromide can be flushed out of the body with salt water alone.

A good example of an iodine-bromine imbalance is illustrated in a study of baby chicks that were fed a very high iodine diet. The chicks exhibited bizarre neurological symptoms and extreme malaise; they would fall over, lie motionless for a few minutes, then stand up for a few minutes, only to fall over again. Food intake and weight gain also decreased as iodine in the diet increased. When bromine was added to their high iodine diet, all their symptoms went away.[86] Other halide salts such as fluoride were tested and did not relieve their symptoms.

A mouse study reported similar findings. A high iodine diet resulted in growth retardation in the mice, but when bromine was added to the diet, growth returned to normal levels.[87] Fluorine was also tested in this study and did not have the same effect as bromine.

Iodism or iodine poisoning sometimes results after high dose iodine treatment. Symptoms include burning in the mouth or throat, severe headache, metallic taste, soreness of teeth and gums, cold symptoms like an inflamed runny nose, coughing, sneezing, eye irritation with eyelid swelling, unusual increase in salivation, confusion, arrhythmias, numbness and weakness. Increased fluid and salt intake may help eliminate the excess iodine. Eliminating or decreasing iodine from any source is also beneficial.[88]

High iodine intake has caused skin lesions that look like boils, called acneiform eruptions. Unfortunately, these often show up on the face and neck area. More severe skin reactions are called *iododerma* and indicate a possibly dangerous response to iodine, so the protocol should be stopped at that point. One case study described an ulcerating iododerma on the cheeks and over the nose caused by oral ingestion of potassium iodide for asthma/bronchitis.[89] *Fatal iododerma* is the medical term used when the skin reaction precedes death. In most cases, the patients had previously used iodine.[90] An underlying systemic disease could also predispose someone to this type of reaction.[91] A fatal case of iododerma in 1931 occurred after the patient was given potassium iodide medication. He passed large quantities of iodide in his urine before his death, and studies after his death revealed large amounts of iodide in his skin, liver, and kidneys.[92] Another fatal case shows a man with iododerma covering his face, arms, and hands after an injection of iodized oil.[93]

Bromoderma is the term for toxic skin reactions to bromine. It tends to be more common on the legs and looks like a large, red, inflamed, crusty area of skin with pustules at the edges.[94] To state the obvious, the case studies for bromoderma reported ingestion of large doses of bromine.[95] Logic says that reactions from large doses of iodine are a display of iodine toxicity, not bromine toxocity. After all, iodine was taken in high doses, not bromine. The high-dose iodine proponents refer to acne on the hands and face as bromoderma, yet there are case studies where those symptoms are called iododerma. Is there a difference? According to a medical manual published in 1907, there is.[96] In the *Intoxication* (poisoning) section, there are separate listings for iodism (iodide poisoning) and bromism (bromide poisoning). Toxic iodine reactions listed include dripping sinuses, frontal headaches, facial swelling, bronchitis, fever and chest congestion resembling pneumonia, and pustular skin eruptions. These symptoms have been reported by quite a few starting the iodine protocol on iodine forums. It does note that sometimes these symptoms are temporary and disappear on their own, as if the person develops a tolerance for the iodine.

The first symptom of bromism is acneiform eruptions, usually on the face and back. Additional symptoms listed are digestive upsets, bronchial secretions, and conjunctivitis. Fatigue, muscular tremor, an unsteady gait, impaired memory, apathy, stammering, mispronunciation of words, and confusion are also listed. Bromine was used as a sleep aid and anti-epileptic drug in the past, and high doses sometimes led to bromism. More recent cases used bromine compounds for pain relief,[97] and saline treatment (without iodine) led to recovery. It appears that other than the acne, the side effects people are describing on the iodine forums better fit the description for iodism rather than bromism. Skin eruptions are also a symptom of iodism. This 1907 medical manual distinguished between iodism and bromism over a century ago, before bromine became commonplace in our environment. Some of the sources of bromine today did not exist back then: flame retardants, agricultural chemicals, brominated flours, and water treatment for hot tubs.[98]

Iodine toxicity symptoms have been reported in other animals. Chronic coughing and profuse nasal discharge affected some calves fed high iodine diets. At lower levels of iodine intake, the nasal discharge abated with time, but at the highest level, the nasal discharge never stopped. Food intake and weight gain also decreased.[99]

Rat studies show that iodide accumulates in the skin during the first few hours after tracer radioactive iodide is ingested. The concentration in the skin exceeds the concentration in the thyroid at any time, although the largest concentration is excreted in urine.[100] The same effect probably occurs in patients following the iodine protocol. The large amounts of ingested iodine/iodide accumulate in the skin, and may be the cause of skin reactions in some people. Bromide can also accumulate in the skin and cause reactions if taken in large doses, but since no bromide is deliberately ingested in the iodine protocol, any effects in the skin would be from an excess of iodine/iodide, not bromine/bromide.

Other symptoms people report are those of someone who is either hypo or hyperthyroid. A rapid pulse, feeling hot when others aren't, bowel movements trending towards diarrhea, and weight loss are some of the first signs that iodine has induced hyperthyroidism. A slow pulse, feeling cold, constipation, and weight gain are some of the first signs that iodine has induced hypothyroidism. Hair loss can be caused by thyroid levels that are either too high *or* too low. Bromine/iodine toxicity and hypothyroidism are two different things. Hypothyroidism results from a lack of thyroid hormone, not lack of iodine. There's a difference. Taking too much iodine can induce the Wolff-Chaikoff effect, so less thyroid hormone is made and/or released. While it's counterintuitive, taking more iodine can result in less thyroid hormone for some. For others predisposed to Graves', even a small increase in daily iodine consumption may exacerbate the hyperthyroid condition.

Bromine's role in the body

Bromide, like the other halides (fluoride, chloride, and iodide), is found in all human bodies. A small amount of each halogen is normal, and iodide is the halide found in the lowest concentration. Fluoride is considered an essential trace element at minute levels because it stimulates bone formation and reduces dental decay. Levels that are too high will cause discoloration of the teeth and skeletal fluorosis.[101] Bromine may also be an essential trace element and is found in blood serum, hair, liver, and breast milk. The average urinary excretion per day is about 5 mg.[102] A bromine compound, 1-methylheptyl γ-bromoacetoacetate, is found in human cerebrospinal fluid, induces REM sleep,[103] and may explain bromine's sedative effects. When samples of serum, urine, and hair from healthy men were analyzed, the bromine levels formed a normal distribution pattern (most values clustered towards the middle of a symmetrical reference range). Serum levels ranged from 3.2 to 5.6 µg/mL, urine between 0.3 to 7.0 µg/mL, and hair from 1.1 to 49.0 µg/mL.[104] The serum levels in this study are in agreement with other bromine analyses, which also found a normal distribution pattern. A normal distribution pattern is often found in essential, rather than non-essential elements.[105]

Explaining why bromide may not the "bad guy" it's made out to be involves some basic chemistry. Bromide belongs to the halogen family, which also includes fluoride, chloride, iodide, and astatide. Even though they all belong to the same chemical group because they have similar properties, they are all different sizes. This is expressed by their atomic mass. Iodide is physically larger than bromide, which is graphically shown in Figure 18-1.

As stated earlier, NIS is a transporter, not a receptor. A transporter moves items through a passageway, like a truck going through a tunnel. NIS is specifically sized for iodide, but other anions (molecules with a single negative charge) may also fit if they are similar enough in size and shape. While bromide can enter tissues through NIS,[106] other anions have a greater affinity (stronger attraction) for NIS than bromide, and even iodide! This simply means that if all the anions that could fit NIS lined up at the same time, bromide would not be picked first, because larger anions are preferred. In fact, radioactive tracer bromide, iodide, and fluoride have been tested to see how they would concentrate in the thyroid gland. The thyroid gland has only a slight affinity for fluoride and bromide,[107] with a much greater affinity, as expected, for iodide.

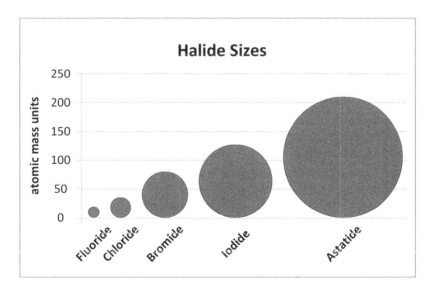

Figure 18-1. Iodide has a higher atomic mass than bromide, chloride, or fluoride.

The affinity of other anions for NIS has been tested, and those that are relevant to this discussion are perchlorate, thiocyanate, nitrate, and bromide. These ions can be ranked by their size (partial molal ionic volume), which correlates with their affinity for NIS. The larger the ion, the stronger the affinity for NIS. As shown in Figure 18-2, perchlorate is larger than iodide, which is larger than bromide. Perchlorate (ClO_4^-) is a component of rocket fuel and is sometimes found in drinking water,[108] thiocyanate (SCN^-) is found in tobacco smoke and cruciferous vegetables,[109] nitrate (NO_3^-) is found naturally in green, leafy vegetables,[110] and bromide (Br^-) is primarily used in flame retardants, brines for oil drilling, pesticides, and water treatment.[111]

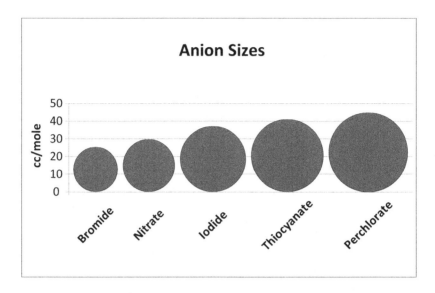

Figure 18-2. Perchlorate and thiocyanate are larger anions with a higher affinity for NIS than iodide.[112]

Perchlorate has the highest affinity for NIS, therefore, it would "win" in a competition with iodide, or any of the other anions listed, for transport by NIS. Iodide has a higher affinity for NIS than bromide, so unless iodide levels are extremely low, bromide cannot force its way in. Studies on iodine-sufficient and iodine-deficient rats confirm this. High levels of bromide in the presence of iodine deficiency enhance bromide's goitrogenic effects,[113] because bromide replaces iodide in the thyroid gland, leaving less iodide available for thyroid hormone production. Excess bromide will also cause an increase in kidney excretion to keep halide equilibrium in the body. Both iodide and bromide will be excreted, again, leaving less iodide available for thyroid hormone production. Note that these studies examined the effect of high dose bromide intake when the blood concentration of bromide was several thousand times greater than that of iodide.[114] This is not analogous to the normal levels found in humans, unless they are purposely ingesting a bromine product. Lower doses of bromide showed little effect if iodine levels were sufficient.

Again, affinity for NIS is greatest for perchlorate, not iodide, and not bromide. Fluoride isn't even on the affinity list because it is physically much smaller than iodide, and may not fit NIS. Fluoride also has different chemical and physical properties than the other halides.[115] The anions that fit all have something in common: they all have a negative charge, similar ionic radius/volume, and similar shape (roughly spherical).[116] Bromide and astatide are the halides closest in atomic mass to iodide, and both can be transported by NIS.[117] Administration of perchlorate can accelerate renal clearance of chloride, bromide, and iodide.[118]   Again, perchlorate "wins" in a competition with the other halides and forces them out. This time, size matters.

Bromide and fluoride may be lesser players contributing to hypothyroidism than perchlorate and thiocyanate.   Thyroxine (T4) concentrations were found to be 12.9% lower in subjects who had high perchlorate, high thiocyanate, and low iodine combined, when compared to subjects with low perchlorate, low thiocyanate, and adequate iodine.[119] This illustrates how well perchlorate and thiocyanate can inhibit iodide uptake, which results in lower thyroid hormone levels.

When lactating rats were given perchlorate, both the mothers and the sucklings exhibited a 50% decrease in thyroidal iodide uptake relative to controls.   The same researchers conducted an *in vitro* study where NIS was expressed on only one side of a tissue. When perchlorate and iodide were added simultaneously, perchlorate was always translocated to the other side first, before iodide.[120]   This illustrates perchlorate's dominance of NIS over iodide. Not surprisingly, perchlorate has been used as a treatment for hyperthyroidism.[121]

Nitrate and thiocyanate are two other NIS uptake inhibitor anions found in our food and water. Nitrates are found naturally in green leafy vegetables, as preservatives in meats and fish, and as contaminants from fertilizers. The precursors to thiocyanates are found in foods like cassava, sweet potatoes, corn, apricots, cherries and almonds. Plants in the *Brassica* family (cabbage, Brussels sprouts, cauliflower and broccoli) also contain chemicals that the body metabolizes into thiocyanates. One woman, after ingesting large amounts of bok choy (Chinese white cabbage) for several months, became severely hypothyroid.   Her FT4 was undetectable.[122] Cigarette smoking is another source of thiocyanate. According to one study, nitrate and thiocyanate are much more prevalent in our environment and their effect as NIS inhibitors far exceeds that of perchlorate.[123] First, thiocyanate has a half-life of about 6 days, while perchlorate's is 8 hours, and nitrate's is 5 hours. This means thiocyanate remains in the body 18 times longer than perchlorate. Second, only a small portion of NIS inhibition from drinking water (< 10%) will be from perchlorate.   Third, perchlorate concentration in food is negligible, though it is how most nitrate and thiocyanate enters our bodies. Less than half a cup of milk (100 ml) will contain 5.76 parts per billion (ppb) of perchlorate, but 4000 ppb of thiocyanate, and 5000 ppb of nitrate.

Only a true iodine deficiency (less than 150 mcg per day) will allow anions with lesser affinity to enter the thyroid instead of iodide, with the end result of decreased thyroid hormone production. The Japanese diet is high in both iodide and bromide, with little negative effect. Bromide does not replace iodide in their thyroid gland because their iodide intake is more than adequate.   Keeping iodide at sufficient levels will probably likewise minimize any NIS inhibiting effects of perchlorate, thiocyanate, or nitrate.

Is an iodine allergy possible?

Delayed reactions to iodinated contrast media have been reported in 2-5% of patients for years. Turning this around, 95-98% of patients have no reaction. What do those small percent of patients have in common? Half those patients reported other drug allergies, and skin biopsies show the presence of T cells, which suggests a true immune reaction.[124]

T cells are white blood cells that act like soldiers and seek out and destroy invaders. They play a major role in immunity. These patients have overactive immune systems, so iodine isn't the only thing they react to. Just like some can have a fatal reaction to peanut butter (which is completely innocuous to others), some can have fatal reactions to iodine.[125] Peanut butter (or iodine) isn't the problem, it's the allergic person's immune system that's the problem.

Patients who had previously reacted to iodinated radio contrast media were given an oral provocation test with Lugol's. Of 19 patients, one reacted with urticaria (hives) and two reacted with exanthema (widespread rash).[126] These reactions to Lugol's confirm that iodine/iodide is the offending substance, and not other compounds in the radio contrast media.

Allergic individuals with atopic symptoms (asthma, hives, runny noses, food allergies, and eczema) may be more prone to reactions to iodine. Iodine is manufactured in a process that uses sulfur dioxide and sulfites,[127] which some people are highly allergic to.[128] Trace amounts of these compounds in the iodine may be inducing reactions in highly sensitive individuals.

Technically, a true allergic reaction involves immunoglobulins or antibodies, which are measurable in the blood. When reactions do not show measurable immunoglobulins, they are called a sensitivity reaction. They are still an adverse reaction and result in extreme discomfort for the patient. One study describes four individuals with a potassium iodide sensitivity who all developed hives after exposure.[129]

Whether it's called a sensitivity or allergy, some people have visible reactions to iodine. Skin lesions that look like boils or a chronic runny nose and cough are signs of toxicity. I happen to have the atopic symptoms of asthma, hives, food allergies, and eczema, and have suffered from allergic symptoms my entire life. Both sulfur dioxide and sulfites make me wheeze. I thought the runny nose, cough, and chest congestion that started after I started the iodine protocol were from the spring pollen season. My symptoms appeared with only one drop of 2% Lugol's. It was only when I started to research the side effects of iodine that I realized I was one of those who could not tolerate iodine, even at low doses. And yes, I'd been taking Vitamin C, selenium, magnesium, and sea salt for years before ever starting on the protocol, and in the recommended amounts. Iodine proponents usually recommend working on liver health in cases like mine, but I don't have hepatitis, cannot drink alcohol (allergic to sulfites and hops), my liver enzymes are normal, and I had rashes on my face even as a newborn (probably allergic to the formula). I may have suboptimal liver detoxification pathways because I lack specific enzymes, but I am unaware of any way to remedy those. Because of unique biochemistries, there are some people who will simply not be able to follow the iodine protocol—it literally makes them sick.

Are we all iodine deficient? How accurate is the iodine loading test?

To determine whether or not someone is deficient in iodine, high-dose iodine proponents direct people to an iodine loading test developed by Dr. Guy Abraham, the owner of the company that sells Iodoral. This test measures the amount of iodine captured in the urine after consuming 50 mg Iodoral. If less than 90% of the 50 mg iodine is collected in a 24-hour urine sample (less than 45 mg), the person is considered iodine deficient, and would benefit from iodine supplementation. The assumption is that the body will retain any iodine it needs and only excrete what it doesn't use, so if the amount collected is less than 90%, a deficiency is implied.[130] Retesting is recommended after three months of supplementation to see if iodine sufficiency has improved, and Iodoral is recommended as the form of iodine supplemented, for comparable test results.

There are serious flaws in the above testing methodology. For one thing, iodine excretion continues for approximately three days after ingestion; secondly, iodine is also excreted in sweat, and this is not accounted for in a 24-hour urine collection. In a study of iodine absorption and excretion in healthy men,[131] iodine was primarily excreted in urine (65-88%), but was also found in sweat (2-9%), and feces (0.35%). The small amount of iodine collected in sweat is enough to push total iodine recovered to 90% for some of the men.

The fact that iodine excretion continues for three days after iodine intake is stopped was an unexpected finding. The men in this study had to walk for five hours each day (except on Sundays) over a period of six weeks. They were free to drink as much water as they wished, but Lugol's had been added to the water. Average daily iodine intake was 88 mg, but ranged between 20-440 mg per day. Because they did not walk on Sundays, they did not consume as much iodinated water on that day, yet they excreted more iodine than they ingested! This could only come from the previous days' higher intake. Knowing that there was a time lag before full iodine excretion, the authors knew they could not calculate an accurate daily yield, so instead used a 7-day moving average. Urine iodine recovery amounted to 74% of all intake when expressed as a 7-day moving average. If this study reflects typical iodine excretion levels, a more realistic passing score for a one-day urinary iodine loading test would be closer to 74% than 90%.

A second study gave very similar results. Urinary iodine excretion was observed over three days after ingestion of 50 mg Iodoral. An average of 70% iodine/iodide was excreted during the first 24 hours, with 16% excreted on days 2 and 3 combined.[132] Total urinary iodine recovery over three days would then amount to 86% of the ingested dose. While the iodine excreted in sweat was not reported in this particular study, only 4% more iodine would need to be recovered from sweat to reach the desired 90%. Based on the first study, that amount is possible. These subjects would then be declared "iodine sufficient," even though none of them had ever supplemented iodine directly or followed the iodine protocol.

These two studies raise serious questions about the validity of this urinary iodine loading test. Some patients pass their first test with a score greater than 90%, only to retake the test later and receive a lower score.[133] How could someone ever score more than 90% when it takes three days to approach 100% elimination, and the two studies above suggest a score in the 70% range would be more likely? The high-dose iodine proponents claim that "iodine receptors" are defective at the time of the first test, so most of the iodine is simply being passed through the body without being used (remember, NIS is a transporter, not receptor). Therefore, iodine supplementation is indicated, even though the patient scored over 90%. With time and daily iodine supplementation, the "iodine receptors" improve, more iodine is absorbed, and a more realistic lower test score is obtained. Let's review. If you score less than 90%, you are iodine deficient and should start the high-dose iodine protocol, supplementing with Iodoral for consistent results. If you score more than 90%, you are iodine deficient because your "iodine receptors" are defective and not absorbing any iodine. You should start the high-dose iodine protocol. Most laboratory tests are performed to determine a course of action based on the results. Since the course of action is always "take Iodoral" regardless of the results, there is really no need for this test.

Blood draws are another way to test iodine levels. One woman who was taking about 30 mg Lugol's reported serum iodine levels that were over nine times higher than the top of the reference range. Her thyroid levels were all trending lower. She was concerned about her high iodine levels on this test, but was told on an iodine forum that the blood test she had taken was useless and not reliable, because it only showed the iodine that was in circulation, and not her saturation levels. She was advised that the only test that would give her accurate information was the 24-hour loading test, which was described in the previous paragraph. When two tests that supposedly measure the same thing give conflicting results, patients should question why that is, and not blindly accept what they are told. They are being given a red flag warning that they should investigate.

How much iodine do we really need?

According to the U.S. RDA, we only need 150 mcg of iodine daily. At the other end of the spectrum are the high-dose iodine proponents who believe iodine intake should be closer to 50 mg (50,000 mcg) for optimal health. Iodine forum members are told that a normal thyroid gland contains 50 mg iodine, even though other studies report much lower numbers. One study found a range of 0.9 – 20.2 mg iodine per gland.[134] Another study found a range of 4 - 37 mg iodine per gland in healthy men, and noted that these values were higher than those reported in other studies.[135] There are other studies with different ranges, but none of them approach 50 mg iodine per gland; in fact, most report averages of 5-15 mg iodine per gland.[136]

Some people are able to take milligram doses of iodine without toxic effects because the body has built-in iodine overdose mechanisms. When too much iodine is taken, the Wolff-Chaikoff effect kicks in so thyroid hormone production by the thyroid gland is (usually) temporarily halted. Dietary iodine normally enters the body through the small intestine and if intake is excessive, a downregulation of NIS in the intestine lowers absorption.[137] Excess iodine is then excreted through the kidneys and sweat. Anyone with a pre-existing kidney condition may need to be cautious with high iodine doses; rising creatinine, sodium, and chloride levels are signs of renal (kidney) insufficiency. Renal clearance is highly dependent on the glomerular filtration rate (GFR), which tends to be lower in those who are hypothyroid.[138] If the GFR is low, then iodine can build up to toxic levels in the body.[139] Low urinary iodine excretion rates may be due to renal insufficiency rather than iodine deficiency, as the iodine loading test presumes. There are also NIS mutation defects which lead to inefficient iodide absorption, and hence insufficient thyroid hormone production.[140]

Iodine is an essential mineral needed in trace (microgram) amounts for thyroid function. Yet iodine has documented, beneficial effects against cancer and tumors when taken in milligram doses. If someone is fighting cancer, iodine should probably be a part of their protocol; but if they have any underlying thyroid condition, supplementation may negatively affect their thyroid function. A daily dose of 2-3 mg iodine for general health is recommended by Dr. David Derry, who says this amount is enough to saturate the thyroid gland with enough left over for the rest of the body. Other thyroid researchers are recommending that iodine intake should be at least 3 mg/day in the presence of cancer, because of its proven, suppressive effect on tumors.[141] One surgeon noted that anything over 6 mg was enough to treat a thyrotoxic gland. Some patients on iodine forums claim to have significant health improvements at doses exceeding 50 mg, while others only end up with toxic symptoms at much lower doses (that don't resolve with any amount of supplemental sea salt and companion nutrients). It may also be that both time and dose are variables in this equation, and a lower dose for a longer period of time may achieve the same positive results. Since some people raise their doses slowly to deal with toxic symptoms, they may not reach a 50 mg dose until a year has passed. At that point, they see an improvement in their symptoms which they attribute to the 50 mg dose they finally worked up to. But it could also be that they finally saw improvement because they'd been on the protocol for a year, and they would have seen improvements even if they'd stayed on a lower dose for that length of time.

Conclusion

If iodine supplementation allows someone's thyroid to return to normal production levels, then that would certainly be preferable to a lifetime of prescription thyroid hormone replacement. The problem is that iodine supplementation reduces the need for prescription thyroid replacement in some, but initiates it in others. There is probably no way to determine what effect iodine supplementation will have on each individual. However, as previously stated, anyone with an underlying thyroid condition prior to starting the iodine protocol is more at risk.

Iodine supplementation may generate the following reactions:
- It improves the health of those who are slightly hypothyroid and not on thyroid medication, possibly correcting the iodine deficiency that prevented their thyroid glands from producing healthy levels of thyroid hormone; these people then do not need thyroid medication.
- It allows patients already on thyroid medication to reduce their dose, again possibly correcting an iodine deficiency; these people report feeling better when taking iodine in addition to their thyroid medication(s).
- It induces hyperthyroidism in those who were not on thyroid medication; because this is a serious condition that must be controlled, they may then need to explore anti-thyroid medications or other remedies, because they may still be hyperthyroid even after discontinuing the iodine.
- It induces hypothyroidism in those who were not on thyroid medication; these patients then need prescription thyroid hormone because they are still hypothyroid after discontinuing the iodine.
- *Iodism* (iodine toxicity) is any toxic reaction from taking too much iodine; *iododerma* (skin lesions that look like boils) is one visible form of iodine toxicity.

- Due to individual biochemistry, some people will have toxic symptoms and cannot tolerate supplemental iodine at any dose.

While the high-dose iodine proponents blame bromide for toxicity symptoms and for "blocked iodine receptors," research shows that other NIS inhibitors like perchlorate, thiocyanate, and nitrate may be more problematic. The toxic symptoms people report while taking iodine in the recommended milligram amounts may be a symptom of iodine toxicity, not bromide toxicity. Even Japanese studies do not support a daily intake of 50 mg/day. Ironically, the reason the salt loading protocol may work to reduce toxic symptoms is because it helps flush out excess iodide. The chloride in salt water will flush out any other halide.

Research confirms that iodine can be highly beneficial in the fight against cancer. Studies show positive effects at only 3 mg, yet there are multiple anecdotal reports of greater benefits at higher doses. It may be individual biochemistry that allows for the higher doses. The body has mechanisms to deal with excessive iodine levels—the thyroid will only accept so much iodine before shutting down, NIS in the intestines will down-regulate to reduce absorption, and the kidneys flush the excess out.

This chapter was written so people are aware that the high-dose iodine protocol is not smooth sailing for everyone and may actually worsen their health. Iodine deficiency contributes to many thyroid abnormalities, from Graves' hyperthyroidism to nodular goiters and hypothyroidism.[142] But iodine supplementation has induced hypothyroidism, hyperthyroidism, and unsightly skin lesions and other toxic symptoms in some people when taken in milligram doses. These are real side effects, experienced by more than a few, even though the high-dose iodine proponents tend to gloss over them. Anyone considering any iodine protocol should do considerable research, from *multiple* sources, before taking any iodine. Profiting from the sale of a product is a direct conflict of interest to providing objective information for that product. In my opinion, many of the "research" articles I've read are actually just propaganda.

Key points

- Both TSH and sodium are essential for NIS function, which transports iodide into the thyroid gland.
- Iodine deficiency can result in goiters.
- A hormone called prolactin can be activated when severely hypothyroid. Prolactin activates NIS. Only women who are breastfeeding should have prolactin and NIS in their breasts. Iodine should not be present in non-lactating women's breasts.
- Prolactin is associated with tumors.
- Iodine normalizes fibrocystic breasts and causes tumor regression.
- Iodine has shown positive effects against breast, colon, and prostate cancer.
- Iodine can exacerbate or induce the hyperthyroid condition
- High iodine intake induces the Wolff-Chaikoff effect, where thyroid production and release temporarily halts. In some, this is temporary, in others it is perma-

nent. If it's permanent, the patient becomes hypothyroid and must take prescription thyroid hormone replacement.

- Some people escape from the Wolff-Chaikoff effect after approximately 21 days; others do not.
- Extended iodine use can backfire in Graves' patients and become ineffective or worsen the condition, although initially, there is usually remarkable improvement.
- Adverse effects from iodine are more likely in those who have been iodine deficient for a while, have underlying thyroid disorders, or who are sensitive to iodine.
- Some studies indicate the Japanese only consume up to 4 mg of iodine daily.
- High iodine intake in the Japanese also results in lower thyroid levels.
- High iodine intake can induce reversible hypothyroidism and goiters.
- Excess iodine intake during pregnancy can result in congenital hypothyroidism for the infant because iodine crosses the placenta, inducing the Wolff-Chaikoff effect.
- Different people, because of different biochemistries, have different reactions to iodine. Some get positive results, others negative.
- Bromine may be an essential trace element that balances iodine. It is found naturally in the ocean at much higher concentrations than iodine.
- The Japanese have higher levels of bromine than those that live inland.
- Bromide can be flushed out of the body with salt water (without iodide).
- Bromide can be transported by NIS, but only when iodide levels are insufficient.
- Iodine toxicity appears to correlate to the dose; lowering the dose usually solves the problem.
- A runny nose, chronic coughing, metallic taste, headaches, facial swelling, and skin lesions that look like boils are signs of iodine toxicity.
- Perchlorate may be the strongest inhibitor of normal NIS function, not bromide.
- Thiocyanate and nitrate are also strong NIS inhibitors.
- Someone is hypothyroid if they have insufficient levels of thyroid hormone. Because of the Wolff-Chaikoff effect, supplementing iodine can actually result in *less* thyroid hormone.
- Those who react to iodine may have oversensitive immune systems; these patients report other drug allergies.
- Iodine (both Lugol's and Iodoral) is manufactured in a process using sulfur dioxide and sulfites. Highly sensitive people may be reacting to traces of these compounds.
- The iodine loading test is based on flawed premises. Since urinary iodine is secreted over a three-day period, it is impossible to capture 90% of any iodine dose in only 24-hours. Only a three-day urinary iodine test will give accurate results.
- The body has mechanisms that downregulate excess iodine ingestion, both in the thyroid and the intestines.

- The iodine protocol should be approached with caution by anyone with pre-existing kidney disease, because excess iodine is flushed out through the kidneys. A low GFR rate could lead to a toxic build-up of iodine in the body.
- Profiting from the sale of a product is a direct conflict of interest to providing objective information for that product.

---

[1] Padmanabhan, Hema. "Amiodarone and thyroid dysfunction." *Southern Medical Journal* 103.9 (2010): 922-930.

[2] Abraham, Guy E. "The historical background of the iodine project." *The Original Internist* 12.2 (2005): 57-66.

[3] Abraham, Guy E., Jorge D. Flechas, and J. C. Hakala. "Optimum levels of iodine for greatest mental and physical health." *The Original Internist* 9.3 (2002): 5-20.

[4] Abraham, Guy E. "The Wolff-Chaikoff Effect: Crying Wolf." *The Original Internist* 12.3 (2005): 112-118.

[5] Abraham, Guy E. "The history of iodine in medicine Part III: thyroid fixation and medical iodophobia." *Original Internist* 13 (2006): 71-78.

[6] Abraham, Guy E., Jorge D. Flechas, and J. C. Hakala. "Orthoiodosupplementation: Iodine sufficiency of the whole human body." *The Original Internist* 9.4 (2002): 30-41.

[7] Di Bernardo, Julie, and Kerry J. Rhoden. "Gene Section: SLC5A5 (solute carrier family 5 (sodium iodide symporter), member 5)." *http://AtlasGeneticsOncology. org* (2010): 581.

[8] Riedel, Claudia, Orlie Levy, and Nancy Carrasco. "Post-transcriptional regulation of the sodium/iodide symporter by thyrotropin." *Journal of Biological Chemistry* 276.24 (2001): 21458-21463.

[9] Colin, Ides M., et al. "Recent Insights into the Cell Biology of Thyroid Angiofollicular Units." *Endocrine reviews* (2013).

[10] Chatterjee, Sushmita, et al. "Quantitative Immunohistochemical Analysis Reveals Association between Sodium Iodide Symporter and Estrogen Receptor Expression in Breast Cancer." *PloS one* 8.1 (2013): e54055.

[11] Rasmussen, Louise Maymann, et al. "Prolactin and oestrogen synergistically regulate gene expression and proliferation of breast cancer cells." *Endocrine-related cancer* 17.3 (2010): 809-822.

[12] Verma, I., et al. "Prevalence of hypothyroidism in infertile women and evaluation of response of treatment for hypothyroidism on infertility." *International Journal of Applied and Basic Medical Research* 2.1 (2012): 17.

[13] Kim, J., S. Lee, and K. H. Oktay. "Effect of BRCA1 gene and estrogen-receptor {alpha} on regulation of serum estradiol levels in women with breast cancer." *J Clin Oncol (Meeting Abstracts)*. Vol. 28. No. 15_suppl. 2010.

[14] Subbaramaiah, Kotha, et al. "Increased levels of COX-2 and prostaglandin E2 contribute to elevated aromatase expression in inflamed breast tissue of obese women." *Cancer Discovery* 2.4 (2012): 356-365.

[15] Muderris, Iptisam Ipek, et al. "Effect of thyroid hormone replacement therapy on ovarian volume and androgen hormones in patients with untreated primary hypothyroidism." *Annals of Saudi medicine* 31.2 (2011): 145.

[16] Komiya, Akira, et al. "Severe oligozoospermia in a patient with myxedema coma." *Reproductive Medicine and Biology* (2012): 1-5.

[17] Mendes, Graziella Alebrant, et al. "Prolactin gene expression in primary central nervous system tumors." *Journal of Negative Results in BioMedicine* 12.1 (2013): 4.

[18] Levina, Vera V., et al. "Biological significance of prolactin in gynecologic cancers." *Cancer research* 69.12 (2009): 5226-5233.

[19] Hekimsoy, Zeliha, et al. "The prevalence of hyperprolactinaemia in overt and subclinical hypothyroidism." *Endocrine journal* 57.12 (2010): 1011.

[20] Carvalho, M. M., and C. Góis. "[Hyperprolactinemia in mentally ill patients]." *Acta médica portuguesa* 24.6 (2011): 1005.

[21] Muench, John, and Ann M. Hamer. "Adverse effects of antipsychotic medications." *Am Fam Physician* 81.5 (2010): 617-22.

[22] Santos, Nadine Correia, et al. "Revisiting Thyroid Hormones in Schizophrenia." *Journal of Thyroid Research* 2012 (2012).

[23] Oh, Jong-Ryool, and Byeong-Cheol Ahn. "False-positive uptake on radioiodine whole-body scintigraphy: physiologic and pathologic variants unrelated to thyroid cancer." *American Journal of Nuclear Medicine and Molecular Imaging* 2.3 (2012): 362.

[24] Ruhla, Stephan, et al. "A high normal TSH is associated with the metabolic syndrome." *Clinical endocrinology* 72.5 (2010): 696-701.

[25] Arroyo-Helguera, O., et al. "Uptake and antiproliferative effect of molecular iodine in the MCF-7 breast cancer cell line." *Endocrine-Related Cancer* 13.4 (2006): 1147-1158.

[26] Elio Torremante, Pompilio, and Harald Rosner. "Antiproliferative Effects of Molecular Iodine in Cancers." *Current Chemical Biology* 5.3 (2011): 168-176.

[27] Stoddard II, Frederick R., et al. "Iodine alters gene expression in the MCF7 breast cancer cell line: evidence for an anti-estrogen effect of iodine." *International journal of medical sciences* 5.4 (2008): 189.

[28] Poor, Alexander E., et al. "Urine Iodine, Estrogen, and Breast Disease." *Journal of Cancer Therapy* 3 (2012): 1164-1169.

[29] Derry, David. "Breast Cancer and Iodine : How to Prevent and How to Survive Breast Cancer." Trafford Publishing, 2001.

[30] Kessler, Jack H. "The effect of supraphysiologic levels of iodine on patients with cyclic mastalgia." *The breast journal* 10.4 (2004): 328-336.

[31] García-Solís, Pablo, et al. "Inhibition of N-methyl- N-nitrosourea-induced mammary carcinogenesis by molecular iodine (I $_2$) but not by iodide (I$^-$) treatment: Evidence that I2 prevents cancer promotion." *Molecular and cellular endocrinology* 236.1 (2005): 49-57.

[32] Thomasz, Lisa, et al. "6 Iodo-δ-lactone: A derivative of arachidonic acid with antitumor effects in HT-29 colon cancer cells." *Prostaglandins, Leukotrienes and Essential Fatty Acids* (2013).

[33] Gärtner, Roland, Petra Rank, and Birgit Ander. "The role of iodine and delta-iodolactone in growth and apoptosis of malignant thyroid epithelial cells and breast cancer cells." *Hormones (Athens)* 9.1 (2010): 60-66.

[34] Aranda, Nuri, et al. "Uptake and antitumoral effects of iodine and 6-iodolactone in differentiated and undifferentiated human prostate cancer cell lines." *The Prostate* (2012).

[35] Tomer, Yaron, et al. "Fine mapping of loci linked to autoimmune thyroid disease identifies novel susceptibility genes." *Journal of Clinical Endocrinology & Metabolism* 98.1 (2013): E144-E152.

[36] Ban, Yoshiyuki, et al. "Association of a C/T single-nucleotide polymorphism in the 5'untranslated region of the CD40 gene with Graves' disease in Japanese." *Thyroid* 16.5 (2006): 443-446.

[37] Starrenburg-Razenberg, A. J., et al. "Four patients with hypothyroid Graves' disease." *The Netherlands journal of medicine* 68.4 (2010): 178-180.

[38] Krishnan, Binu, and Emma Bingham. "'Health supplements'-not always good for your health!" *Endocrine Abstracts*. Vol. 19. 2009.

[39] Phillppou, George, et al. "The effect of iodide on serum thyroid hormone levels in normal persons, in hyperthyroid patients, and in hypothyroid patients on thyroxine replacement." *Clinical endocrinology* 36.6 (1992): 573-578.

[40] Fountoulakis, Stelios, George Philippou, and Agathocles Tsatsoulis. "The role of iodine in the evolution of thyroid disease in Greece: from endemic goiter to thyroid autoimmunity." *HORMONES-ATHENS-* 6.1 (2007): 25.

[41] Garrod, Oliver. "Thyrotoxicosis." *British medical journal* 1.5179 (1960): 1123-1125.

[42] Fahrni, Gordon S. "Important Factors in the Management Of Hyperthyroidism." *Canadian Medical Association Journal* 21.5 (1929): 511.

[43] Robertson, J. Douglas. "Disordered Metabolisms in Thyrotoxicosis and Myxœdema: Lecture delivered at the Royal College of Surgeons of England on 13th December, 1948." *Annals of The Royal College of Surgeons of England* 4.1 (1949): 3.

[44] Goetsch, Emil. "Correct and incorrect use of iodine in the treatment of goiter." *The American Journal of Surgery* 26.3 (1934): 417-430.

[45] DeCourcy, Joseph L. "The Use of Lugol's Solution in Exophthalmic Goitre: An Explanation for the Beneficial Results of Pre-Operative Medication." *Annals of Surgery* 86.6 (1927): 871.

[46] Marine, David. "Studies on the Etiology of Goiter Including Graves' Disease.*." *Annals of Internal Medicine* 4.5 (1930): 423-432.

[47] Fitzgerald, R. R. "The Dangers of the Incorrect Use of Iodine in Goitre Treatment." *Canadian Medical Association Journal* 51.6 (1944): 527.

[48] Pennington, J. A. "A review of iodine toxicity reports." *Journal of the American Dietetic Association* 90.11 (1990): 1571.

[49] Reported by Dr. Lauren Browne, "Japan Tops List of Healthiest Countries," http://abcnews.go.com/blogs/health/2012/12/13/japan-tops-list-of-healthiest-countries/, December 13, 2012.

[50] Zava, Theodore T., and David T. Zava. "Assessment of Japanese iodine intake based on seaweed consumption in Japan: A literature-based analysis." *Thyroid Research* 4.14 (2011): 1-7.

[51] Fuse, Y., et al. "Is Japan an iodine excess country? Current iodine status assessed by urinary iodine and food frequency questionnaire." *Endocrine Abstracts*. Vol. 29. 2012.

[52] Katamine, Shinichiro, et al. "Iodine content of various meals currently consumed by urban Japanese." *Journal of nutritional science and vitaminology* 32.5 (1986): 487.

[53] Sohns, Chun Young, and Jae June Oh. "Dietary iodine intake and urinary iodine excretion in normal Korean adults." *Yonsei medical journal* 39.4 (1998): 355-362.

[54] Konno, N., et al. "Screening for thyroid diseases in an iodine sufficient area with sensitive thyrotrophin assays, and serum thyroid autoantibody and urinary iodide determinations." *Clinical endocrinology* 38.3 (2008): 273-281.

[55] Konno, Norimichi, et al. "Association between dietary iodine intake and prevalence of subclinical hypothyroidism in the coastal regions of Japan." *Journal of Clinical Endocrinology & Metabolism* 78.2 (1994): 393-397.

[56] Nagata, Koji, et al. "Urinary iodine and thyroid antibodies in Okinawa, Yamagata, Hyogo, and Nagano, Japan: the differences in iodine intake do not affect thyroid antibody positivity." *Endocrine journal* 45.6 (1998): 797.

57 Suzuki, M., and T. Tamura. "Iodine intake of Japanese male university students: urinary iodine excretion of sedentary and physically active students and sweat iodine excretion during exercise." *Journal of nutritional science and vitaminology* 31.4 (1985): 409.

58 Ishizuki, Y., Y. Hirooka, and Y. Murata. "[Urinary iodide excretion in Japanese people and thyroid dysfunction]." *Nihon Naibunpi Gakkai Zasshi* 68.5 (1992): 550.

59 Markou, K., et al. "Iodine-induced hypothyroidism." *Thyroid* 11.5 (2001): 501-510.

60 Rubinstein, Herbert M., and Leo Oliner. "Myxedema induced by prolonged iodide administration." *New England Journal of Medicine* 256.2 (1957): 47-52.

61 Hoang, Thanh D., et al. "Over-the-Counter-Drug-Induced Thyroid Disorders." *Endocrine Practice* (2013): 1-18.

62 Yoshinari, Mototaka, et al. "Clinical importance of reversibility in primary goitrous hypothyroidism." *British medical journal (Clinical research ed.)* 287.6394 (1983): 720-722.

63 Mizukami, Y., et al. "Iodine-induced hypothyroidism: a clinical and histological study of 28 patients." *Journal of Clinical Endocrinology & Metabolism* 76.2 (1993): 466-471.

64 Namba, H., et al. "Evidence of thyroid volume increase in normal subjects receiving excess iodide." *Journal of Clinical Endocrinology & Metabolism* 76.3 (1993): 605-608.

65 Connelly, Kara J., et al. "Congenital Hypothyroidism Caused by Excess Prenatal Maternal Iodine Ingestion." *The Journal of Pediatrics* (2012).

66 Vicens-Calvet, Enric, et al. "Diagnosis and treatment in utero of goiter with hypothyroidism caused by iodide overload." *The Journal of pediatrics* 133.1 (1998): 147-148.

67 Carswell, F., M. M. Kerr, and J. H. Hutchison. "Congenital goitre and hypothyroidism produced by maternal ingestion of iodides." *The Lancet* 295.7659 (1970): 1241-1243.

68 Nishiyama, Soroku, et al. "Transient hypothyroidism or persistent hyperthyrotropinemia in neonates born to mothers with excessive iodine intake." *Thyroid* 14.12 (2004): 1077-1083.

69 Pagan, J. D. "Micromineral requirements in horses." *Proceedings*. 2000.

70 Hassan, Abdelhadi I., Galal H. Aref, and A. Samir Kassem. "Congenital iodide-induced goitre with hypothyroidism." *Archives of disease in childhood* 43.232 (1968): 702-704.

71 Dixon, Theodore Frederic. "Bromine in the tissues." *Biochemical Journal* 29.1 (1935): 86.

72 Channer, DM DeR, C. E. J. De Ronde, and E. T. C. Spooner. "The Cl- Br- I- composition of~ 3.23 Ga modified seawater: implications for the geological evolution of ocean halide chemistry." *Earth and planetary science letters* 150.3 (1997): 325-335.

73 Wan, Yi, et al. "Contribution of synthetic and naturally occurring organobromine compounds to bromine mass in marine organisms." *Environmental science & technology* 44.16 (2010): 6068-6073.

74 Kawai, T., et al. "Comparison of urinary bromide levels among people in East Asia, and the effects of dietary intakes of cereals and marine products." *Toxicology letters* 134.1 (2002): 285-293.

75 Romarís-Hortas, Vanessa, et al. "Speciation of the bio-available iodine and bromine forms in edible seaweed by high performance liquid chromatography hyphenated with inductively coupled plasma-mass spectrometry." *Analytica chimica acta* (2012).

76 Saenko, G. N., et al. "Concentration of Iodine and bromine by plants in the seas of Japan and Okhotsk." *Marine Biology* 47.3 (1978): 243-250.

77 Zhang, Z-W., et al. "Urinary bromide levels probably dependent to intake of foods such as sea algae." *Archives of environmental contamination and toxicology* 40.4 (2001): 579-584.

78 Dolphin, Alexis E., et al. "Bromine in Teeth and Bone as an Indicator of Marine Diet." *Journal of Archaeological Science* (2012).

79 Forbes, Gilbert B. "The adult." *Human Body Composition*. Springer New York, 1987. 169-195.

80 Allain, Pierre, et al. "Determination of iodine and bromine in plasma and urine by inductively coupled plasma mass spectrometry." *Analyst* 115.6 (1990): 813-815.

81 Shani, J., et al. "Serum bromine levels in psoriasis." *Pharmacology* 25.6 (2008): 297-307.

82 Hollister, Leo E. "The pre-benzodiazepine era." *Journal of psychoactive drugs* 15.1-2 (1983): 9-13.

83 Pavelka, Stanislav. "Metabolism of bromide and its interference with the metabolism of iodine." *Physiological research* 53 (2004): S81-90.

84 Hand, Commander Eugene A. "Temporary unilateral loss of vision associated with ioderma." *Archives of Dermatology* 54.1 (1946): 29.

85 Burgess, J. F. "Some Recent Researches On Iodide and Bromide Eruptions." *Canadian Medical Association Journal* 15.2 (1925): 178.

86 Baker, David H., Theresa M. Parr, and Nathan R. Augspurger. "Oral iodine toxicity in chicks can be reversed by supplemental bromine." *The Journal of nutrition* 133.7 (2003): 2309-2312.

87 Huff, Jesse W., et al. "A nutritional requirement for bromine." *Proceedings of the Society for Experimental Biology and Medicine. Society for Experimental Biology and Medicine (New York, NY)*. Vol. 92. No. 1. Royal Society of Medicine, 1956.

88 Hassan, Iffat, and Abid Keen. "Potassium iodide in dermatology." *Indian Journal of Dermatology, Venereology, and Leprology* 78.3 (2012): 390.

89 Khan, F., J. M. Einbinder, and N. S. Seriff. "Suppurative ulcerating iododerma—a rare manifestation of inorganic iodide hypersensitivity." *New England Journal of Medicine* 289.19 (1973): 1018-1020.

90 Hollander, Lester, and George H. Fetterman. "Fatal iododerma the eleventh case reported in the literature." *Archives of Dermatology* 34.2 (1936): 228-241.

91 Soria, Caridad, et al. "Vegetating iododerma with underlying systemic diseases: report of three cases." *Journal of the American Academy of Dermatology* 22.3 (1990): 418-422.

92 Eller, Joseph Jordan, and Everett C. Fox. "Fatal iododerma." *Archives of Dermatology* 24.5 (1931): 745-757.

93 Goldstein, D. W. "Fatal iododerma following injection of iodized oil for pulmonary diagnosis." *Journal of the American Medical Association* 106.19 (1936): 1659-1660.

94 Smith, Stephen Z., and S. Randolph Scheen. "Bromoderma." *Archives of Dermatology* 114.3 (1978): 458.

95 Maffeis, Laura, Maria Carmela Musolino, and Stefano Cambiaghi. "Single-plaque vegetating bromoderma." *Journal of the American Academy of Dermatology* 58.4 (2008): 682-684.

96 Wilcox, Reynold Webb. The Treatment of Disease: a Manual of Practical Medicine. P. Blakiston's Son & Co., Philadelphia, 1907, p. 295-296.

97 Hsieh, P. F., et al. "Bromism caused by mix-formulated analgesic injectables." *Human & experimental toxicology* 26.12 (2007): 971-973.

[98] Gay-Lussac, Joseph-Louis. "The history of bromine from discovery to commodity." *Indian journal of chemical technology* 9 (2002): 263-271.

[99] Newton, G. L., et al. "Iodine toxicity. Physiological effects of elevated dietary iodine on calves." *Journal of Animal Science* 38.2 (1974): 449-455.

[100] Brown-Grant, K., and G. Pethes. "Concentration of radio-iodide in the skin of the rat." *The Journal of Physiology* 148.3 (1959): 683-693.

[101] Sunitha, V., and M. Ramakrishna Reddy. "Medical Geology: A Globally Emerging Discipline." *Krishna Rao, KSV.* 1.1 (2012): 57-64.

[102] Iyengar, V. , and J. Woittiez. "Trace elements in human clinical specimens: evaluation of literature data to identify reference values." *Clinical chemistry* 34.3 (1988): 474-481.

[103] Yanagisawa, Isamu, and Shizuo Torii. "A Bromine Compound Existing in Blood." *The Tohoku Journal of Experimental Medicine* 196.3 (2002): 111-121.

[104] Cuenca, R. E., W. J. Pories, and J. Bray. "Bromine levels in human serum, urine, hair." *Biological trace element research* 16.2 (1988): 151-154.

[105] Liebscher K., and Smith, H. "Essential and nonessential trace elements. A method of determining whether an element is essential or nonessential in human tissue." *Arch. Environ. Health* 17.6 (1968): 881–890.

[106] Eskandari, Sepehr, et al. "Thyroid Na+/I− symporter Mechanism, stoichiometry, and specificity." *Journal of Biological Chemistry* 272.43 (1997): 27230-27238.

[107] Baumann, Emil J., et al. "Behavior of the thyroid toward elements of the seventh periodic group." *American Journal of Physiology–Legacy Content* 185.1 (1956): 71-76.

[108] MacAllister, Irene E., et al. "Use of the thyrocyte sodium iodide symporter as the basis for a perchlorate cell-based assay." *Analyst* 134.2 (2009): 320-324.

[109] Erdoğan, Murat Faik. "Thiocyanate overload and thyroid disease." *Biofactors* 19.3 (2003): 107-111.

[110] Gilchrist, Mark, et al. "Effect of dietary nitrate on blood pressure, endothelial function, and insulin sensitivity in type 2 diabetes." *Free Radical Biology and Medicine* (2013).

[111] Guerra, P., et al. "Introduction to Brominated Flame Retardants: Commercially Products, Applications, and Physicochemical Properties." *Brominated Flame Retardants*. Springer Berlin Heidelberg, 2011. 1-17.

[112] Wolff J. "Transport of iodide and other anions in the thyroid gland." *Physiol Rev 44 (1964):45–90.*

[113] Pavelka, Stanislav. "Use of 82 Br and 131 I radionuclides in studies of goitrogenic effects of exogenous bromide." *Journal of Radioanalytical and Nuclear Chemistry* 291.2 (2012): 379-383.

[114] Pavelka, Stanislav. "Metabolism of bromide and its interference with the metabolism of iodine." *Physiological research* 53 (2004): S81-90.

[115] Ullberg, Sven, et al. "A comparison of the distribution of some halide ions in the body." *Biochemical pharmacology* 13.3 (1964): 407-412.

[116] Jauregui-Osoro, Maite, et al. "Synthesis and biological evaluation of [18F] tetrafluoroborate: a PET imaging agent for thyroid disease and reporter gene imaging of the sodium/iodide symporter." *European journal of nuclear medicine and molecular imaging* 37.11 (2010): 2108-2116.

[117] Carlin, Sean, et al. "Sodium-iodide symporter (NIS)-mediated accumulation of [211At] astatide in NIS-transfected human cancer cells." *Nuclear medicine and biology* 29.7 (2002): 729-739.

[118] Seyfert, S. "Accelerated fall in serum bromide level after administration of perchlorate to man." *European Journal of Clinical Pharmacology* 16.5 (1979): 351-353.

[119] Steinmaus, Craig, et al. "Combined effects of perchlorate, thiocyanate, and iodine on thyroid function in the National Health and Nutrition Examination Survey 2007–08." *Environmental Research* (2013).

[120] Dohan, Orsolya, et al. "The Na+/I− symporter (NIS) transports two of its substrates, I− and ClO 4−, with different stoichiometries." (2007).

[121] Leung, Angela M., Elizabeth N. Pearce, and Lewis E. Braverman. "Perchlorate, iodine and the thyroid." *Best Practice & Research Clinical Endocrinology & Metabolism* 24.1 (2010): 133-141.

[122] Chu, Michael, and Terry F. Seltzer. "Myxedema coma induced by ingestion of raw bok choy." *New England Journal of Medicine* 362.20 (2010): 1945-1946.

[123] De Groef, Bert, et al. "Perchlorate versus other environmental sodium/iodide symporter inhibitors: potential thyroid-related health effects." *European Journal of Endocrinology* 155.1 (2006): 17-25.

[124] Kanny, Gisèle, et al. "T cell–mediated reactions to iodinated contrast media: Evaluation by skin and lymphocyte activation tests." *Journal of allergy and clinical immunology* 115.1 (2005): 179-185.

[125] Sumner, John, A. I. Lichter, and E. Nassau. "Fatal acute iodism after bronchography." *Thorax* 6.2 (1951): 193-199.

[126] Scherer, K., et al. "The role of iodine in hypersensitivity reactions to radio contrast media." *Clinical & Experimental Allergy* 40.3 (2010): 468-475.

[127] Faust, John B. "The Production of Iodine in Chile." *Industrial & Engineering Chemistry* 18.8 (1926): 808-811.

[128] Yang, William H., and Emerson CR Purchase. "Adverse reactions to sulfites." *Canadian Medical Association Journal* 133.9 (1985): 865.

[129] Curd, John G., et al. "Potassium iodide sensitivity in four patients with hypocomplementemic vasculitis." *Annals of internal medicine* 91.6 (1979): 853-857.

[130] The Iodine/Iodide Loading Test, available at http://www.optimox.com/pics/Iodine/loadTest.htm Accessed 4/19/2013.

[131] Nelson, Norton, et al. "The absorption, excretion, and physiological effect of iodine in normal human subjects." *Journal of Clinical Investigation* 26.2 (1947): 301.

[132] Zava, Theodore. "Evaluation of the Iodine Loading Test: Urine Iodine Excretion Kinetics after Consumption of 50 mg Iodine/Iodide." *Townsend Letter*, (January 2013).

[133] Guy, E., and David Brownstein. "A Simple Procedure Combining the Evaluation of Whole Body Sufficiency for Iodine With the Efficiency of the Body to Utilize Peripheral Iodide: The Triple Test."

[134] Milakovic, M., et al. "Determination of intrathyroidal iodine by X-ray fluorescence analysis in 60-to 65-year olds living in an iodine-sufficient area." *Journal of internal medicine* 260.1 (2006): 69-75.

[135] Zabala, José, et al. "Determination of normal human intrathyroidal iodine in Caracas population." *Journal of Trace Elements in Medicine and Biology* 23.1 (2009): 9-14.

[136] Zaichick, V. Ye, and Yu Ya Choporov. "Determination of the natural level of human intra-thyroid iodine by instrumental neutron activation analysis." *Journal of radioanalytical and nuclear chemistry* 207.1 (1996): 153-161.

[137] Nicola, Juan Pablo, et al. "Dietary iodide controls its own absorption through post-transcriptional regulation of the intestinal Na+/I− symporter." *The Journal of Physiology* 590.23 (2012): 6013-6026.

[138] Basu, Gopal, and Anjali Mohapatra. "Interactions between thyroid disorders and kidney disease." *Indian Journal of Endocrinology and Metabolism* 16.2 (2012): 204.

[139] Cruz, Francine Dela, et al. "Iodine absorption after topical administration." *Western Journal of Medicine* 146.1 (1987): 43.

[140] Mostofizade, Neda, et al. "The G395R Mutation of the Sodium/Iodide Symporter (NIS) Gene in Patients with Dyshormonogenetic Congenital Hypothyroidism." *International journal of preventive medicine* 4.1 (2013): 57.

[141] Aceves, Carmen, Brenda Anguiano, and Guadalupe Delgado. "The extrathyronine actions of iodine. Antioxidant, apoptotic and differentiator factor in iodine-uptake tissues." *Thyroid* ja (2013).

[142] Bürgi, Hans. "Iodine excess." *Best Practice & Research Clinical Endocrinology & Metabolism* 24.1 (2010): 107-115.

19

Osteoporosis, Gum Disease & Bad Teeth can be from Low or High Thyroid Levels (not low TSH)

You'll get osteoporosis if your TSH is too low.

—common misconception

Thyroid's effect on bones

Bones are living tissues that are constantly remodeled (repaired) by two types of cells: osteoclasts dissolve old bone (bone resorption), while osteoblasts produce new bone (bone formation). These two opposing processes are controlled by several hormones, including thyroid hormone. Thyroid levels that are too high *or* too low can contribute to osteoporosis by affecting the rates of these two processes. An excess of thyroid hormone will speed up both bone resorption and bone formation, but bone resorption predominates, resulting in decreased bone mass. In contrast, a deficiency of thyroid hormone slows down the process of bone resorption, but also slows down bone formation, which results in fragile, brittle bones. Triiodothyronine (T3) is essential for bone matrix formation and collagen maturation (bone generation), so if T3 levels are too low, bone generation is impaired.[1] Healthy bone metabolism requires thyroid levels that are neither too high nor low. The bone remodeling cycle can be as short as 100 days in thyrotoxicosis (high thyroid levels) and over 1,000 days in the case of myxedema (extremely low thyroid levels).[2]

A low Thyroid Stimulating Hormone (TSH) level may be an indicator of high thyroid levels and can be diagnostic for hyperthyroidism. This is why doctors are reluctant to prescribe more thyroid hormone when the TSH drops too low. They cite the possibility of osteoporosis as the reason not to prescribe more hormone, because high thyroid levels can indeed cause osteoporosis. They will only prescribe enough to bring the TSH into the reference range. Unfortunately, some people with a low TSH actually have low thyroid levels. Because of the misleading TSH test, patients may be kept on a thyroid replacement dose that is so low they still remain hypothyroid, and with time, they eventually develop low thyroid symptoms that include osteoporosis, osteopenia, gingivitis, perio-dontitis, high cholesterol, heart disease, and depression.

A study of mice that lacked thyroid hormone receptors illustrates the dangers of thyroid levels that are too high or too low. A receptor is like a lock that is opened with a key—in this case, thyroid hormone. Without specific thyroid receptors, thyroid hormone (T3 or T4) may have no effect. Mice that were thyroid receptor alpha deficient developed osteosclerosis (abnormal hardening of the bone) and reduced osteoclastic bone resorp-tion, a form of skeletal hypothyroidism, even though thyroid hormone and TSH levels were normal. Mice that were thyroid receptor beta deficient had elevated TSH and thyroid hormone levels, and developed osteoporosis with evidence of increased bone resorption. These mice displayed skeletal thyrotoxicosis without a suppressed TSH, which means elevated thyroid hormone levels, not a low TSH, caused osteoporosis.[3] This is another reason why both Free T3 and Free T4 should be monitored, not the TSH.

To determine the relative importance of T3 and TSH in bone, the skeletal properties of two mouse models with congenital hypothyroidism were compared. One type of mouse had a 1900-fold increase in TSH (certainly not deficient), a normal TSH Receptor, and undetectable T3 and T4 levels. The other had a 2300-fold elevation of TSH, a nonfunc-tional TSH Receptor, and a T4 level that was 95% lower than wild mice. Both types of mice displayed skeletal hypothyroidism: delayed ossification (new bone formation), reduced cortical bone (the stronger, outer part), a trabecular bone remodeling defect (old bone must be resorbed to make way for new bone), reduced bone mineralization (where calcium is added to bone), and impaired osteoblast T3 target gene expression (bone building cells are not activated).[4] Because one type of mouse had a normal TSH receptor and the other did not, it stands to reason that TSH is not the major determinant of skele-tal development, since both types of mice had skeletal hypothyroidism with ample TSH. The lack of T3 and/or T4 would be more likely. Also, TSH did not influence primary osteoblast (bone formation) or osteoclast (bone resorption) differentiation and functional activity *in vitro* (in a lab). Earlier mice studies support these conclusions: low T3 levels caused reduced bone mineralization and delayed ossification.

Female human thyroid cancer patients who received thyroidectomies and then sup-pressive doses of T4 medications (their TSH was nearly zero) were compared to normal controls to examine the effects on bone mineral density. When the patients were sepa-rated into premenopausal and postmenopausal groups, bone mineral density in both the femoral neck (top of the thigh bone that fits into the hip socket) and lumbar spine (lower back) was similar between patients and controls. The proportion of women with normal bone mass density, osteopenia and osteoporosis in patient and control groups was similar in the pre- and postmenopausal groups. Long-term TSH suppressive T4 treatment did not appear to affect skeletal integrity in these women.[5] In other words, even though TSH was kept at an undetectable level in the thyroid cancer patients, their bone health was not different from normal women *of their age*. This study points to age and menopausal status as the primary determinants of bone health, not TSH. Lower levels of estrogen are normal in menopause, and there are numerous studies that implicate estrogen deficiency in osteoporosis.[6] Progesterone, which also declines once ovulation stops, has also been shown to help build and maintain bones.[7] In this case, lack of TSH cannot be said to be the primary cause of poor bones.

Thyroid's effect on teeth

Gingivitis, periodontitis, gum disease, bad teeth, dentures at age 25, and root canals at age 12 have been reported by members of thyroid internet forums. Like bones, there is a definite connection between dental health and optimal thyroid levels.

Periodontitis is the inflammation/infection of the gums (gingivitis) that leads to inflammation/infection of the bones and ligaments that support the teeth, which can cause the teeth to become loose and eventually fall out. A study of nearly 14,000 people in the U.S. who had received a periodontal exam found that severe periodontitis is associated with the metabolic syndrome in middle-aged subjects. Interestingly, the five symptoms of the metabolic syndrome are similar to the symptoms of hypothyroidism: abdominal obesity, high triglycerides, low HDL cholesterol, hypertension, and insulin resistance.[8] If low thyroid levels are the root cause of the metabolic syndrome, then they would also be implicated in periodontitis. In fact, one study found that low normal Free T4 levels were significantly associated with increased insulin resistance and all the other metabolic syndrome traits except hypertension.[9]

In postmenopausal women with periodontitis, there is an increased proportion of osteopenia and osteoporosis cases of the lumbar spine and femur. This suggests an association between bone mineral density and periodontitis.[10] It appears that the condition that is affecting the teeth is also affecting the bones, and this condition could be low thyroid levels, as discussed in the first section.

Tooth loss that results from root resorption is an occasional unfortunate side effect of orthodontia (braces). Rats treated with thyroid hormone (who had orthodontic appliances inserted) displayed significantly less force-induced root resorptive lesions compared with a control group.[11] In other words, thyroid hormone treatment resulted in less root resorption. Another study confirmed these findings—hypothyroidism significantly increased periodontitis-related bone loss, as a function of an increased number of resorbing cells.[12] In other words, low thyroid levels can negatively affect the bones that support your teeth. The results from the rats suggest that orthodontia is not a good idea for someone who is hypothyroid, because it may result in tooth loss.

To see what effect thyroid levels had on titanium implants, rat tibiae (leg bones) were implanted with titanium screws. The hyperthyroid rats had significantly more newly formed bone around the implants, whereas the hypothyroid rats had significantly less.[13] This suggests that dental implants may not be successful if the patient is still hypothyroid, which could be the cause of tooth loss in the first place.

Thyroid treatments such as T3-only and hydrocortisone (HC) may cause osteoporosis

Osteoporosis can be caused by thyroid hormone deficiency, as discussed earlier in this chapter. At the other end of the spectrum, excessive thyroid hormones, especially T3, can lead to elevated sex hormone binding globulin (SHBG) levels,[14] and elevated SHBG levels are a major risk factor for osteoporosis.[15] SHBG can be affected by other factors like age, weight, sex steroids, and insulin, to name just a few, but there is a strong positive correlation of high T3 with high SHBG, and high SHBG is correlated with poor bone mineral density and osteoporotic fractures of the vertebra and peripheral bones, especially the femur (thigh bone).[16] Hip fractures are also associated with higher levels of SHBG, independent of bioavailable estradiol and testosterone levels.[17] SHBG appears to have a bone wasting effect on post-menopausal women, while estradiol has a bone preserving effect.[18] SHBG levels, in conjunction with symptoms and other thyroid lab tests (like Free T3), could be used to determine when thyroid levels are too high.

Hydrocortisone (HC) supplementation to treat adrenal insufficiency, at excessive levels, can also lead to osteoporosis. Hydrocortisone is the bioidentical replacement for the hormone cortisol, but because cortisol has a circadian rhythm and rises and falls on its own in response to stress, it is nearly impossible to replicate by manual dosing. If cortisol levels throughout the day were depicted graphically, it would look like a downward sloping curve--highest in the early morning, and lowest at night. Manual HC dosing would show as multiple, decreasing mountain peaks, with cortisol levels above the normal level immediately after a dose, and then below the normal level before the next dose. These high cortisol peaks are behind the physical high cortisol signs of moon face, buffalo hump, "Buddha belly," and general weight gain. Bones may also be adversely affected, because corticosteroids not only decrease bone formation, they also increase bone resorption.[19] A hydrocortisone dose no higher than 20 mg/day is sufficient for daily life, according to some studies. In fact, one study had patients reduce their 20-30 mg daily hydrocortisone doses to 10-15 mg/day. None of the patients reported low cortisol symptoms. Instead, 10 out of 11 subjects lost weight (specifically abdominal fat), total cholesterol and triglycerides decreased, and Quality of Life scores improved.[20] Another study that compared the effects of 15, 20, and 30 mg of daily hydrocortisone found no difference in Quality of Life between the doses, but a negative correlation with osteocalcin (a protein involved with bone formation) as the hydrocortisone dose was increased. In other words, as the HC dose increased, bone formation decreased. Since bone loss would be induced at a daily hydrocortisone dose of 30 mg, the study recommended 15 to 20 mg of HC instead.[21] Bone density scans are recommended while on hydrocortisone, and Vitamin D levels should also be tested and treated if low.[22]

Conclusion

Osteoporosis is a real risk when a thyroid patient is either over or undermedicated. Since TSH is not a reliable marker of thyroid levels, it cannot be used to gauge the correct dose for an individual. But there are other lab tests that may indicate when thyroid levels are too high. High SHBG levels are correlated with poor bone health, and tend to rise when thyroid levels are too high, especially on the T3-only protocol. Hydrocortisone supplementation may also have adverse effects on bone health, and someone who is on both T3 and HC should have regular bone density scans. Calcium levels rise in some hyperthyroid patients. Serum concentrations of alkaline phosphatase, osteocalcin, osteoprotegerin, and FGF-23 correlate with the severity of biochemical hyperthyroidism.[23] In other words, these serum markers will rise as the thyroid dose rises, which is a bad sign for bone health. In another study, high levels of four bone resorption markers were associated with an increased fracture risk: urinary-free deoxypyridinoline (D-Pyr), urinary type I collagen N-telopeptides (NTX), and urinary and serum type I collagen C-telopeptides

(CTX). Low serum levels of estradiol and dehydroepiandrosterone-sulfate (DHEA-S) were also associated with a higher risk of fracture.[24]

Some patients believe that the calcitonin found in desiccated thyroid is protective to their bones, but in one study, no dose of intranasal calcitonin appeared to offer any benefit to bone mineral density or bone resorption in those who were biochemically hyperthyroid.[25] Calcitonin is also not well absorbed orally; prescription calcitonin is given nasally or through injection.[26] In reality, an overdose of T3 and/or T4 from any source, whether it's desiccated thyroid, synthetic T3 or T4, or overproduction from one's own gland, can result in high bone turnover osteoporosis with an increased susceptibility to fractures. In one study, doses of 3 grains or higher of natural desiccated thyroid resulted in a lower combined cortical thickness (CCT), which is a measure of bone health (a higher value is desirable). Subjects on 4 grains had a lower CCT than the subjects on 3 grains, while those on 2 grains had a higher CCT.[27]

Likewise, insufficient levels of T3 and/or T4 can result in reduced bone turnover and formation and cause brittle bones. Healthy bones should obtain the majority of their T3 energy from the conversion of T4 (through the D2 deiodinase enzyme).[28] This may explain why bone loss is found in patients taking high doses of T4.[29] Or it may be that those on T4-only lack the benefits of T3 in bone generation. Likewise, those on desiccated thyroid have a relative T4 deficiency until they approach 3 grains, because humans produce, on average, about 100 mcg T4 daily.[30] The T4 content in desiccated thyroid only rises above 100 mcg at a dose of 2.75 grains, but that dose contains too much T3 for some patients.

If someone has been hypothyroid and undermedicated for years (with low T3 levels) because they have been dosed by TSH, they may suffer from brittle bones, because healthy bone was not produced for years. If they then transition to desiccated thyroid or the T3-only protocol and take too high a dose, it may cause high bone turnover on already weak bones and increase the susceptibility to fractures. This is not a good scenario. As with most hormones, levels that are either too high or low can be detrimental, and patients should strive for balance.

Key points

- Osteoporosis can be caused by thyroid levels that are too high *or* too low.
- A low TSH is not always an indicator of high (hyperthyroid) thyroid hormone levels.
- High thyroid levels increase bone resorption and bone loss.
- Low thyroid levels decrease bone generation.
- Studies in mice show that TSH had no effect on bone health, but an excess or deficiency of T3 and/or T4 did.
- Age and menopausal status in women are the primary determinants of bone health.
- Both estrogen and progesterone may keep bones healthy, not the presence of TSH.
- Low thyroid levels are associated with periodontitis.
- Thyroid hormone keeps the bones that support teeth healthy.

- Orthodontia may be unsuccessful in severely hypothyroid patients; it may result in root resorption which could result in tooth loss.
- Dental implants may be unsuccessful in severely hypothyroid patients because new bone formation around the implants is impaired.
- High thyroid levels, especially T3, may raise SHBG, which is strongly correlated with osteoporosis.
- The use of hydrocortisone is correlated with osteoporosis.
- Some studies report bone loss on a daily HC dose of 30 mg.
- Bone turnover markers like elevated calcium and alkaline phosphatase may be indicators that the thyroid dose is too high.
- The calcitonin in desiccated thyroid probably has a minimal effect on bones, since calcitonin cannot be absorbed orally.
- Doses of 3 grains or more of desiccated thyroid had a negative effect on bones in one study.

---

[1] Varga, F., et al. "T3 affects expression of collagen I and collagen cross-linking in bone cell cultures." *Biochemical and biophysical research communications* 402.2 (2010): 180-185.

[2] Eriksen, Erik Fink. "Cellular mechanisms of bone remodeling." *Reviews in Endocrine and Metabolic Disorders* 11.4 (2010): 219-227.

[3] Bassett, JH Duncan, et al. "A lack of thyroid hormones rather than excess thyrotropin causes abnormal skeletal development in hypothyroidism." *Molecular endocrinology* 22.2 (2008): 501-512.

[4] Bassett, JH Duncan, et al. "Thyroid hormone excess rather than thyrotropin deficiency induces osteoporosis in hyperthyroidism." *Molecular Endocrinology* 21.5 (2007): 1095-1107.

[5] Reverter, J. L., et al. "Lack of deleterious effect on bone mineral density of long-term thyroxine suppressive therapy for differentiated thyroid carcinoma." *Endocrine-Related Cancer* 12.4 (2005): 973-981.

[6] Khosla, Sundeep, L. Joseph Melton, and B. Lawrence Riggs. "The unitary model for estrogen deficiency and the pathogenesis of osteoporosis: is a revision needed?" *Journal of Bone and Mineral Research* 26.3 (2011): 441-451.

[7] Schmidmayr, M., et al. "Progesterone enhances differentiation of primary human osteoblasts in long-term cultures." *Geburtshilfe und Frauenheilkunde* 68.07 (2008): 722-728.

[8] D'Aiuto, Francesco, et al. "Association of the metabolic syndrome with severe periodontitis in a large US population-based survey." *Journal of Clinical Endocrinology & Metabolism* 93.10 (2008): 3989-3994.

[9] Roos, Annemieke, et al. "Thyroid function is associated with components of the metabolic syndrome in euthyroid subjects." *Journal of Clinical Endocrinology & Metabolism* 92.2 (2007): 491-496.

[10] Suresh, Snophia, et al. "Periodontitis and bone mineral density among pre and post menopausal women: A comparative study." *Journal of Indian Society of Periodontology* 14.1 (2010): 30.

[11] Vázquez-Landaverde, Luis Andrés, et al. "Periodontal 5′-deiodination on forced-induced root resorption—the protective effect of thyroid hormone administration." *The European Journal of Orthodontics* 24.4 (2002): 363-369.

[12] Feitosa, D. S., et al. "The influence of thyroid hormones on periodontitis-related bone loss and tooth-supporting alveolar bone: a histological study in rats." *Journal of periodontal research* 44.4 (2009): 472-478.

[13] Feitosa, Daniela da Silva, et al. "Thyroid hormones may influence cortical bone healing around titanium implants: a histometric study in rats." *Journal of periodontology* 79.5 (2008): 881-887.

[14] Staub, J. J., et al. "[Sex hormone binding globulin (SHBG), a new metabolic in vitro thyroid function test]." *Schweizerische medizinische Wochenschrift* 108.48 (1978): 1909-1911.

[15] Lormeau, C., et al. "Sex hormone-binding globulin, estradiol, and bone turnover markers in male osteoporosis." *Bone* 34.6 (2004): 933-939.

[16] Hoppé, Emmanuel, et al. "Sex hormone-binding globulin in osteoporosis." *Joint Bone Spine* 77.4 (2010): 306-312.

[17] Lee, Jennifer S., et al. "Associations of serum sex hormone-binding globulin and sex hormone concentrations with hip fracture risk in postmenopausal women." *Journal of Clinical Endocrinology & Metabolism* 93.5 (2008): 1796-1803.

[18] Hemert, Albert M., et al. "Sex hormone binding globulin in postmenopausal women: a predictor of osteoporosis superior to endogenous oestrogens." *Clinical endocrinology* 31.4 (1989): 499-509.

[19] Basak, Ramen C., Manas Chatterjee, and Mahmoud W. Rassem. "A Case of Severe Primary Hyperthyroidism, Secondary Hyperparathyroidism, Adrenal Insufficiency and Osteoporosis with Multiple Fractures." *Kuwait Medical Journal* 41.2 (2009): 152-155.

[20] Danilowicz, Karina, et al. "Correction of cortisol overreplacement ameliorates morbidities in patients with hypopituitarism: a pilot study." *Pituitary* 11.3 (2008): 279-285.

[21] Wichers, Maria, et al. "The influence of hydrocortisone substitution on the quality of life and parameters of bone metabolism in patients with secondary hypocortisolism." *Clinical endocrinology* 50.6 (1999): 759-765.

[22] Quinkler, Marcus, and Stefanie Hahner. "What is the best long-term management strategy for patients with primary adrenal insufficiency?" *Clinical endocrinology* 76.1 (2012): 21-25.

[23] Gorka, Jagoda, Regina M. Taylor-Gjevre, and Terra Arnason. "Metabolic and Clinical Consequences of Hyperthyroidism on Bone Density." *International Journal of Endocrinology* 2013 (2013).

[24] Garnero, Patrick, et al. "Biochemical markers of bone turnover, endogenous hormones and the risk of fractures in postmenopausal women: the OFELY study." *Journal of Bone and Mineral Research* 15.8 (2000): 1526-1536.

[25] Jódar, Esteban, et al. "Antiresorptive therapy in hyperthyroid patients: longitudinal changes in bone and mineral metabolism." *Journal of Clinical Endocrinology & Metabolism* 82.6 (1997): 1989-1994.

[26] Lee, Yong-Hee, and Patrick J. Sinko. "Oral delivery of salmon calcitonin." *Advanced drug delivery reviews* 42.3 (2000): 225-238.

[27] Ettinger, Bruce, and John Wingerd. "Thyroid supplements: effect on bone mass." *Western Journal of Medicine* 136.6 (1982): 473.

[28] Bassett, JH Duncan, et al. "Optimal bone strength and mineralization requires the type 2 iodothyronine deiodinase in osteoblasts." *Proceedings of the National Academy of Sciences* 107.16 (2010): 7604-7609.

[29] Ross, Douglas S., et al. "Subclinical hyperthyroidism and reduced bone density as a possible result of prolonged suppression of the pituitary-thyroid axis with L-thyroxine." *The American journal of medicine* 82.6 (1987): 1167-1170.

[30] Wiersinga, Wilmar M., et al. "2012 ETA Guidelines: The Use of L-T4+ L-T3 in the Treatment of Hypothyroidism." *European Thyroid Journal* 1.2 (2012): 55-71.

20

Prescription Thyroid Choices & Dosing Protocols

*Treatment of hypothyroidism is best accomplished using
synthetic T4 sodium preparations.*

—debatable statement from the 2012 Clinical
Practice Guidelines for Hypothyroidism in
Adults: Co-sponsored by the American Associ-
ation of Clinical Endocrinologists and the
American Thyroid Association

The different types of prescription thyroid hormone

There are three different types of thyroid hormone prescriptions for hypothyroid patients, and each has pros and cons. Levothyroxine or synthetic thyroxine (T4) is the Standard of Care that endocrinologists have been taught to prescribe. Synthroid is the oldest brand name, and generics are also available at a lower cost. Tirosint is a fairly new brand of T4 in gel cap form, with no food colors in any dose. The problem with taking just T4 is that a normal thyroid secretes a little triiodothyronine (T3) in addition to T4. In fact, a normal thyroid *produces*, on average, about 100 mcg T4 and 6 mcg T3 daily,[1] though it *secretes* closer to 10 mcg of T3, because some conversion from T4 to T3 is performed in the thyroid gland before release. Therefore, to truly replicate a normal thyroid, both T4 *and* T3 should be taken.[2] In fact, the presence of T3 induces the D1 deiodinase enzyme that converts T4 to T3 in the liver, kidney, thyroid, and pituitary gland. It is responsible for the T3 found in plasma.[3] This is an extremely important point that is often overlooked, and may be why those on T4-only replacement tend to have lower T3 levels and a higher FT4/FT3 ratio (despite similar TSH values), when compared to normal controls.[4]

Cytomel or liothyronine (synthetic T3) is the second type of prescription thyroid hormone, but difficult to get prescribed. Most doctors have been taught that T4 is all that is necessary, so that's what most will prescribe.

Natural desiccated thyroid (NDT), which is made from dried (desiccated) pig thyroid glands, is available in the U.S. as Armour Thyroid and Nature-Throid, but both have had an availability problem in the last few years. NDT contains both T4 and T3. Many patients reported that a reformulation of Armour in 2009 made the medication ineffective for them. NP Thyroid, a new desiccated thyroid brand, became available in

November 2010. Availability problems were reported by patients in 2013. Another new brand, WP Thyroid, was introduced in spring 2013. Erfa Thyroid, which is most like Armour before it was reformulated, can be ordered from Canadian pharmacies, but shortages were reported early in 2014. A doctor's prescription is required to place an order, ample lead time is required to get through customs, and it may not be reimbursed by insurance. Shipment time from Canada has varied from four days to five weeks for me. The five-week delay did not appear to be a customs issue; it was likely a local postal problem because we have had other problems with other U.S. packages that never arrived.

Over the years, several prescription thyroid formulations have disappeared, new ones have been introduced, and availability problems have become commonplace. The list above does not include every available brand of thyroid hormone that exists worldwide, but was meant to give an overview of the three different types: T4, T3, or NDT.

What's the difference between T4, T3, and desiccated thyroid?

Which type of prescription should a patient choose? Well like most things medical, it depends. There are some who are militant that desiccated thyroid is the only way to go. But it is contraindicated in some. A few people on Graves' forums have reported that their Thyroid Stimulating Immunoglobulin (TSI) antibodies increased and their thyroid eye disease worsened after they started desiccated thyroid. The theory is that their anti-bodies recognized the antigens in the pork thyroid glands and mounted an attack. Returning to synthetic T4 and/or T3 often resolved the problem. Yet others with Graves' take desiccated thyroid successfully. And others without Graves' have had negative reactions too. The bottom line is that individual responses vary to the three different thyroid formulations.

T4 prescriptions like levothyroxine usually result in a free and total T4 in the upper half of the reference range, but a free and total T3 in the lower half. When patients report lingering hypothyroid symptoms to their doctors, they are usually prescribed additional T4. Not surprisingly, this can cause the T4 levels to go over range, without much of an increase in T3, nor much improvement in symptoms. This does not match normal thyroid production. Both T4 *and* T3 must be taken to simulate healthy thyroid gland output. One study compared the Total T3/T4 ratios of healthy people to the ratios of T4-medicated patients and found a lower ratio in the T4-medicated patients. A very simple way to equalize the ratios would be to add some T3.[5]

Most people who have switched from synthetic T4 to desiccated thyroid report feeling better, especially if they have no thyroid gland. It's a popular medication; it's just difficult to find a doctor to prescribe it. Desiccated thyroid is made from whole pig thyroid glands and therefore contains all the components found in a thyroid gland: T4, T3, reverse T3 (rT3), diiodotyrosine (DIT), monoiodotyrosine (MIT), thyroglobulin, thyroperoxidase enzyme (TPO), hydrogen peroxide (H_2O_2), iodide, tyrosyl residues, and calcitonin (a hormone involved in calcium and bone metabolism).[6] Calcitonin is not a thyroid hormone, but another hormone produced by the parafollicular cells, which just happen to be located within the thyroid. Prescription calcitonin is administered by nasal spray, rectally, or by injection, because it is not absorbed well orally,[7] so its effect in desiccated thyroid may be minimal. However, there is probably a synergy in all these components that makes it more complete and effective than synthetic replacements. People on desiccated thyroid tend to have healthier bones, but that may be from the T3, not the calcitonin. Studies show that some T3 is essential to bone health.[8]

Some thyroid patients claim that T2 and T1 are the special ingredients in desiccated thyroid, but thyroid physiology textbooks say that only T4, T3, MIT, and DIT are produced in the thyroid gland. T2 has only been measured in trace amounts in thyroglobulin in the thyroid,[9] and T1 cannot be formed by combining the iodotyrosine building blocks MIT (1 iodine) and DIT (2 iodine). Thyroid hormone (also known as an iodothyronine) is produced when two iodotyrosines (MIT or DIT) couple together, forming a compound with two tyrosyl residues. MIT and DIT, in any combination, cannot form T1. Therefore, T2, T3, and T4 are the only possible thyroid hormones that could be manufactured *within* the thyroid gland, though T2 production may be accidental, since it is only found in trace amounts. Perhaps the confusion is because one of the thyroid precursors is called diiodo*tyrosine* (DIT), while T2 is also known as diiodo*thyronine*. The words are similar but they refer to two different things: DIT is a precursor with only one tyrosine ring, while T2 has two tyrosine rings and has measurable effects as a thyroid hormone. Diiodotyrosine (DIT), like T4 and T3, has been found in the thyroid and in serum.[10]

The following eight charts illustrate how thyroid hormone is produced and dispel some well-entrenched internet myths. Figures 20-6, 20-7, and 20-8 illustrate the common misconceptions. My apologies to real chemists; I have grossly simplified the molecules in order to show only the relevant parts. Thyroid hormone is primarily composed of iodide and tyrosine. The hexagon represents the tyrosine ring, and the *I* represents iodide.

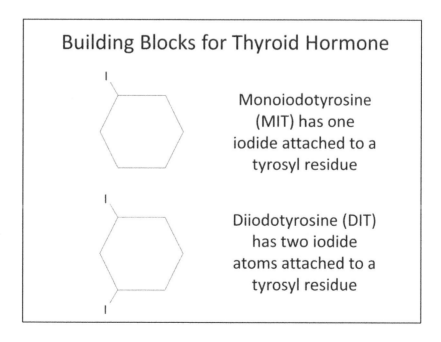

Figure 20-1. There are only two building blocks that make T4 and T3: MIT and DIT.

3,3'-Diiodothyronine or T2

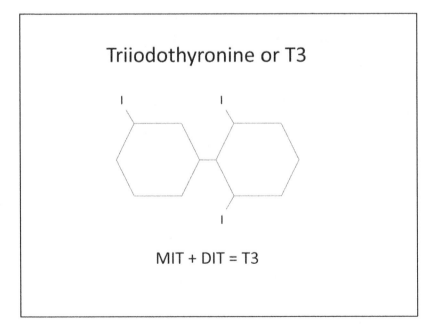

MIT + MIT = T2

Figure 20-2. MIT + MIT = T2

Triiodothyronine or T3

MIT + DIT = T3

Figure 20-3. MIT + DIT = T3

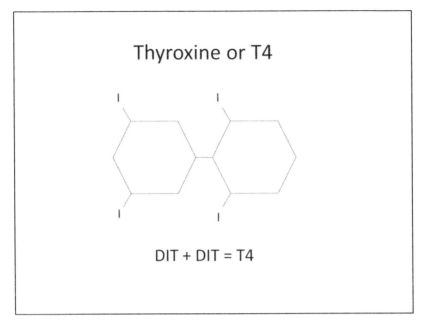

Figure 20-4. DIT + DIT = T4

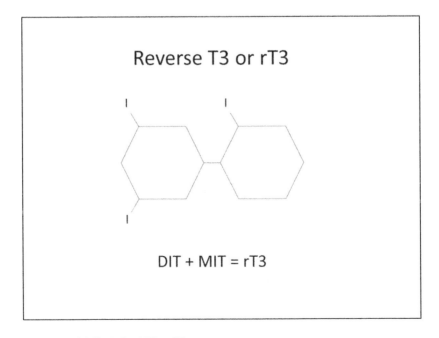

Figure 20-5. DIT + MIT = rT3

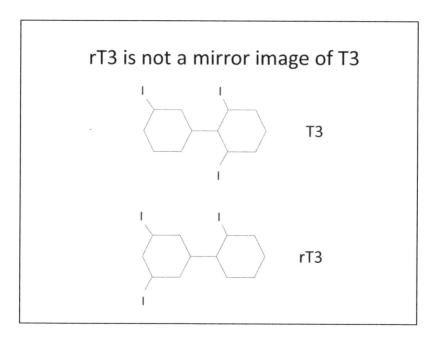

Figure 20-6. rT3 is not a mirror image of T3

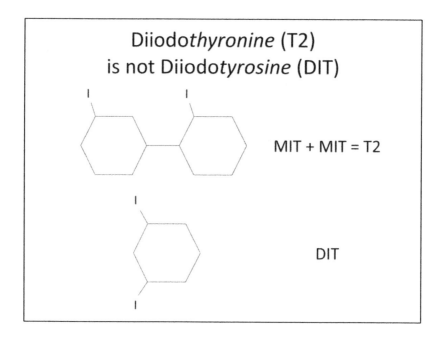

Figure 20-7. T2 and DIT are two different molecules, even though their scientific names sound alike.

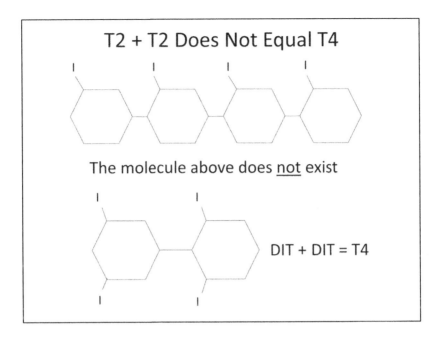

Figure 20-8. T4 is made from DIT + DIT, not T2 + T2.

Where do T2 and T1 come from, if they're not made within the thyroid gland? They are produced from deiodination *outside* of the thyroid gland.[6] Deiodination is the process where an enzyme strips off one iodine from T4, resulting in T3 (or rT3). The process of deiodination continues and another iodine is stripped off forming T2 (there are three types of T2), then T1 (there are two types of T1), and eventually T0, otherwise known as a non-iodinated thyronine.[11] The production rate of T2 is very close to the combined T3 + rT3 production rate. In other words, T2 came from deiodination of T3 or rT3.[9] Desiccated thyroid cannot be considered a major source of T2 or T1, since it would only contain the hormones normally found in a thyroid gland (T4, T3, rT3, and the precursors MIT and DIT).

In one laboratory experiment, thyroid hormone production was found to be pH dependent. The higher the pH, the more hormone was formed.[12] The majority of the hormone produced was T4, followed by rT3, T3, and negligible amounts of T2. No T2 was produced if the pH was below 6, though the other hormones were still produced at a pH of 5. Another study referenced in this report determined that thyroglobulin from actual human thyroid glands contained approximately 90% T4, 7.4% T3, 2.2% rT3, and 0.4% T2, as illustrated in Figure 20-9.

If rT3 is made in the thyroid gland, then it will be a component of desiccated thyroid. Anyone taking desiccated thyroid would then be ingesting some amount of rT3, which is a normal metabolite of thyroid conversion, as discussed in Chapter 23 on rT3. They should not be surprised if their rT3 levels rise as their desiccated thyroid dose rises.

Does T2 have any biological activity? Studies show that it does. In one study, rats were fed a high fat diet, and some rats were given T2 for 30 days, while the control rats were not. The T2 group showed reduced fat accumulation, triglycerides, cholesterol, fat content of the liver, and body weight, when compared to the control rats fed the same high fat diet, that were not given T2.[13]

The T3 in desiccated thyroid stimulates an enzyme that converts T4 to T3 in the liver, kidneys, and thyroid, and contributes to circulating T3 in the body. The same enzyme also converts rT3 to T2.[14] T3 and rT3 are the precursors to T2, and desiccated thyroid provides both, so the essential raw material for T2 is more readily available. Interestingly, enzymes convert both T3 and rT3 to T2, but the conversion is rapid from rT3, but slow from T3.[15]

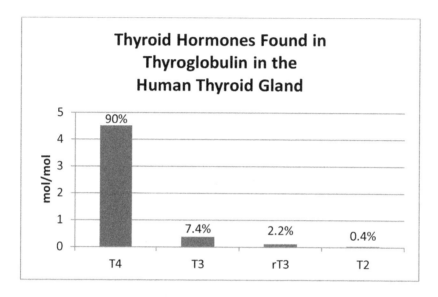

Figure 20-9. Thyroglobulin content from thyroid glands shows that T4 is the primary hormone made, with much lower amounts of T3 and rT3, and only negligible amounts of T2.

Many on desiccated thyroid show a low in range Total and Free T4 even though their Free T3 may be closer to the middle of the reference range or higher. This is because desiccated thyroid is approximately 80% T4, and 20% T3, while a normal human's thyroid output is closer to 90% T4 and 10% T3. The simple remedy for people who test low in T4 is to take both synthetic T4 *and* desiccated thyroid. Studies show that both T4 and T3 need to be optimal for mental and physical well-being. The brain and body are in two different compartments, and some functions prefer T4, others T3.[16]

Other people do not convert their T4 to T3 as readily, so their labs will look fine on desiccated thyroid, with Total T4 (or Free T4) *and* Free T3 roughly in the same part of the reference range. In other words, their T3 and T4 values rise together, at about the same rate. Really poor converters will show Total T4 in the upper half, but Free T3 in the lower half. These people have underlying conversion problems that should be addressed. Are ferritin and cortisol optimal? Are other drugs such as beta blockers being taken that may interfere with conversion? Is the patient diabetic? If all factors have been addressed, then the ideal dose might be desiccated thyroid + additional T3. Desiccated thyroid could be used as the base, with additional T4 or T3 added as necessary to bring the person's thyroid labs into the optimal range, or to a point where they feel best. This is usually accomplished through trial and error.

Is there an optimal dose or type of thyroid prescription patients should ask for?

Is there an optimal dosage that patients should aim for? Is any type of prescription thyroid replacement better than others? My personal opinion is an emphatic NO! First person testimonies show that people are successfully taking T4-only, T4 + T3, T3-only, desiccated thyroid, and combinations of all the above. I have read case studies of people with myxedema (severest hypothyroid state) taking 15 grains,[17] which would be an overdose for most other people. The wide variation in doses between individuals is due to different absorption rates (gut health), different conversion rates (liver health), and whether a systemic illness is present (which increases enzymes that "fritter away" any T3, keeping T3 levels low). Even some foods (coffee, high fiber foods), medical conditions (celiac disease, lactose intolerance, *Helicobacter pylori* infection), and supplements (calcium, iron) will affect absorption.[18] Graves' patients may have higher conversion rates because of their TSI antibodies, which stimulate T4 to T3 conversion, and may fare better on T4-only.[19]

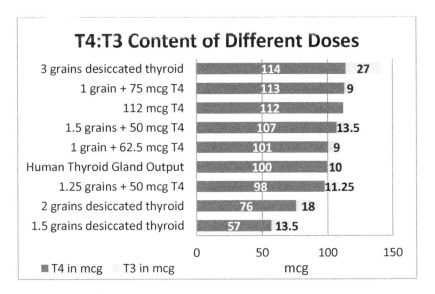

Figure 20-10. Only the combinations of NDT + T4 provide a T3/T4 ratio that is comparable to a normal thyroid gland. NDT has a much higher T3/T4 ratio than is found in humans. At 2 grains, the T3 content of 18 mcg is already almost 2x that of a normal human thyroid gland's daily output of 10 mcg.

Because of the TSH feedback loop, it is very difficult to just "supplement" thyroid hormone; any external dose usually suppresses the patient's own thyroid hormone production because the decrease in TSH means less stimulation to their own thyroid gland. Once thyroid production is suppressed, the dose must then be raised high enough for hypothyroid symptoms to disappear. For some, 3 grains of desiccated thyroid is a serious overdose (because it has too much T3 for them) and can result in typical hyper-thyroid symptoms like fatigue, muscle weakness, shortness of breath, hair loss, etc. which can be mistaken for hypothyroid symptoms. Someone who has never been on desiccated thyroid should have lab work once they have worked up to 1.5 grains and held the dose for six weeks. At that point, some people are already at optimal levels, while others are still in the lower part of the thyroid reference ranges. Or, like me, they will have an imbalance in their FT3 and FT4 levels, with FT3 much higher in the reference range than FT4, because of desiccated thyroid's higher T3 content (Figure 20-10). Testing at this point allows them to fine-tune their dosage before overshooting. In my case, it was a mistake to raise to 2 grains, and I feel much better combining 1-1.5 grains NDT + somewhere between 25-75 mcg T4.

My observation from reading thousands of posts on thyroid forums is that quite a few people optimize on less than 3 grains of desiccated thyroid, but that doesn't mean some won't need more, and some less. Some may benefit from adding T4 to their dose if their thyroid lab results show them high in T3 and low in T4. Likewise, others might do better adding some T3 to their dose if their lab results show them high in T4 and low in T3. They might also want to look into conversion problems. The optimal thyroid dosage for each individual varies; age, weight, and gender having nothing to do with an optimal dose. To insist that only one type of medication will work for everyone, be it synthetic T4, natural desiccated thyroid, or synthetic T3-only, is illogical, given that everyone's bio-chemistry is different. Symptoms should be used in conjunction with thyroid reference ranges to determine the optimal dose. If thyroid lab results (either Free T3 or Free T4) are below the midpoint of the range and the patient still exhibits multiple, common hypothyroid symptoms (like fatigue and feeling cold all the time), it would make sense to increase the thyroid hormone that is deficient by adding either a little more T4 or T3, or both. Few people feel well when their thyroid hormone levels are at the bottom of the reference range. There are literally thousands of hypothyroid patients on the forums who will attest to that. T3 and T4 reference ranges are both negatively skewed curves (a statistical description that means the majority of the healthy values *start* just below the middle of the range; in other words, there are few values at the bottom of the range).

Why do some people do so well on desiccated thyroid and so poorly on T4?

Some people have reactions (dizziness, nausea, diarrhea[20]) to the extra filler ingredients found in levothyroxine, but some of the same ingredients (lactose monohydrate, corn-starch) are also found in some desiccated thyroid pills. Food colors are in every strength of levothyroxine except the 50 mcg pill. T4 pills contain levothyroxine sodium; when stomach acid cleaves the sodium off, what is left is a molecule that is bioidentical in molecular structure to human T4. It may be that some patients don't produce enough stomach acid to cleave off the sodium, so never realize the benefit of the T4. It is not that levothyroxine sodium is "crap" (a term used by patients who did poorly on T4), but possibly that they are unable to utilize it in pill form. In fact, some gastric bypass patients who had a normal TSH on levothyroxine pills prior to surgery developed an elevated TSH after surgery, which suggests malabsorption. When these patients were placed on an oral liquid form of T4, their TSH reverted back to normal levels, which suggests that levothyroxine itself was not the problem, but that lack of absorption of the pill form was. These patients had Roux-en-Y gastric bypass (RYGB), which bypasses almost the entire stomach, which is the source of stomach acid. This is why levothyroxine ingestion is recommended on an empty stomach before breakfast, to benefit from gastric acidity.

Other contents in the stomach that can interfere with levothyroxine absorption include coffee, aluminum hydroxide (antacids), sucralfate (ulcer and gastroesophageal reflux disease medications), ferrous sulphate (iron supplement), cholestyramine (lowers cholesterol in the blood), calcium carbonate (calcium supplement), and fiber supplements.[21] *Helicobacter pylori* infection, which causes chronic gastritis and decreases gastric acid secretion in the stomach, also lowers oral thyroxine absorption. Once the *Helicobacter pylori* was successfully treated in some patients, the same dose of levothyroxine, which previously had no effect on an elevated TSH, then lowered TSH below the reference range.[22]

Hashimoto's disease patients may also have autoimmune atrophic gastritis, celiac disease, inflammatory small bowel disease, and lactose intolerance, which would all affect absorption.[23] Lactose monohydrate is an ingredient in Synthroid.[24]

A woman who became hypothyroid after a thyroidectomy displayed severe malabsorption and at one point, and was taking 400 mcg levothyroxine and 20 mcg thyronine (T3) with no improvement in symptoms. Her TSH was elevated and her FT4 was below the reference range. She weighed 300 pounds (150 kg) and had a body temperature of 96°F (35.6°C). Even after her dose was slowly raised to 2200 mcg levothyroxine and 80 mcg thyronine, her TSH remained elevated, her FT4 was below the reference range, and there was no improvement in symptoms. At that point, she was switched to subcutaneous injections of 500 mcg thyroxine weekly, which finally brought her FT4 up and lowered her TSH. Because her symptoms would return before the week was over, she was then given her 500 mcg thyroxine shots every four days.[25] This patient could rightfully declare levothyroxine, in pill form, "crap." It did not work for her. However, she suffered from antral gastritis, which means she probably had very little gastric acid. Would taking the levothyroxine with a little vinegar or hydrochloric acid (an over-the-counter supplement) allow the T4 to become bioavailable? That idea was never tested. It's possible that desiccated thyroid would have had better results, but it was not tested either. Because desiccated thyroid comes from a pig's thyroid gland, it would contain thyroxine or T4, not levothyroxine sodium; in other words, no sodium molecule needs to be cleaved off for the T4 to become bioavailable. That may explain why desiccated thyroid works better for some patients—specifically, those who do not have enough stomach acid.

Isn't desiccated thyroid better because it's bioidentical?

The word *bioidentical* means the structure of the molecule is identical to the naturally produced one. Desiccated thyroid is bioidentical and natural, because it was not synthesized in a laboratory, and came from a living thing.

Levothyroxine sodium, on the other hand, is synthetic, but it's also bioidentical. As stated earlier, gastric acid in the stomach should cleave off the sodium molecule, and what remains is a bioidentical thyroxine molecule. I personally take both types of hormones to give me both T4 and T3 in a ratio that's suitable for my body.

How often should thyroid hormone be taken?

Levothyroxine or T4 has a half-life of about one week, which means it takes days before it is completely eliminated from the body, even if another dose isn't taken the next day. It is usually taken once per day and works fine that way. Liothyronine or T3 has a half-life of about one day, so many doctors and patients recommend that it be taken more than once per day. T3 is also fast acting, which means it creates a spike in T3 levels about 2-4 hours after a dose.[26] Therefore, smaller doses at more frequent intervals are recommended. The number of daily doses may boil down to individual preference and ability to maintain the schedule. I know of a woman who has no thyroid function because of radioactive iodine treatment that destroyed her thyroid; she takes a small dose of desiccated thyroid or T3 every hour and uses a digital watch that beeps every hour to keep her on this schedule. I find that a little too much to deal with and depending on my dose, take some desiccated either three or four times a day (before breakfast, lunch, dinner, and bedtime), which are natural breaks in my day, so fairly easy for me to remember. I do not use an alarm system of any kind. I also supplement my desiccated thyroid hormone with T4, so I'm not that dependent on constant T3 dosing. I have heard of patients who take desiccated once a day, though it seems that would create an unnatural daily spike in T3 levels.

Thyroid hormone has a natural circadian rhythm in the body, with TSH and T3 levels both peaking overnight, sometime after midnight.[27] Knowing this, it makes sense to replicate this by taking some T3 before bedtime. I've heard that a bedtime dose keeps some patients awake, but it may be that they just have to work up to a bedtime dose, just like any other dose increase. The adrenals also have a natural circadian rhythm and start firing up about 3 a.m. One hypothesis is that the T3 spike overnight gives the adrenals the energy they need to start producing in those early hours. If a patient has been on a T4-only protocol for years, then they may not have had much T3 overnight for some time, and consequently, the adrenals may have lowered their daily cortisol output. Taking T3 at night may initially use up more cortisol than the body can provide, and keep them awake. For this reason, it may be prudent to start with the smallest possible dose of desiccated thyroid or T3 at bedtime, and then slowly work on increasing that dose. I sleep much deeper and have more detailed dreams when I take a bedtime dose. I have only taken ¼ or ½ grain at bedtime. When my overall dose is too low, I have scary dreams, where things attack me: dogs lunge at me, people startle me, and I wake with my heart racing. Any small bedtime dose of T3 should be beneficial to the body, and patients should experiment with different doses.

Conclusion

The three options for thyroid hormone replacement should be combined to fit the needs of the individual. If a normal human thyroid gland secretes about 10 mcg of T3 daily, then any dose should provide something close to that; at a bare minimum, at least ½ grain of NDT or 5 mcg T3 could be added to whatever amount of T4 makes a patient feel well. Both doctors and patients tend to be dogmatic and intransigent in thinking that only one type of prescription can work for everyone. This is simply *not true* and has caused a great deal of grief for many people.

Hopefully, this chapter clarifies *why* T3 is essential, while also dispelling some internet myths.

Key points

- Three different types of prescription thyroid hormone are available to patients: levothyroxine (T4), liothyronine (T3), or natural desiccated thyroid (NDT).
- A normal thyroid secretes both T4 and T3, so both hormones should be replaced to replicate normal physiology.
- T3 induces the D1 enzyme that converts T4 to T3 in the liver, kidney, thyroid, and pituitary. It contributes to circulating plasma T3.
- Patients have different reactions to the different prescriptions, and some may even react to different brands. Finding the right dose may involve some trial and error.
- Patients on T4-only may have upper range T4 levels with lower range T3 levels. Adding some T3 will improve this ratio.
- Patients on desiccated thyroid may have upper range T3 levels with lower range T4 levels, because of the higher T3 content in desiccated thyroid. Adding some T4 will improve this ratio.
- There are many misconceptions about desiccated thyroid:
  1) It really doesn't contain much T2 or T1
  2) rT3 is a component of desiccated thyroid, because it's in a normal thyroid gland
  3) Calcitonin cannot be absorbed orally
  4) the ratio of T3/T4 is much higher than found in a human thyroid gland
- rT3 is not a mirror image of T3
- T2 and DIT are two different molecules
- T2 + T2 does not equal T4
- T2 and T1 are both made from deiodination (conversion) outside of the thyroid gland
- T2 appears to have biological activity, and is a metabolite of T3 and rT3
- Age, weight, and gender have nothing to do with a patient's optimal dose.
- 3 grains of NDT can be a serious overdose for some patients, and no one should blindly work up to that, or any dose they read about on the internet. Periodic lab work should be performed and used in conjunction with physical symptoms to determine the optimal dose.
- T4 can be dosed once daily, because of its long half-life.
- T4 pills will not work if the patient does not produce enough gastric acid.
- Desiccated thyroid is bioidentical and natural.
- Levothyroxine is bioidentical, but synthetic.
- T3 peaks within 4 hours, so smaller doses more often are more physiological.
- T3 has a circadian rhythm and peaks overnight. Taking a very small bedtime dose of T3 mimics normal physiology and may help the adrenal glands produce cortisol, which is essential for thyroid metabolism.

[1] Pilo, Alessandro, et al. "Thyroidal and peripheral production of 3, 5, 3'-triiodothyronine in humans by multicompartmental analysis." *American Journal of Physiology-Endocrinology And Metabolism* 258.4 (1990): E715-E726.

[2] Escobar-Morreale, H. F., et al. "Only the combined treatment with thyroxine and triiodothyronine ensures euthyroidism in all tissues of the thyroidectomized rat." *Endocrinology* 137.6 (1996): 2490-2502.

[3] Koenig, Ronald J. "Regulation of type 1 iodothyronine deiodinase in health and disease." *Thyroid* 15.8 (2005): 835-840.

[4] Woeber, K. A. "Levothyroxine therapy and serum free thyroxine and free triiodothyronine concentrations." *Journal of endocrinological investigation* 25.2 (2002): 106-109.

[5] Mortoglou, A., and H. Candiloros. "The serum triiodothyronine to thyroxine (T3/T4) ratio in various thyroid disorders and after Levothyroxine replacement therapy." *HORMONES-ATHENS-* 3 (2004): 120-126.

[6] Miot, Françoise, et al. "Thyroid hormone synthesis and secretion." *Thyroid disease manager* (2010).

[7] Buclin, Thierry, et al. "Bioavailability and biological efficacy of a new oral formulation of salmon calcitonin in healthy volunteers." *Journal of Bone and Mineral Research* 17.8 (2002): 1478-1485.

[8] Feigerlova, Eva, et al. "Thyroid Disorders and Bone Mineral Homeostasis." (2012).

[9] Gavin, Laurence A., et al. "3, 3'-Diiodothyronine production, a major pathway of peripheral iodothyronine metabolism in man." *Journal of Clinical Investigation* 61.5 (1978): 1276.

[10] Benker, G., et al. "Effects of small doses of bovine TSH on serum levels of free and total thyroid hormones, their degradation products, and diiodotyrosine." *Acta endocrinologica* 108.2 (1985): 211-216.

[11] Hulbert, A. J. "Thyroid hormones and their effects: a new perspective." *Biological Reviews* 75.4 (2000): 519-631.

[12] De Vijlder, J. J., and Marcel T. den Hartog. "Anionic iodotyrosine residues are required for iodothyronine synthesis." *European journal of endocrinology* 138.2 (1998): 227-231.

[13] Lanni, Antonia, et al. "3, 5-diiodo-L-thyronine powerfully reduces adiposity in rats by increasing the burning of fats." *The FASEB journal* 19.11 (2005): 1552-1554.

[14] Larsen, P. Reed, and Ann Marie Zavacki. "Role of the Iodothyronine Deiodinases in the Physiology and Pathophysiology of Thyroid Hormone Action." *European thyroid journal* 1.4 (2012): 232-242.

[15] Höffken, B., et al. "Conversion of T3 and rT3 to 3, 3'-T2: pH dependency." *Clinica chimica acta; international journal of clinical chemistry* 90.1 (1978): 45.

[16] Kansagra, Shayri M., Christopher R. McCudden, and Monte S. Willis. "The challenges and complexities of thyroid hormone replacement." *Lab Medicine* 41.6 (2010): 338-348.

[17] Gardner, J. Addyman, and Hugh Gainsborough. "The relationship of plasma cholesterol and basal metabolism." *British medical journal* 2.3542 (1928): 935.

[18] Ward, Laura S. "The difficult patient: drug interaction and the influence of concomitant diseases on the treatment of hypothyroidism." *Arq Bras Endocrinol Metabol* 54.5 (2010): 435-442.

[19] Brown, Rosalind S. "Graves' Disease (GD) in childhood and adolescence: current concepts and controversies." *Rev Esp Endocrinol Pediatr* 4.1 (2013): 7-14.

[20] El-Houni, A., et al. "Diarrhoea soon after levothyroxine replacement therapy." *QJM* 95.2 (2002): 125-126.

[21] Pirola, Ilenia, et al. "Oral Liquid l-Thyroxine (l-T4) May Be Better Absorbed Compared to l-T4 Tablets Following Bariatric Surgery." *Obesity surgery* 23.9 (2013): 1493-1496.

[22] Bugdaci, Mehmet Sait, et al. "The role of Helicobacter pylori in patients with hypothyroidism in whom could not be achieved normal thyrotropin levels despite treatment with high doses of thyroxine." *Helicobacter* 16.2 (2011): 124-130.

[23] Ward, Laura S. "The difficult patient: drug interaction and the influence of concomitant diseases on the treatment of hypothyroidism." *Arq Bras Endocrinol Metabol* 54.5 (2010): 435-442.

[24] Synthroid Prescribing Information. http://www.rxabbvie.com/pdf/synthroid.pdf accessed 11/12/13.

[25] Groener, Jan B., et al. "Subcutaneous application of levothyroxine as successful treatment option in a patient with malabsorption." *The American journal of case reports* 14 (2013): 48.

[26] Saberi, Mansour, and Robert D. Utiger. "Serum thyroid hormone and thyrotropin concentrations during thyroxine and triiodothyronine therapy." *Journal of Clinical Endocrinology & Metabolism* 39.5 (1974): 923-927.

[27] Russell, Wanda, et al. "Free triiodothyronine has a distinct circadian rhythm that is delayed but parallels thyrotropin levels." *Journal of Clinical Endocrinology & Metabolism* 93.6 (2008): 2300-2306

21

Reference Ranges:
Why "Normal" Does not Equal "Optimal"

Your TSH and Free T4 are normal;
therefore, you're not hypothyroid

—the statistical definition of "normal" prevents hypothyroid patients from being diagnosed and treated

How is it possible that so many people with obvious hypothyroid symptoms (fatigue, cold hands and feet, dry skin, thin hair, and constipation) are declared "normal" by their laboratory tests? The answer has to do with reference ranges, which are statistical interpretations of the data. To form a reference range for any variable, whether it's free thyroxine (Free T4 or FT4), free triiodothyronine (Free T3 or FT3), or cholesterol, measurements from a large sample of people are taken, and the results are plotted in a graph. Two different data distribution shapes are relevant to this discussion and will be explained: normal (symmetrical bell-shape) and negatively-skewed (more values in the upper half).

To explain these concepts, I created (completely fabricated, this is *not* real data) some graphs to illustrate the points. My apologies to any true statisticians—my explanations are greatly simplified in order to explain my points.

A normal distribution

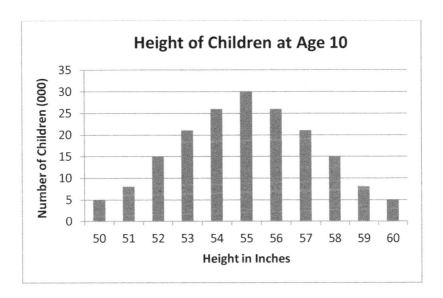

Fig. 21-1. A normal distribution is symmetrical, with the largest number of values in the middle of the range, with equal numbers falling on either side. This hypothetical graph plots both boys and girls, so even though more boys may fall into the upper half of the range, more girls fall into the lower half, and plotted together, the graph is symmetrical. The middle of the range (midrange, midpoint, average, or *mean*) is calculated by adding the highest and lowest values together, and then dividing by two. In this example, the mean is (60 + 50)/2 = 55. The *mode* is the most common value, which in this case is also 55 inches. In a normal distribution, the mean and mode are identical; in other words, the average of the values (55") is also the most common value (55").

A negatively skewed distribution

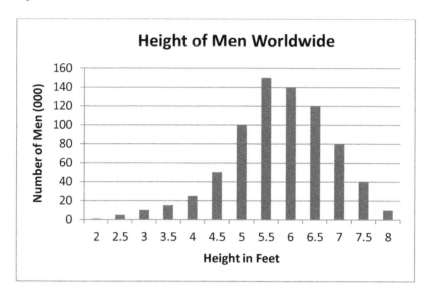

Figure 21-2. A negatively skewed distribution has a "tail" on the left, or negative side of the graph, with more values to the right of the midpoint. According to Wikipedia, the shortest man in history was 21", or almost 2 feet tall, and the tallest 8'11". For simplicity's sake, this graph starts at 2 feet and ends at 8 feet. In this example, the mean = (8+2)/2 = 5. Most men are taller than midrange, or 5 feet, so this is not a normal distribution, but a negatively skewed distribution. The mode, or most common value (5.5 feet) is higher than the mean (5 feet).

The distribution of the data says a lot about what is considered common in that data set, and what is not, because data tends to aggregate. In Figure 21-2 depicting the height of men worldwide, 5 feet is the mean (average) height. But that is not the most common height. The most common height, 5' 6", is actually higher than the mean. I know quite a few men who are close to that height. Now move just one value lower than the mean on this graph, and that is for someone 4'6". I do not personally know any man of that stature, though I know they exist. And yet, both 5'6" and 4'6" are just one value away from the mean. In this particular graph, there are three times as many men that are 5'6" than 4'6". According to the data presented on this chart, any man I meet will more than likely be 5 feet or taller. In other words, most men have a height that's above the average, or to the right of the midpoint on this graph.

Now compare this to Figure 21-1, which depicts the normal distribution of the height of 10-year-olds. The average height is 55 inches, or 4' 7". The most common height *is* the average height. Moving one value either way gives an equal chance of being either slightly taller or shorter. According to the data presented on this chart, any 10-year-old I meet has an equal chance of being either taller or shorter than the mean. Unlike men's height, there is no skew to this data; the points are equally distributed.

Free T3 distribution

What shape does a Free T3 graph form? Would the distribution of values affect how a reference range should be interpreted? (Note: I did not have access to real data; the data and graphs were created just to illustrate the points.)

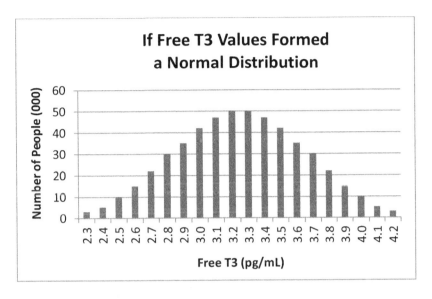

Figure 21-3. If Free T3 values formed a normal distribution, this is what it would look like. Midrange is between 3.2 and 3.3, and there would be an equal chance of testing above or below this midpoint. These are the ranges my laboratory uses; any value between 2.3-4.2 pg/mL would be considered "normal" and is not flagged on the lab report. Only values that are outside of the reference range are flagged.

When I asked the Director of Quality Assurance at my laboratory how T3 reference ranges were determined, he told me that healthy people were tested and their values plotted. "Healthy" meant these people were not on any medication, they were not complaining of any ailments, and no other lab values were out of range. The data formed a negatively skewed curve, with far fewer values on the lower end than on the higher end. He described the curve as having a tail on the left, with a steep ascent to a peak to the right of the midpoint, and then a much more gradual descent to the right. I plotted what he described in Figure 21-4. Seeing that it was a negatively skewed distribution, I asked why they didn't just choose the higher part of the range as normal and eliminate the lower values. Well, different medical directors from different specialties argue about what "normal" should be, and they all have input on the final ranges. An endocrinologist would have a different opinion from an ob-gyn, for example. Therefore, all designated ranges are a compromise of statistics, medical directors' input, and someone's analysis at the lab. Unfortunately, many people are not formally diagnosed as hypothyroid (because their Thyroid Stimulating Hormone or TSH is "normal"), and their lab results may become the lower part of the thyroid reference ranges. If Figure 21-4 (negatively skewed graph of FT3) is laid over Figure 21-2 (negatively skewed graph of the height of men), the FT3 numbers towards the bottom of the range are analogous to men that are less than 4 feet tall. It doesn't make sense to call that "normal," in my opinion. It makes much more sense to define "normal" as values that start just below midrange, if the distribution is negatively skewed.

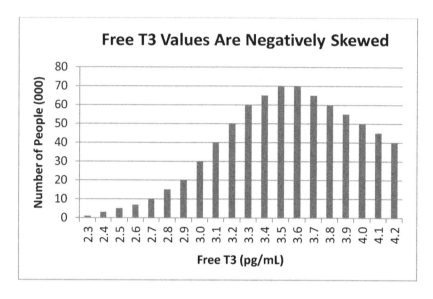

Figure 21-4. Free T3 values form a negatively skewed curve, with the majority of the values above the midpoint of 3.25. A healthy person has a greater chance of testing above the midpoint than below.

Since Free T3 is a negatively skewed curve, patients should aim for a lab value that is about midrange or higher. There may be some individuals who feel best with levels just below midrange, but the majority of people will feel better as their levels approach the middle of the range and higher. That's what the curve of this statistical data says. This graph also explains why people may be told they are "normal," when they are obviously hypothyroid and have every symptom in the book. "Normal" is a statistical term that refers to whether their lab values fall into the arbitrary reference range determined by the lab. And as just shown, they could have a Free T3 value that is analogous to a 2 foot tall man, but that would still be "normal," statistically, if that value was included in the range.

The graph of men's height included *all* men, from the shortest to tallest in the world. But does it make sense to define "normal" as a range from 2 feet to 8 feet tall? Of course not. Just looking at the graph, it would make much more sense to tighten up the reference range for normal by bringing in both ends of the range. The mode, or most common value, 5 feet 6 inches, could be used as the center point, and the range could extend outward equally either way from that point. How loose or tight to make that range is an arbitrary decision, as the lab director explained. If the reference range was defined as three values above and below the mode, then any man between 4 and 7 feet tall would be statistically "normal." This makes much more sense than a range from 2 feet to 8 feet tall!

Thyroid reference ranges

It appears that Total T4, Free T4, Total T3, and Free T3 are all negatively skewed curves, based on the assessment of patients on multiple thyroid forums who say they only feel well when their values are close to midrange or higher, the *optimal* part of the reference range. In a negatively skewed curve, the upper half will always represent the majority of values. But *how* high in the range should a patient aim? Both high *and* low levels are detrimental to the body and may contribute to osteoporosis[1] or insulin resistance,[2] so care must be taken to find the correct dose. After a certain point, continuing to raise T4 seems to have diminishing returns, and it may be that T3 needs to be added instead. The reasons for this are explained in Chapter 25, The TSH and T3 Dilemma. In some patients, high FT4 seems to correlate with high reverse T3 and different illnesses (poor physical function[3] or mood disorders[4]). Certain drugs like aspirin[5] and heparin[6] can artificially elevate FT4, but the Total T4 will show the true deficiency, because it will be close to the bottom of the range. Some people have a condition called resistance to thyroid hormone, and their levels need to be above the thyroid reference ranges for them to feel well.[7] Some bipolar patients have shown improvement taking extremely high doses of levothyroxine (320 mcg T4 daily, on average) that raises their Total T4 above the reference range.[8] This is rare, however, and where someone feels best in the reference range is very individual; other signs and symptoms should be used to find the optimal dose. Here are some physical signs that may indicate someone is still hypothyroid:

- dry skin and rough, cracked heels
- thin hair (hair loss is also common with too much thyroid)
- thin eyebrows; outer third of eyebrow thin or missing
- pulse below 70 or sometimes, over 90 beats per minute
- respiration (breaths per minute) less than 12
- morning basal temperature below 97.8
- cold hands or feet when others feel fine
- constipation: bowel movements come out as hard pellets after heavy pushing
- nightmares/disturbed sleep

Research shows that T3 is a much better predictor of thyroid status than T4. One study using levothyroxine showed that patients with T4 levels over the reference range did not show signs of being clinically hyperthyroid unless their T3 levels were also over range.[9]

The term *subclinical hypothyroidism* is used when TSH is elevated, but FT4 is "normal." There is a mismatch between the two values, because TSH is above the reference range, while FT4 is within. Since many disease states are associated with subclinical hypothyroidism (infertility and pregnancy loss,[10] heart disease,[11] memory deficits[12]), it seems that the TSH is a valid indicator in these cases, and that low values of FT4 that are labeled "normal" are the cause of the discrepancy. Subclinical hypothyroidism may just be another indicator that reference ranges for FT4 start far too low.

A healthy person who is not on any thyroid medication will more than likely have thyroid lab results (FT4, Total T4, FT3, Total T3) in the upper half of the reference range, because that's where the majority of the values are. But for thyroid patients who are manually replacing their thyroid hormone, there are several confounding factors that need to be mentioned. First, all of these lab values are measurements of what's found in a person's serum. It does not reflect what happens at the cellular level. Someone can have a FT3 or FT4 at the top of the reference range and feel terrible. That level may be too high for them, while it may be fine for someone else. Conversely, someone may have a FT3 or FT4 that is just below midrange and feel fine. We each have our own optimal sweet spots. Some people may have good levels of thyroid hormone in their serum, but are still hypothyroid because their T4 doesn't make it into their cells to be converted into T3. They are deficient at the cellular level. In other cases, FT4 may be in the upper half of the range, while FT3 may be at the bottom of the reference range, or vice versa. *Both* levels are found at midrange or higher in healthy people. That's what the negatively skewed curves show. The human body uses both hormones in different processes, and neither a T4-only or T3-only protocol mimics normal thyroid physiology.

Conclusion

Knowing whether a reference range is based on a normal distribution or negatively skewed distribution makes a huge difference in how it's interpreted. In a normal distribution, the bottom half of the range is equally as likely as the top half of the range. Not so with a negatively skewed distribution. Few people feel well when their thyroid hormone levels are at the bottom of the reference range because T3 and T4 levels are both negatively skewed curves. The values at the bottom of the range in a negatively skewed curve are so few that in statistics it's referred to as a "tail."

Doctors are often faulted for seeing lab results in black or white—if the patient's lab values are within the reference range, they're often told they're fine, and the patient wonders if they're imagining how poorly they feel. Only if their lab values fall outside of the reference range will the doctor even consider making any dosing changes. Is this really the doctor's fault? It seems that the problem originates with the lab ranges. Ideally, the references ranges should be modified, and the bottom of the range brought up closer to the mode, or most common value, so that the lowest values, the ones that are analogous to two foot tall men, are dropped. Then, a lab result that low would automatically be flagged, and the doctor would know that the patient needs a dose increase. As it stands now, doctors can rightfully say that the lower values in the range are "normal," although patients would passionately disagree.

Key points

- In statistics, any value within a reference range is called *normal*.
- When lab results from a large number of people are plotted on a graph, they form a shape or curve. Two common shapes are the normal, bell-shaped, completely symmetrical curve, and a negatively skewed curve, where there are so few values at the beginning of the range that it looks like a tail.
- The distribution curves for measurable thyroid hormones (FT3, FT4, Total T3, Total T4) are negatively skewed, meaning most of the values are in the upper half of the range.

- Reference ranges are arbitrarily defined by the lab; they may include a long tail with few values.
- The point in the reference range where someone feels well is very individual, and other physical symptoms should be used in conjunction with lab values to determine whether a dose is too low or too high.
- For some people, being at the top of the reference range is an overdose, because their body requires less hormone, or makes more efficient use of the hormone at the cellular level.
- Other people only feel well when their dose is significantly above the range; bipolar patients are one example of a group that feels better when their Total T4 is above the reference range.
- Lab values do not reflect what happens at the cellular level; someone may have "optimal" lab values but still feel poorly for other reasons.
- Generally, both FT4 and FT3 should be close to mid-range or higher to mimic healthy thyroid gland output.
- It would benefit both doctors and patients if current thyroid reference ranges were modified so that the lowest levels were dropped from the reference range.

---

[1] Flynn, Robert W., et al. "Serum thyroid-stimulating hormone concentration and morbidity from cardiovascular disease and fractures in patients on long-term thyroxine therapy." *Journal of Clinical Endocrinology & Metabolism* 95.1 (2010): 186-193.

[2] Lambadiari, Vaia, et al. "Thyroid hormones are positively associated with insulin resistance early in the development of type 2 diabetes." *Endocrine* 39.1 (2011): 28-32.

[3] Van den Beld, Annewieke W., et al. "Thyroid hormone concentrations, disease, physical function, and mortality in elderly men." *Journal of Clinical Endocrinology & Metabolism* 90.12 (2005): 6403-6409.

[4] Sokolov, Stephen TH, Stanley P. Kutcher, and Russell T. Joffe. "Basal thyroid indices in adolescent depression and bipolar disorder." *Journal of the American Academy of Child & Adolescent Psychiatry* 33.4 (1994): 469-475.

[5] Lim, Chen-Fee, et al. "Drug and fatty acid effects on serum thyroid hormone binding." *Journal of Clinical Endocrinology & Metabolism* 67.4 (1988): 682-688.

[6] Jaume, Juan Carlos, et al. "Extremely low doses of heparin release lipase activity into the plasma and can thereby cause artifactual elevations in the serum-free thyroxine concentration as measured by equilibrium dialysis." *Thyroid* 6.2 (1996): 79-83.

[7] Weiss, Roy E., and Samuel Refetoff. "Resistance to thyroid hormone." *Reviews in Endocrine and Metabolic Disorders* 1.1-2 (2000): 97-108.

[8] Bauer, M., et al. "Supraphysiological doses of levothyroxine alter regional cerebral metabolism and improve mood in bipolar depression." *Molecular psychiatry* 10.5 (2005): 456-469.

[9] Rendell, M., and D. Salmon. "'Chemical hyperthyroidism': the significance of elevated serum thyroxine levels in l-thyroxine treated individuals." *Clinical endocrinology* 22.6 (1985): 693-700.

[10] Khalid, Azriny Shaziela, Caroline Joyce, and Keelin O'Donoghue. "Prevalence of subclinical and undiagnosed overt hypothyroidism in a pregnancy loss clinic." *Instructions for Authors* 106.5 (2013).

[11] Rodondi, Nicolas, et al. "Subclinical hypothyroidism and the risk of coronary heart disease and mortality." *JAMA: the journal of the American Medical Association* 304.12 (2010): 1365-1374.

[12] Correia, Neuman, et al. "Evidence for a specific defect in hippocampal memory in overt and subclinical hypothyroidism." *Journal of Clinical Endocrinology & Metabolism* 94.10 (2009): 3789-3797.

22

Reproductive Problems Caused by Thyroid Dysfunction: Pregnancy, Infertility, PCOS, Delayed Ejaculation, Erectile Dysfunction

PCOS is a common cause of infertility

—infertility clinic, unaware that hypothyroidism causes PCOS (polycystic ovary syndrome)

Healthy thyroid levels are essential for all reproductive functions. Females need energy to ovulate and successfully complete all of the steps of pregnancy—this energy comes from adequate thyroid levels. Men also need thyroid energy for normal sperm production and ejaculation. Anyone who has been labeled infertile should have their thyroid levels checked, which should include more than a TSH (Thyroid Stimulating Hormone) test (a routine screening test that does not identify all cases of hypothyroidism).

Thyroid hormone's effect on female fertility

Thyroid hormone is essential for a normal pregnancy. A normal menstrual cycle is approximately 28 days long. The uterine lining should build up each month in preparation for fertilization and an egg should be released (ovulation). If that does not occur, a woman should have a period to shed the lining. When a woman is hypothyroid, her body does not have enough energy to complete the cycle in 28 days. Cycles become infrequent and intermittent, or more than 28 days apart (oligomenorrhea). Marathon runners, who expend a lot of energy running, often have no periods (amenorrhea). They may have cycles in which ovulation simply does not occur (anovulation). Oligomenorrhea is also common in women with polycystic ovary syndrome (PCOS). These women have very irregular cycles, ranging from amenorrhea (no period) to oligomenorrhea (occasional periods) to menorrhagia (heavy periods). In one profoundly hypothyroid woman, periods were so severe that they induced life-threatening anemia and medical procedures had to be taken to stop the bleeding. Thyroid hormone replacement resolved this symptom and she delivered a healthy baby three years later.[1]

Women with PCOS have higher levels of androgens or male hormones, and their prolactin (a pituitary hormone) will also be higher than normal. In one study, levothyroxine (T4) replacement given to women with PCOS lowered elevated prolactin, free and total testosterone, estradiol, and ovarian volume and cysts.[2] The polycystic appearance of the ovaries disappeared in all patients. Laboratory testing confirmed that an increase in thyroid hormones, Free T3 (FT3) and Free T4 (FT4), correlated with these positive changes. TSH also decreased, as expected. In another study, pregnancy resulted within a year in the majority of women with a high TSH and high prolactin who were given levothyroxine.[3] Lack of thyroid hormone can cause the whole reproductive system to be dysfunctional.

Both thyroid autoimmunity and subclinical hypothyroidism (high TSH with normal Free T4) are associated with early miscarriage, though a high TSH seems more predictive of pregnancy loss than the presence of autoimmune antibodies. In women who had miscarried before the 12th week, those with a TSH above the reference range miscarried at an average of 6.5 weeks, while those who were positive for thyroid antibodies miscarried on average at 8.2 weeks.[4] In another study, placental abruption (the separation of the placenta from the uterus before birth) was three times more likely in women who were subclinically hypothyroid. Preterm birth (delivery before 34 weeks) was also almost two times higher in these women.[5]

Women who are positive for TPO (thyroid peroxidase) antibodies fare better if given levothyroxine replacement during their pregnancy, even if TSH is in the normal range. In one experiment, T4 supplementation in these women resulted in fewer miscarriages and fewer premature deliveries. Since most miscarriages happen during the first trimester, testing and supplementation should be started as soon as pregnancy is confirmed. A TSH greater than 2.0 mIU/liter and/or high TPO antibodies (> 2000 kIU/liter) were predictive of overt hypothyroidism during pregnancy. Maternal complications from hypothyroidism during pregnancy include anemia, postpartum hemorrhage, cardiac dysfunction, preeclampsia (high blood pressure), and placental abruption. Fetal complications include fetal distress, premature birth and/or low birth weight, congenital malformations, and fetal/perinatal death.[6]

Reproductive problems in woman with thyroid dysfunction range from zero conception, to conception then miscarriage, to conception and birth of children with developmental or cognitive defects. This is because after conception, ample thyroid hormone, specifically T4, is necessary for fetal brain development. If T4 is insufficient because the mother is hypothyroid, iodine deficient, or on the T3-only protocol (taking T3 with no T4), the baby's brain may not develop correctly. A fetus doesn't have a working thyroid until the second trimester. Up until that point, all of its T4 comes from the mother, whose levels rise during the first trimester until the fetus can supply its own T4. In contrast to rising T4 levels, maternal Free T3 is fairly constant throughout the entire pregnancy.[7]

Fetal brain development is dependent on adequate T4 levels, not T3. When a pregnant hypothyroid rat is given only T4, both T4 and T3 rise, and T3 in the fetal brain reaches normal levels. But if high doses of T3 are given instead, fetal brain T3 remains below normal because fetal brain T3 is the sum of direct T3 + T3 converted from T4. T3 alone cannot meet the level of T3 required for normal brain development. No dose of either T4 or T3 alone was able to achieve normal concentrations of T4 and T3 in all tissues; different tissues appear to have different requirements for T3 and T4. Even when T4 of the mother was considerably below that of controls, fetal brain T3 was normal. This can only be explained by the deiodinase enzymes that convert T4 to T3, raising or lowering conversion as needed to create sufficient T3 based on available T4. The enzymes work both ways—fetal brain T3 was also normal when the mother's T4 was excessive.[8] During pregnancy, T4 is critical to the fetus; therefore, the mother's T4 levels must be monitored. The deiodinase enzymes will convert T4 to T3 as needed.

Brain development in the fetus is exceedingly complex. Actin polymerization is a process in the developing brain where protein microfilaments combine to form chainlike molecules. This process is dependent on the presence of T4 and reverse T3 (rT3). Actin polymerization does not occur with T3, only T4 or rT3. Insufficient T4 and the presence of T3 will hinder specific nerve cell formation processes in the brain that follow actin polymerization.[9] This may cause the structural deficits in the brain that have been observed in cretins (a mentally deficient person born to a hypothyroid mother).[10] Again, T4 is critical for normal brain development in a fetus.

Pregnancy raises estrogen levels, which raises thyroxine binding globulin (TBG) levels, which binds up more thyroid hormone, leaving less free. Therefore, more T4 needs to be produced to compensate for this temporary condition. Iodine requirements also increase during pregnancy (50% or more), because more thyroid is produced and transferred to the fetus, and the clearance rate through the kidneys increases.[11]

Studies show that women who were low in T4 during their first trimester (maternal hypothyroxinemia) had children with delayed language development and delayed nonverbal cognitive function. Low FT4, not high TSH, is the principal factor that correlates with poor neurodevelopment in these children. The lower the FT4 levels, the higher the risk for verbal and cognitive dysfunction.[12]

Low T4 can also result from iodine deficiency, since iodine is a component of thyroid hormones. Mothers who were iodine deficient throughout their pregnancies had a higher percentage of children with problems with motor coordination and socialization skills.[13] Severe iodine deficiency can result in cretinism, or stunted growth and mental retardation. This is more common in inland, mountainous areas, like China near the Himalayas, not westernized countries. Of course, too much iodine is just as bad as too little. High dose iodine supplementation (12.5 mg Iodoral) in the mother has resulted in newborns that were born hypothyroid.[14] In other cases, the newborns are born with goiters.[15]

Elevated T4 can be problematic in pregnancy, and appears to correlate with the morning sickness, nausea and vomiting that some women experience.[16] Some studies suggest that a transient form of hyperthyroidism is responsible for these symptoms.[17] I had morning sickness and threw up for most of my first trimester, and I later developed Graves'. My own thyroid was able to adjust to the increased needs of this pregnancy, and while I was sick, I wasn't tired. In my second pregnancy I was both sick and tired. I'd had the radioactive iodine treatment that killed my thyroid by then, so even though my need for thyroid hormone had increased (because of the pregnancy), my body was limited to whatever my daily dose was, since I no longer produced any thyroid hormone on my own. I was grossly undermedicated on 75 mcg of levothyroxine during the first trimester and miscarried. The difference in my appearance between the two pregnancies was striking. In the first pregnancy, my own thyroid was able to adjust its output as needed for the pregnancy. While I did throw up every morning, I looked good and had that "pregnant glow" people talk about. I also had enough energy to work full-time while taking an evening computer programming class at the local university. I don't remember being any more tired than usual and had my baby on a Monday after working through Friday the previous week. During the second pregnancy, I was so exhausted that I was afraid of falling asleep while driving to work every morning. I still threw up, but I don't believe I looked well; I think I looked ragged. I certainly felt ragged!

If a woman taking thyroid hormone becomes pregnant, her T4 dose should be increased to meet the energy demands of pregnancy. An average levothyroxine dose increase of 50% kept TSH in the normal range in one study.[18] In another study, the median thyroxine dose was 100 mcg during the first trimester, 125 mcg the second, and 150 mcg the third.[19] A third study showed an average pre-pregnancy levothyroxine dose of 102 mcg daily, which was increased to 148 mcg per day to bring TSH back down into the reference range, a roughly 50% increase. After pregnancy, doses were decreased to bring a low TSH back up into the normal range.[20] The bottom line is that the T4 dose should be increased once pregnancy is confirmed. Patients on desiccated thyroid should especially not be dosed by their TSH, because the T3 in the desiccated thyroid can suppress TSH, even while T4 levels may be quite low. My TSH is "normal" on 1.5 grains, but suppressed on 1.75 grains. However, 1.5 grains of desiccated thyroid has only 57 mcg of T4, far short of a normal thyroid's daily production rate of 100 mcg of T4,[21] or some pregnant women's requirement of approximately 150 mcg mentioned earlier. Therefore, a pregnant woman taking only 1.5 grains (to keep her TSH normal) could actually suffer from maternal hypothyroxinemia (low T4), and her fetus would be at risk for cognitive and developmental problems. The mother may appear clinically normal because of adequate T3, but the child could have cognitive and motor problems because of the mother's low T4 levels, not her T3 or TSH levels.[22]

High doses of T3 can be toxic to a developing fetus and may cause brain function abnormalities in the hypothalamic-pituitary-thyroid axis, along with impaired hearing and vision, because the fetus was not designed to handle high levels of T3.[23] In fact, umbilical cord blood has significantly higher levels of rT3 and T4, but lower levels of T3 than adult serum.[24] Type 3 iodothyronine deiodinase (D3), the enzyme that inactivates T4 to rT3, and T3 to T2, is high in the pregnant uterus and placenta and most fetal and newborn tissues, probably to protect the fetus from excessive T3 levels. Type 2 iodothyronine deiodinase (D2) is the deiodinase enzyme that converts T4 to T3. In a developing fetus, D2 and D3 work closely together to modulate T3 levels when the cochlea (ears) and retina (eyes) are being formed. T3 levels must be reduced at certain stages of cochlea and retina development, and conversion of T4 to rT3, or T3 to T2 accomplishes this. Likewise, when an influx of T3 is needed, D2 kicks in to raise T3 levels. Both premature exposure to T3 or failure to reach a minimal threshold of T3 at a different point in time can result in hearing or visual impairment. This has been demonstrated in animal experiments.[25]

Thyroid hormone's effect on male fertility

Thyroid hormone affects men's performance; too little or too much thyroid hormone can negatively affect erections. Hyperthyroidism (defined as a suppressed TSH and elevated T4) is associated with severe erectile dysfunction.[26] Premature ejaculation was a problem for 50% of hyperthyroid men in one study. When treatment brought thyroid levels down this number dropped to 15%, which is close to the percentage found in the normal population of men.

Very few hypothyroid (defined as an elevated TSH) men suffered from premature ejaculation; delayed ejaculation was more common in this group. Thyroid treatment resolved the delayed ejaculation and erectile dysfunction for half of these patients. Prolactin, a pituitary hormone, can inhibit arousal, and the hypothyroid men had higher serum prolactin levels that dropped significantly after levothyroxine treatment.[27]

In a group of hypothyroid men, Luteinizing Hormone (LH) and Follicle Stimulating Hormone (FSH) were elevated, while testosterone and Sex Hormone Binding Globulin (SHBG) were low. LH and FSH are the signals that together regulate sperm production. These values normalized after treatment with levothyroxine, and sperm count (number of sperm) and motility (ability to move) also improved.[28]

Compared to normal men, hypothyroid men in another study had higher serum prolactin and more severe erectile dysfunction, while sperm count, sperm motility, and sperm morphology (normal form and structure) were lower.[29] The negative effects on sperm quality reduce fertility in these men. Interestingly, there was no correlation between TSH and the severity of erectile dysfunction, serum free testosterone, and sperm parameters; in other words, TSH would not be a useful diagnostic measure for male fertility problems.

In hyperthyroid men, sperm motility decreases, but rises back to normal levels when thyroid levels are brought down into the normal range. Semen volume and sperm density were also lower in thyrotoxic (hyperthyroid) men.[30]

Androgen deficiency (being low in the male hormone testosterone) is experienced by both hyperthyroid and hypothyroid men. Thyrotoxic men may have increased total testosterone levels, but they have decreased free and bioavailable testosterone. Their SHBG and estrogen levels are also elevated. This can result in gynecomastia (male breasts), decreased libido, erectile dysfunction, spider angiomas (spider web pattern on the skin, often caused by high estrogen levels), and reduced sperm count/motility. These symptoms can be induced by the T3-only protocol or overmedication by any form of thyroid hormone replacement. Hypothyroid men may have decreased SHBG levels, decreased libido, erectile dysfunction, and delayed ejaculation.[31]

Thyroid hormone is essential to healthy testicle formation that starts in the fetus. Thyroid receptors are found in the Sertoli cells in the testes that are involved in sperm production. The number of Sertoli cells is established before puberty and correlates with adult testicular size and sperm output. Hypothyroidism before puberty delays Sertoli cell maturation, resulting in an increased number of Sertoli cells, and consequently, larger testes in the adult. Conversely, hyperthyroidism before puberty results in premature Sertoli cell maturation, smaller testes, and decreased sperm production.[32]

Conclusion

Thyroid hormone plays a major role in the health of the reproductive system of both men and women. It is unfortunate that so many with low thyroid levels are never diagnosed because of "normal" TSH test results, and then need fertility treatments. Infertility can be emotionally and financially devastating, but if hypothyroidism is the cause of infertility, it *is* treatable.

Key points

- Low thyroid levels may cause reproductive problems in both men and women.
- In women, thyroid dysfunction affects the menstrual cycle; periods may become infrequent or intermittent, more than 28 days apart, and flow may become very heavy, often leading to anemia.
- Polycystic ovary syndrome (PCOS) and high androgen levels in women may be a symptom of low thyroid levels.
- A TSH above the reference range is associated with early miscarriage, placental abruption, and preterm births.
- Women with TPO antibodies have fewer miscarriages and preterm births on levo-thyroxine (T4) treatment, even if their TSH is within the normal range.
- T4 is essential for fetal brain development and T3 alone will not meet the needs of a developing brain. Lack of T4 may cause structural deficits in the fetal brain.
- A pregnant woman on thyroid hormone replacement may need to increase her dose by 50% to compensate for the higher estrogen levels (which bind more thyroid hormone), and to fulfill the baby's need for T4.
- Low Free T4 in the pregnant mother, not high TSH, correlates with verbal and cognitive dysfunction in the children.
- Pregnant women on desiccated thyroid may need to add T4 to their dose if FT4 is low. Those taking desiccated thyroid cannot be dosed by TSH because T3 has a suppressive effect on TSH and the woman's T4 levels may be kept too low for fetal health.
- High T3 levels may be toxic to a developing fetus, causing hearing and visual impairment.
- Hyperthyroid men may suffer from severe erectile dysfunction and premature ejaculation.
- Hypothyroid men suffer from delayed ejaculation, lower sperm count and sperm motility, and sperm that are structurally different from normal sperm.
- Hyperthyroid men have decreased sperm motility, semen volume, and sperm density.
- TSH has no correlation with erectile dysfunction, serum free testosterone, or sperm quality.

- Both hyperthyroid and hypothyroid men experience androgen deficiency because free testosterone decreases. Thyrotoxic men can have elevated SHBG and estrogen levels, decreased libido, erectile dysfunction, and reduced sperm count and motility.
- Hyperthyroidism before puberty will result in smaller testes and decreased sperm production.

---

[1] Moragianni, Vasiliki A., and Stephen G. Somkuti. "Profound hypothyroidism-induced acute menorrhagia resulting in life-threatening anemia." *Obstetrics & Gynecology* 110.2, Part 2 (2007): 515.

[2] Muderris, Iptisam Ipek, et al. "Effect of thyroid hormone replacement therapy on ovarian volume and androgen hormones in patients with untreated primary hypothyroidism." *Annals of Saudi medicine* 31.2 (2011): 145.

[3] Verma, I., et al. "Prevalence of hypothyroidism in infertile women and evaluation of response of treatment for hypothyroidism on infertility." *International Journal of Applied and Basic Medical Research* 2.1 (2012): 17.

[4] De Vivo, Antonio, et al. "Thyroid function in women found to have early pregnancy loss." *Thyroid* 20.6 (2010): 633-637.

[5] Casey, Brian M., et al. "Subclinical hypothyroidism and pregnancy outcomes." *Obstetrics & Gynecology* 105.2 (2005): 239-245.

[6] Negro, Roberto, et al. "Levothyroxine treatment in euthyroid pregnant women with autoimmune thyroid disease: effects on obstetrical complications." *Journal of Clinical Endocrinology & Metabolism* 91.7 (2006): 2587-2591.

[7] Patel, Jatin, et al. "Delivery of maternal thyroid hormones to the fetus." *Trends in Endocrinology & Metabolism* 22.5 (2011): 164-170.

[8] Calvo, Rosa, et al. "Congenital hypothyroidism, as studied in rats. Crucial role of maternal thyroxine but not of 3, 5, 3'-triiodothyronine in the protection of the fetal brain." *Journal of Clinical Investigation* 86.3 (1990): 889.

[9] Farwell, Alan P., et al. "Regulation of cerebellar neuronal migration and neurite outgrowth by thyroxine and 3, 3′, 5′-triiodothyronine." *Developmental brain research* 154.1 (2005): 121-135.

[10] Leonard, Jack L. "Non-genomic actions of thyroid hormone in brain development." *Steroids* 73.9 (2008): 1008-1012.

[11] Zimmermann, Michael B. "The effects of iodine deficiency in pregnancy and infancy." *Paediatric and Perinatal Epidemiology* 26.s1 (2012): 108-117.

[12] Henrichs, Jens, et al. "Maternal thyroid function during early pregnancy and cognitive functioning in early childhood: the generation R study." *Journal of Clinical Endocrinology & Metabolism* 95.9 (2010): 4227-4234.

[13] Berbel, Pere, et al. "Delayed neurobehavioral development in children born to pregnant women with mild hypothyroxinemia during the first month of gestation: the importance of early iodine supplementation." *Thyroid* 19.5 (2009): 511-519.

[14] Connelly, Kara J., et al. "Congenital hypothyroidism caused by excess prenatal maternal iodine ingestion." *The Journal of pediatrics* (2012).

[15] Ayromlooi, Jahangir. "Congenital goiter due to maternal ingestion of iodides." *Obstetrics & Gynecology* 39.6 (1972): 818-822.

[16] Mansourian, Azad R. "Thyroid function tests during first-trimester of pregnancy: A review of literature." *Pak. J. Biol. Sci* 13 (2010): 664-673.

[17] Tan, Jackie YL, et al. "Transient hyperthyroidism of hyperemesis gravidarum." *BJOG: An International Journal of Obstetrics & Gynaecology* 109.6 (2002): 683-688.

[18] Alexander, Erik K., et al. "Timing and magnitude of increases in levothyroxine requirements during pregnancy in women with hypothyroidism." *New England Journal of Medicine* 351.3 (2004): 241-249.

[19] Idris, Iskandar, et al. "Maternal hypothyroidism in early and late gestation: effects on neonatal and obstetric outcome." *Clinical endocrinology* 63.5 (2005): 560-565.

[20] Mandel, Susan J., et al. "Increased need for thyroxine during pregnancy in women with primary hypothyroidism." *New England Journal of Medicine* 323.2 (1990): 91-96.

[21] Bunevičius, Robertas, et al. "Effects of thyroxine as compared with thyroxine plus triiodothyronine in patients with hypothyroidism." *New England Journal of Medicine* 340.6 (1999): 424-429.

[22] de Escobar, Gabriella Morreale, María Jesús Obregón, and Francisco Escobar del Rey. "Is neuropsychological development related to maternal hypothyroidism or to maternal hypothyroxinemia?" *Journal of Clinical Endocrinology & Metabolism* 85.11 (2000): 3975-3987.

[23] Hernandez, Arturo, et al. "Type 3 deiodinase deficiency causes spatial and temporal alterations in brain T3 signaling that are dissociated from serum thyroid hormone levels." *Endocrinology* 151.11 (2010): 5550-5558.

[24] Chopra, I. J., J. Sack, and D. A. Fisher. "Circulating 3, 3', 5'-triiodothyronine (reverse T3) in the human newborn." *Journal of Clinical Investigation* 55.6 (1975): 1137.

[25] Germain, Donald L. St, Valerie Anne Galton, and Arturo Hernandez. "Defining the roles of the iodothyronine deiodinases: Current concepts and challenges." *Endocrinology* 150.3 (2009): 1097-1107.

[26] Corona, G., et al. "Thyroid hormones and male sexual function." *International journal of andrology* 35.5 (2012): 668-679.

[27] Carani, Cesare, et al. "Multicenter study on the prevalence of sexual symptoms in male hypo-and hyperthyroid patients." *Journal of Clinical Endocrinology & Metabolism* 90.12 (2005): 6472-6479.

[28] Kumar, B. Jaya, et al. "Reproductive endocrine functions in men with primary hypothyroidism: effect of thyroxine replacement." *Hormone Research in Paediatrics* 34.5-6 (2008): 215-218.

[29] Nikoobakht, Mohammad Reza, et al. "The role of hypothyroidism in male infertility and erectile dysfunction." *Urology Journal* 9.1 (2012): 405-409.

[30] Krassas, G. E., et al. "A prospective controlled study of the impact of hyperthyroidism on reproductive function in males." *Journal of Clinical Endocrinology & Metabolism* 87.8 (2002): 3667-3671.

[31] Singh, Rajender, and A. Agarwal. "Thyroid hormones in male reproduction and fertility." *Open Reprod Sci J* 3 (2011): 98-104.

[32] Wagner, Márcia Santos, Simone Magagnin Wajner, and Ana Luiza Maia. "The role of thyroid hormone in testicular development and function." *Journal of Endocrinology* 199.3 (2008): 351-365.

23

Reverse T3: Side Effects of T3-only (or why you need T4 too)

*We are all free to believe what we wish to believe,
and to reject what we don't like*

—T3-only proponent

Reverse T3 and the T3-only protocol

Thyroxine (T4) is the primary hormone produced by the thyroid gland. It is called T4 because it is composed of four iodine atoms attached to tyrosyl residues (from the amino acid tyrosine). When one of the iodine atoms is removed by an enzyme in a process called deiodination, it becomes triiodothyronine (T3). Since there are four iodine atoms attached to T4, there are really four different iodine atoms that could be removed. Removal of an iodine atom from one position creates the T3 molecule, removal from another position creates the reverse T3 (rT3) molecule. Thyroid receptors are found in every cell, within the nucleus, and are designed for T3, so T3 is considered the active hormone. T4 and rT3 are relatively inactive and do not generate energy through the thyroid receptor, nor do they fit. The term *inactive metabolite* is used to describe rT3 in medical literature. Both T4 and rT3 do, however, initiate actions outside of the cell nucleus, referred to as non-genomic actions. Some of these actions occur at the cell membrane, others occur within the cell, just not at the nucleus. If someone has no T4 in their body, then some biological processes cannot occur.

The T3-only protocol was intended to rid the body of high levels of reverse T3, based on the belief that all rT3 is "bad." Since rT3 can only be made from T4, no T4 is taken, only T3. The body then is forced to function solely on T3. To determine if someone might benefit from the T3-only protocol, a rT3 ratio is calculated. If FT3/rT3 < 20 (Free T3 divided by rT3 is less than 20), then that person is said to have reverse T3 dominance and would benefit from the T3-only protocol. If an alternative calculation, Total T3/rT3 < 10 (Total T3 divided by rT3 is less than 10), then that person is also considered to be rT3 dominant. Reverse T3 is said to be the cause of stubborn hypothyroid symptoms because rT3 is "blocking" the T3 receptors. (The terms "blocking" or "clogging" are used by T3-only proponents to explain their concept; it will be disproved later in this chapter.)

The protocol recommends 75-125 mcg of T3 split throughout the day, and no T4 whatsoever. No human being produces that amount of T3 daily unless they have a hyperthyroid condition like Graves' disease. Some people can tolerate these high doses of T3, others cannot.

Why do so many experience side effects on the T3-only protocol? The reasons are explained in detail in this chapter, but here is a quick summary, which basically proves that the reverse T3 ratio theory is based on faulty premises. Recent research in cellular and molecular biology shows that:

- rT3 does *not* block the receptor at all; neither rT3 nor T3 is bound to the receptor and *that* is the cause of hypothyroid symptoms
- T4 is more than a prohormone and is essential for healthy hair, brain, and other functions
- Excess T3 may cause osteoporosis, muscle wasting, insulin resistance, hair loss, and memory loss.
- Excess T3 will cause an imbalance in other hormones (it raises estradiol, which can be problematic, especially for men)
- Excess T3 (desiccated thyroid has relatively high amounts of T3) can trigger high reverse T3
- Desiccated thyroid contains rT3, because rT3 is found in a normal thyroid gland, and desiccated thyroid is made from normal pig thyroid glands.
- A low reverse T3 ratio can be caused by either high *or* low Free T3 levels. A high FT3 and a low FT3 are different conditions and should not be treated the same way.

Reverse T3's role in the body

Normal, healthy people produce reverse T3, it is not poison, and it is a normal pathway for the breakdown of T4. It is actually abnormal to have *no* reverse T3![1]

One purpose of reverse T3 is to reduce metabolism, to prevent starvation in cases of famine. Anyone on a severe calorie restricted diet will reach a weight plateau at some point because reverse T3 naturally rises in this condition.[2]

Marathon athletes can also have high reverse T3 levels for the same reason—the body is trying to conserve energy to prevent starvation. Strict dieting and excessive exercise will raise reverse T3 levels.[3]

Studies show that there are many other causes of high reverse T3 levels: [4]

- aging
- burns/thermal injury
- chemical exposure
- cold exposure
- chronic alcohol intake
- free radical load
- hemorrhagic shock (often from severe blood loss)
- insulin-dependent diabetes mellitus
- liver disease

- kidney disease
- severe or systemic illness
- severe injury
- stress
- surgery
- toxic metal exposure
- certain drugs like amiodarone[5] and beta blockers[6]
- and high cortisol[7]

It's much healthier to address and correct the conditions just listed, than to take only T3. Diabetics typically have high reverse T3 levels that drop once their glucose is controlled.[8]

Reverse T3 levels can appear high in someone whose liver is not healthy because reverse T3 is processed and eliminated in the liver.[9] [10] There are anecdotal accounts from people who have a suboptimal reverse T3 ratio, with both FT3 and reverse T3 over mid-range, but who feel fine. As long as the FT3 was optimal for them, it didn't matter what the reverse T3 level was. This would not be possible if rT3 truly blocked the T3 receptor.

Aiming for a reverse T3 ratio greater than 20 (or 10) is like aiming for a normal TSH. Having an optimal ratio does not indicate good health any more than a normal TSH does.

Reverse T3, like cholesterol, is a natural substance found in everyone, and has a purpose. When it is high, it indicates an imbalance in the body, but to try to eliminate rT3 from the body is unnatural, and analogous to taking statins to bring cholesterol levels down. Many have suffered permanent damage from taking statins,[11] and people have suffered serious side effects from taking T3-only. The rule that the reverse T3 ratio should be greater than 20 is analogous to saying one's TSH should be a certain number. Both are arbitrary numbers that fluctuate and should not dictate treatment.

A low rT3 ratio has been found in patients with heart failure[12] and severe illnesses,[13] but there is no scientific evidence that says that any ratio below 20 (FT3/rT3) or below 10 (Total T3/rT3) indicates a disease state. Everyone has T3 and rT3, so everyone will have a ratio. However, whether or not being greater or less than 20 indicates health vs. disease is questionable. Just like some feel fine with a low TSH (and not hyperthyroid), others may feel fine with a ratio lower than 20. If they then start taking T3-only in an attempt to "correct" their normal ratio, they may suffer from the dangerous side effects of too much T3.

Here are three different lab profiles where the reverse T3 ratio can be low (in patients already taking thyroid medication). Each has a different cause and requires a different treatment, which is not accounted for with the simplistic reverse T3 ratio formula, which is: *if FT3 divided by rT3 is less than 20, then one should only take T3.* This is called *nonsense math,* where an equation gives an appearance of credibility, even though it makes no sense.[14] If a low ratio can be from either high *or* low Free T3, then the ratio is useless, because it can mean two different things; this makes it mathematically invalid. BMI or Body Mass Index is an example of a valid ratio. Weight is divided by height. The higher the BMI ratio, the more overweight the person. A high BMI ratio does not mean overweight in some cases, but underweight in others. But a low rT3 ratio can mean either too much *or* too little T3. As explained below, it is the level of rT3 (relative to the reference range) that matters, not the ratio.

- Profile I: mid-range to high Free T3, below mid-range Free T4
  Reverse T3 may be slightly high (a few points above the reference range) due to high T3. This lab profile is often found in those taking desiccated thyroid because of the high T3/T4 ratio in the pills. The body senses the high T3 levels, and converts some T4 to rT3 to compensate for those high levels. Desiccated thyroid also contains rT3, so reverse T3 levels should rise as the desiccated dose is increased. Lowering the desiccated thyroid dose and adding T4 has lowered rT3 levels in some patients. These people report improved reverse T3 ratios on higher levels of T4 and say they feel more "balanced" with the additional T4. The T3-only protocol does not work well for these patients because it compounds the problem that caused the high reverse T3 in the first place—too much T3. In fact, a low ratio has been documented in hyperthyroid patients.[15] The people in this group feel best with a higher proportion of T4 to T3, and may suffer severe side effects on the T3-only protocol. The rT3 ratio is too simplistic to differentiate between these people and those found in Profile III.

- Profile II: below mid-range Free T3, mid-range to high Free T4
  Reverse T3 may be high relative to FT3 due to poor conversion and lack of essential cofactors like selenium. This lab profile is often found in those who only take T4. Reverse T3 levels may actually be within the reference range, but the calculated rT3 ratio is low because T3 levels are low. Changing to desiccated, which has T3, or adding T3 to a lower dose of T4 often helps. Addressing factors that impede conversion, such as high cortisol or low iron, is also recommended. These people do best when their T4/T3 ratio is closest to that found in desiccated thyroid. This ratio can also be attained with synthetic T3 and T4, or customized by adding additional T3 to the desiccated thyroid dose. These people feel better once they add some T3 to their dose.

- Profile III: below mid-range Free T3, below mid-range Free T4, over range reverse T3
  If reverse T3 is significantly over the reference range (sometimes hundreds of points over the range), and the patient's Free T3 and Free T4 do not rise with increasing doses of any type of thyroid hormone, this could indicate something more serious that should be investigated. Iron labs may point to Anemia of Chronic Disease, rather than Iron Deficiency Anemia. Serious infections (infected root canals, for example) can cause this. Uterine fibroid or other tumors, as well as damaged heart muscle could also cause high reverse T3. The high reverse T3 is a sign of a problem, not the cause of the problem. Reverse T3 itself does not physically block the receptor. Surgical removal of the infected part has often brought a relief in symptoms. These are the patients that must take extremely high doses of T3 to overcome an overactive D3 enzyme, which not only

converts T4 to reverse T3, but also inactivates any T3 to T2, resulting in minimal T3 for the body's functions. These people do best with a higher proportion of T3 to T4, but may have a hard time tolerating it due to the iron problems. Some of these patients do not tolerate any T4 because of their underlying condition and only feel functional on T3-only. However, they are not immune from the side effects of too much T3, and their T4 deficiency may affect other parts of the body that depend on T4, especially the brain.

D3, the deiodinase enzyme that makes reverse T3 (*not* vitamin D3)

There are three deiodinase enzymes (D1, D2, D3) that convert thyroid hormones by removing various iodine atoms. D3 is the deiodinase enzyme that converts T4 to reverse T3 *and* inactivates T3 to T2. Its purpose is to keep T3 levels low. D3 is absent from most adult tissues, though it is found in the skin and certain parts of the brain. It is also found in fetal tissues, the uterine endometrium, and placenta, where it serves to protect the fetus from the mother's adult levels of thyroid hormones.[16]

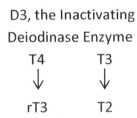

D3, the Inactivating
Deiodinase Enzyme

T4	T3
↓	↓
rT3	T2

Nonthyroidal Illness Syndrome (NTIS), also known as euthyroid sick syndrome (ESS) or low T3 syndrome, presents with high reverse T3, low T3, and normal T4 and TSH. In NTIS, the three deiodinase enzymes work together to lower T3 and raise reverse T3, making the patient more hypothyroid. The illness itself causes the derangement in thyroid levels.[17] This is an important concept to understand—the thyroid itself has not gone bad (as in autoimmune disease), but a serious illness has taken control of, and downregulated thyroid levels. These are the patients that can take the high doses of T3 recommended in this protocol without any hyperthyroid symptoms because their extremely high D3 levels inactivate much of their T3.

The brain and spinal cord prefer stable blood serum T3 levels and the deiodinase enzymes work together to maintain this stability. If T3 becomes too high, for example, D3 rises, increasing T3 clearance to T2, which lowers T3. Simultaneously, D2 levels decrease, decreasing T3 production from T4. The rise in D3 would also shunt more T4 to the reverse T3 pathway, so less T3 would be made.[18] In other words, too high a dose of T3 can cause high reverse T3 by increasing the D3 enzyme. Desiccated thyroid has a higher proportion of T3 than a human thyroid, so as some raise their desiccated dose, their reverse T3 also increases. Desiccated thyroid also contains reverse T3, so while it raises Free T3, it also raises reverse T3. A large dose of T3 taken all at once (when T4 is also present) could also have the same effect and raise reverse T3 levels.

D3 is reactivated in certain medical conditions in adults. After a heart attack, the heart muscle itself expresses D3. Mice who suffered heart attacks were found to have increased D3 activity in the heart muscle, with a corresponding 50% decrease of T3 in left ventricular tissues.[19]   This implies that patients who have had cardiac episodes may always have high reverse T3 levels, and there are some people on the thyroid internet forums that fit this profile.

High D3 activity has been found in vascular (blood vessel), brain, and other tumors, and some malignant cancers.[20] It has been found in basal cell carcinomas, colon cancer, and other solid tumors.[21] There is even a condition called consumptive hypothyroidism, where D3 activity from a tumor is so pronounced that it literally consumes any thyroid hormone, resulting in profound hypothyroidism. Blood serum T4 and T3 levels do not increase even with increasing doses of T4 medication, though reverse T3 stays high.[22] In one case, high levels of D3 were found in a woman's liver tumor, and her elevated TSH returned to normal after the mass was surgically removed.[23]

D3 can also be reactivated when cell proliferation is desired, to lower T3, which stimulates cell differentiation and inhibits cell growth. Healing from a burn is an example where cell proliferation is necessary to regenerate new tissue. When livers were partially removed in rats and mice, D3 activity increased 40-fold in the mice 36 hours after surgery. In the rats, blood serum and liver T3 and T4 levels decreased 2- to 3-fold 20 to 24 hours after the surgery.[24] Other studies show high D3 activity in various states of tissue injury: starvation, cryolesion (frostbite or medical procedures that purposely freeze tissue to destroy it), cardiac hypertrophy (thickened heart muscle, usually due to high blood pressure), infarction (heart attack), and chronic inflammation.[25] High reverse T3 should be expected anytime there is tissue damage that needs repair.

During acute bacterial infections, granulocytes (a type of white blood cell) in infected organs express D3, and serum thyroid hormones decrease proportionately to the severity of the illness. In other words, the more severe the illness is, the lower the T3 levels. D3 is also highly expressed in response to chemical inflammation (such as a turpentine induced abscess).[26] Infections and abscesses would then be expected to cause high reverse T3.

Perhaps those with high reverse T3 have an underlying condition, like those just listed in the paragraphs above. Quite a few thyroid patients have reported tonsillectomies (infection/inflammation), hysterectomies (fibroid tumors), heart conditions, problem root canals (infection), and various cancers. Sinus infections and gut inflammation (celiac) are other possible causes.

Recent research shows individual genetic differences in many aspects of thyroid physiology, and these can all impact T3 and reverse T3 levels. Genetic variations have been found in the TSH receptor, thyroid hormone receptors, thyroid transporters (that take hormone into the cells), and the deiodinase enzymes (a variation in D2 correlates with diabetes, and diabetics have high reverse T3).[27]

T4's role in the body

While T3 appears to be the most metabolically active, all thyroid hormones (T4, T3, T2, T1, T0) have non-genomic effects many are not aware of. Non-genomic means the hormone can exert an effect on the cell at the plasma membrane (surface) or in the cytoplasm (cell interior), whereas the primary effects of T3 are at the cell's nucleus (after conversion from T4). In other words, T4 exerts these non-genomic effects outside of the nucleus, and before its conversion to T3. So to say T4 is a prohormone (storage hormone) with no effect is incorrect, because it does have an effect in its unconverted state.[28]

Hair needs T4, because it lengthens the hair growth phase. Tests on various hair parameters showed that T4 and T3 had different effects, which suggests that both T4 *and* T3 are essential for healthy hair. Both the D2 and D3 deiodinase enzymes are expressed in human hair follicles, which means hair follicles can convert T4 to either T3 *or* rT3. When T4 was added to hair follicles in a medium, measurable T3 was generated in the medium.[29] My Free T3 has been below the reference range, mid-range, and over-range, but my hair was never quite right at any of those levels. The addition of T4 combined with a reduction in my desiccated dose finally raised my Free T4 above mid-range, and both my hair texture and volume improved. It should be noted that hair loss is a symptom of both too much *and* too little thyroid.

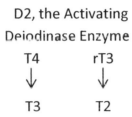

D2, the Activating
Deiodinase Enzyme

In one experiment on dogs, T4 was administered both topically and orally. In either case, there was an increase in both the rate of hair growth and in the number of hair follicles entering the growth (anagen) phase of the hair cycle.[30]

T4 converts into other essential metabolites besides T3. These cannot be made from T3. Just like T4 is deiodinated (converted) to T3, T4 can also be deaminated (converted) to tetraiodothyroacetic acid (tetrac). Tetrac has been shown to inhibit tumor growth, while T3 and T4 stimulate it.[31] If T4 is eliminated, then there is no source from which to make tetrac, which may be just one of several metabolites that can only be created from T4.

T(1)AM (3-iodothyronamine) is another biologically active T4 metabolite which has nongenomic cardiac effects. This metabolite induces opposite effects from those stimulated by T3 and T4, such as decreased heart muscle contractions and decreased heart rate. Both T3 and T4 have multiple nongenomic cardiac effects, and an equilibrium between T3, T4, and T(1)AM levels is essential for heart health.[32]

T3 and T4's role in the brain

There are two different transporters for T3 and T4 into the brain. One (OATP1c1) transports only T4, the other (MCT8) transports T3 and T4. T4 is then converted locally to T3 by the D2 deiodinase enzyme. The total T3 in the brain comes from what was converted locally (from T4), plus what was transported in as T3.[33]

Deiodinase activity is different in specific regions of the brain. Thyroid hormone levels in the brain are kept in tight ranges because the brain requires that stability. D3 expression increases in hyperthyroidism (when T3 levels are too high), to keep T3 levels from rising even higher. The T4 to reverse T3 pathway is enhanced, as well as the T3 to T2 pathway. Likewise, D2 expression is suppressed, lowering T4 to T3 conversion, while also limiting rT3 to T2 conversion. Reverse T3 levels appear higher because more is made and less is cleared out. The D2 and D3 deiodinase enzymes work together to lower high T3 levels. Conversely, in hypothyroidism (when T3 levels are too low), D2 expression is increased, which raises T4 to T3 conversion, to raise T3 levels in the brain. When someone takes T3-only and no T4, they may lose this important regulatory feature of reverse T3 (to lower high T3 levels), and T3 levels may exceed the brain's optimal range, since there is no T4 to inactivate. It's analogous to running too much voltage through a low-voltage appliance. This can result in what is called hyperthyroid dementia or fresh amnesia, where recall of events minutes earlier is impaired.[34] [35] I suffered from this fresh amnesia and could not recall things I'd done two minutes earlier when taking too much T3. I was also completely unable to perform simple math in my head, which I do routinely. My memory and math skills returned once my T3 dose was reduced. In another case, the person lost their foreign language fluency.

A study of rats treated with T3 supports these observations. After T3 treatment, their brains showed a 50% decrease in specific membranes of the cerebral cortex, which is the part of the brain involved with memory, attention, and language.[36]

Thyroid hormone levels of healthy women (all thyroid labs within normal range) were analyzed for any correlation of their performance in neuropsychological tests to their thyroid levels. High Free T3 levels were positively associated with slower completion times for certain cognitive tests; in other words, the higher the Free T3, the longer it took the subject to complete three tests. In Trail Making Test-A, subjects draw a line connecting numbered circles, which are randomly placed on the page. In other words, after finding circle 1, they draw a line to circle 2, etc. until they reach circle 25. In Trail Making Test-B, subjects have to connect both numbers and letters in order: 1-A-2-B-3-C etc. This test can cause extreme confusion and will take longer to complete if the brain isn't working correctly. The third test that subjects with high Free T3 took longer to complete is the Tower of London test. In this test, subjects rearrange stacked, colored beads on three posts into a new configuration they're shown. A bead that was formerly on the bottom of a post in the old configuration may need to be on the top of a different post in the new configuration. Getting the beads in the correct order involves thought and planning. Because high Free T3 was consistently correlated with slower performance test times, the authors concluded that elevations in thyroid hormones (within the normal range) may negatively affect frontal cortex executive functions in the brain, where memory, attention and language are located.[37]

Female thyroid cancer patients who had undergone thyroidectomies followed by radioactive iodine (who were on suppressive doses of levothyroxine), were studied when their levothyroxine doses were stopped for an upcoming radioactive iodine whole body scan. They were tested at three points in time:

- before stopping their dose, when they were considered mildly hyperthyroid (suppressed TSH, over range FT4, normal to high FT3)
- 4-7 days after stopping their dose, when considered euthyroid (FT3 and FT4 normal, but TSH still suppressed for most), and

- about 30 days later, when considered profoundly hypothyroid (TSH high, FT3 and FT4 below range). Controls of similar ages and backgrounds were also measured for comparison.

A visual scanning test that measures distractibility and visual inattentiveness gave interesting results. Subjects had to locate a particular symbol in a paper filled with a matrix of symbols, and there were 60 correct matches. While nearly all symbols were found each time (59/60), the subjects took the longest time to perform the task when they were mildly hyperthyroid, longer even than when they were profoundly hypothyroid![38] This suggests that too much thyroid hormone causes some type of brain dysfunction and may actually be a mild form of hyperthyroid dementia. In fact, Graves' hyperthyroid patients frequently exhibit deficits in attention, memory, and complex problem solving.[39]

The hippocampus and temporal cortex areas of the brain, which affect memory and cognitive functions, exhibit the highest D3 concentrations, the enzyme that inactivates T3. This suggests that these two areas of the brain are the most sensitive to high T3 levels, and the studies just mentioned appear to confirm that statement. In one experiment, D3 could not be detected in hypothyroid brains, and D3 levels were found to correlate with thyroid status in the central nervous system. In other words, D3 would rise as thyroid levels rose, so reverse T3 could be made if T3 levels became too high.[40][41]

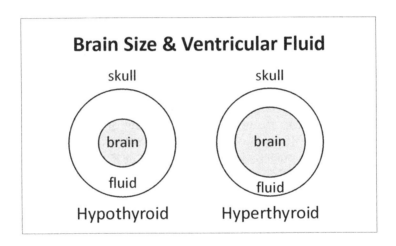

Figure 23-1. Thyroid hormone levels affect the size of the brain and the surrounding fluid. In hypothyroid patients, the brain is smaller while the fluid space is larger. The opposite state is found in hyperthyroid patients, who have larger brains with less fluid. Note: this is a graphical depiction and is not drawn to any scale.

Brain size physically changes when thyroid levels are too high or too low. The hyperthyroid brain is larger than normal, and the hypothyroid brain is smaller than normal. Conversely, ventricular size (which contains the cerebrospinal fluid) is smaller than normal in hyperthyroid patients, and larger than normal in hypothyroid patients. The reduction in brain size and increase in ventricular size found in hypothyroid patients significantly correlated to reduced T4 levels. In other words, as T4 levels rose, brain size increased and ventricular size decreased towards normal. Interestingly, brain size did not correlate with T3 levels. However, ventricular size decrease strongly correlated with rising T3 levels.[42] People starting on the T3-only protocol often report headaches and the decrease in ventricular size may be a factor.

In the brain, T3 that is deiodinated (converted) from T4 accounts for more than 80% of the total T3 specifically bound to nuclear receptors in the cerebral cortex, and approximately 67% of that in the cerebellum. In other words, T4 is the major source of intracellular T3 in the central nervous system.[43] If 80% of the T3 in the brain came from T4, then a higher than normal dose of T3 would be necessary to compensate for the loss of T4 in a T3-only protocol. But a dose that high could have adverse effects on other systems that are more sensitive to T3, like the cardiovascular system, and may cause problems like tachycardia (rapid heart rate) and high blood pressure.

EEGs (brain electrical activity) of hypothyroid patients (thyroidectomy followed by radioactive iodine) were compared at three points in time: while they were still hypothyroid, after supplementation with T3, and after supplementation with T3 + T4. The EEGs only normalized when T4 was added to the T3, and correlated significantly with the rise in serum T4 levels. Patients may appear clinically normal, but increased serum T3 with low T4 is called *hypothyroxinemia* in medical literature. EEGs of these patients will confirm abnormalities indicative of brain hypothyroidism. T4 appears to be essential for normal brain function.[44][45]

The psychological well-being of patients on thyroid hormone replacement was compared to their Free T3, Free T4, and reverse T3 levels. There was a strong positive correlation of higher FT4 levels with well-being; in other words, patients with higher FT4 levels (even above the reference range) just felt better mood-wise. But there was no correlation of psychological well-being to Free T3, rT3, rT3/FT4, or FT3/rT3. The authors noted that all measures are serum measures and do not reflect intracellular levels, and that many tissues obtain their T3 by conversion from T4.[46] As stated earlier, with ample T4, the brain can create the optimal amount of T3 it needs with the appropriate deiodinase enzymes. If T4 levels are too high, more will be shunted to rT3. If T4 levels are low, nearly all T4 will be converted to T3. But if T4 is extremely low, then T3 in the brain will be insufficient.

T3's negative effect on other hormones

Apparently some people remain on T3-only indefinitely and actually feel fine, or certainly better than they ever did on T4 medications. Others, however, become worse, because the high T3 levels have side effects and create imbalances in other hormones. In men, high T3 levels will cause sex hormone binding globulin (SHBG) to increase,[47] the production rate of estradiol to rise, and the metabolic clearance rate of estradiol to fall.[48] The net effect is higher estradiol levels, which can have a disastrous effect on men's health and well-being. In men, a hyperthyroid state can elevate estradiol and result in gynecomastia (male breasts).[49] Premature ejaculation seems to be a problem for hyperthyroid men, and delayed ejaculation a problem for hypothyroid men.[50] High SHBG in men also correlates with osteoporosis and a higher fracture risk.[51]

SHBG also rises in women taking excessive T3.[52] Plasma estrogen levels may be two to threefold higher because the metabolic clearance rate of estradiol decreases.[53] This may be the cause of painful breasts that some women have reported on the T3-only protocol. Women's testosterone levels also decrease on this protocol. This may be desirable if a woman exhibits high androgen symptoms like facial hair, infertility, etc., but undesirable if levels become too low.[54]

In women, estrogen and progesterone can also raise SHBG if taken orally,[55] so a woman on these other hormones following the T3-only protocol can become quite imbalanced. Hormonal imbalance is often the cause of both physical and emotional symptoms.

T3-only side effects

The problem with T3-only treatment is that one must usually go over the reference range on T3 levels to compensate for the lack of T4 in the body. People on thyroid internet forums that have been on T3-only protocols have reported the following side effects:

- erythrocytosis[56]—thick blood or high RBC, hematocrit, and hemoglobin
- osteoporosis[57]—subjects given 50-75 µg of T3 showed increased bone resorption and fecal calcium loss
- muscle weakness[58][59]—especially thigh or upper arm muscles: difficulty climbing stairs or rising from sitting; also difficulty holding arms above head to wash hair. T3 doses greater than 60 µg/day enhanced muscle catabolism (breakdown) during fasting. In other words, high T3 can cause muscle wasting. The heart is a muscle and is not immune from this effect.
- insulin resistance[60][61]—Both plasma glucose and insulin increase after T3 ingestion, which is not a desirable effect. A correlation was found between higher Free T3 and Free T4 levels and insulin resistance in the early stages of Type 2 diabetes.[62]
- fast heart rate or palpitations[59]
- intolerance to exercise[59]
- shortness-of-breath[59]
- insomnia[59]
- hair loss/thinning[59]
- elevated liver enzymes (AST and/or ALT)[63]
- brain fog or hyperthyroid dementia—can't remember things that just happened, or trouble solving problems (math, scheduling, etc.) [64][65][35]

These are symptoms that anyone on T3-only therapy should be aware of, and are actually classic symptoms of hyperthyroidism. Hypothyroidism presents with some of these same symptoms, so it can be difficult for patients to tell whether they are over or under-medicated. Like hydrocortisone, there are side effects to this therapy that anyone undertaking this protocol should know about. Many have ended up feeling worse than before they started. Because hydrocortisone helps a person to tolerate thyroid hormone, there is the potential problem of taking more and more hydrocortisone to tolerate more and more T3, ultimately resulting in a serious overdose of both hormones. In fact, high T3 levels have been observed to lower cortisol levels to the point of adrenal insufficiency in hyperthyroid Graves' patients. Cortisol levels returned to normal when thyroid levels were brought back into the normal range with antithyroid medications.[66]

Another danger of T3-only therapy is the potential to "run out" of thyroid hormone in the event of an emergency. The half-life of T3 is approximately 10-15 hours, while the half-life of T4 is about 5 days.[67] Without any T4 reserves, constant T3 dosing is essential. An incident where one was rendered unconscious or could not access their medication (natural disasters) would result in rapidly declining thyroid levels in the body after only 24 hours. This severe hypothyroid state would hinder any recovery.

Do thyroid receptors really get blocked and take 12 weeks to clear? Is T4 really the problem?

Proponents of T3-only therapy believe that reverse T3 "blocks" or "clogs" the T3 receptors, therefore only T3 should be taken for 12 weeks until the reverse T3 is "cleared." Yet others who have not changed their dose to T3-only (and continued to take some T4) have reported reduced reverse T3 levels in subsequent test results, by addressing problems like low iron, or increasing their caloric intake and eating more frequently. A study in Calcutta, India illustrates that reverse T3 is indeed dynamic. Patients who suffered from malnutrition had reverse T3 values that were above the values of normal subjects, but their reverse T3 fell once they were fed, so the condition is dynamic, not static.[68] In another experiment on fasting obese subjects, reverse T3 levels rose significantly by day 7, but returned to normal after 4 days of refeeding.[69] In both studies, the subjects' reverse T3 levels returned to normal without being put on a T3-only regimen. The rT3 proponents argue that rT3 may have cleared from the blood, but it's still "stuck" in the receptors for 12 weeks. Cellular biology shows that rT3 does not bind to the cell nuclear receptor. It is also highly improbable that any hormone can last for 12 weeks or 84 days. As previously stated, the half-life of T3 is less than a day, and the half-life of T4 is less than a week.

Reverse T3 inhibits the D2 enzyme that converts T4 to T3 in the rat brain cortex and pituitary. Rats were infused daily with four increasing levels of reverse T3, and D2 enzyme activity decreased (so T4 to T3 conversion decreased) as the reverse T3 levels increased. Tracers on the reverse T3 showed the reverse T3 was not detectable in the cell nuclei, and only 1% was found elsewhere in a homogenized mixture of the rat brain and pituitary tissue. The infused reverse T3 was no longer present, which means reverse T3 did not "clog" these receptors, nor would it be present 12 weeks later.[70] Reverse T3 has a much higher clearance rate than FT3.[71]

A study was performed to observe the effects of reverse T3 vs. T3 on cellular metabolism in vitro (in a lab). As expected, cells incubated with reverse T3 showed a decrease in metabolism, and those incubated with T3 showed an increase. The later addition of T3 to the cells that had been incubated with reverse T3 completely reversed the metabolic reduction. There was no 12-week delay for "clearing." This suggests that the lack of T3, not the blocking by reverse T3, is the cause of reduced cellular metabolism.[72]

T4 is not always to blame for high reverse T3. High levels of T4 will lower D2 enzyme activity, which lowers T4 conversion to T3. But high levels of T3 will raise D3 enzyme activity, so more T4 is converted to reverse T3 to keep T3 levels normal. In other words, neither T4 nor T3 can become too high, or the appropriate enzymes are invoked to keep the levels where the body deems appropriate. Several studies that compared reverse T3 levels of hyperthyroid patients to normal or hypothyroid patients showed high reverse T3 levels in the hyperthyroid patients. The reverse T3 levels of hyperthyroid patients were high whether measured in urine,[73] blood serum,[74] or production rate.[75] Urinary excretion of reverse T3 was 6.4 times higher in hyperthyroids than hypothyroids, up to 43 times higher in blood serum in hyperthyroids vs. hypothyroids, and the production rate was 63 times higher in hyperthyroids vs. hypothyroids. In addition, reverse T3 has a metabolic clearance rate that is almost three times faster than FT3,[71] so as long as there is adequate FT3, there should be sufficient thyroid energy reaching the cells.

If the hyperthyroid state causes high reverse T3 levels, and reverse T3 really does "clog" receptors, then no one could ever become hyperthyroid. The enhanced reverse T3 pathway in hyperthyroid patients lowers Free T3 levels somewhat, but apparently enough T3 is still getting to the cells to create hyperthyroid symptoms. This is the strongest argument against the "clogged receptors" theory. The receptors are not clogged at all; there is no reverse T3 or T3 in the receptors if someone is still hypothyroid. In those with high reverse T3, there is simply not enough T3 available to fill the receptors, and that is why the person still has hypothyroid symptoms.

The T3-only protocol is actually modeled after the hyperthyroid condition, where T3 levels are so high, that they exhaust the capacity of the D3 enzyme to inactivate any T3 to T2. What is left gets through to the open receptor. There is no reverse T3 to "unclog." Corepressors silence the receptors when T3 is not available, not rT3. This concept is discussed in the next section.

The following charts illustrate how two of the deiodinase enzymes (D2 and D3) work. It's an oversimplified diagram to depict the key concepts. The circle represents a cell, which is floating in plasma, where thyroid hormones like T4, T3, rT3, and T2 can be found. The squares represent the cell's nucleus, where the thyroid receptors are located.

T4's Two Potential Cellular Pathways

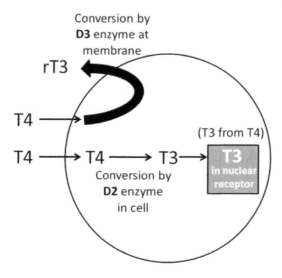

Figure 23-2. T4 can take two different pathways upon entering a cell. In normal conditions, T4 from the plasma enters the cell through a transporter, is converted by the D2 deiodinase enzyme into T3, and then enters the nuclear thyroid receptor. In cases such as non-thyroidal illness, as T4 enters the cell, the D3 deiodinase enzyme at the cell membrane inactivates the T4 by converting it to rT3 and bounces it back out.[76] Reverse T3 does not stay inside the cell to "block" the receptor.

T3's Two Potential Cellular Pathways

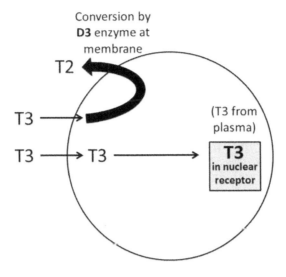

Figure 23-3. T3 can take two different pathways upon entering a cell. In normal conditions, T3 from the plasma enters the cell through a transporter, and then enters the nuclear thyroid receptor. In cases such as non-thyroidal illness, as T3 enters the cell, the D3 deiodinase enzyme at the cell membrane converts T3 to T2 and bounces it back out. No T3 would reach the thyroid receptor in this case.

Source of T3 for Thyroid Receptors

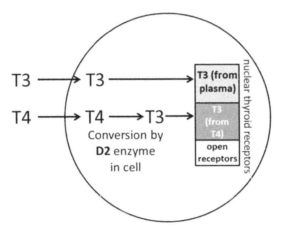

Figure 23-4. In normal conditions, nuclear thyroid receptors are filled with T3 from two different sources: T3 from the plasma, and newly converted T3 from T4 in the cell. In non-thyroidal illness, neither source of T3 reaches the thyroid receptors because the D3 deiodinase enzyme at the cell membrane converts T4 to rT3, and T3 to T2, and bounces it back out. There is no reverse T3 blocking the receptor. The receptors remain unfilled with no source of T3 and the cell would have no energy.

If reverse T3 doesn't block the receptor, what is this "clearing" people experience?

Activating a cell's thyroid receptor with T3 is just one of several steps in thyroid hormone metabolism. Problems can result at any step in the process.

- Transport into the cell: Transporters take T3 or T4 across the cell membrane. Mutations have been identified in these transporters which would affect whether thyroid hormone even enters the cell.[77]
- Conversion within the cell: The three deiodinase enzymes work together and determine whether T4 is activated to T3 or inactivated to rT3. T3 production by D2 varies depending on T4, rT3 and T3 levels; these feedback mechanisms allow different tissues to produce the specific amount of T3 needed. Genetic variations have been found in the deiodinase enzymes which may account for the vastly different thyroid hormone doses required for different people.[78]
- Binding with the nuclear thyroid receptor: Thyroid receptors do not work alone. There are nuclear corepressors and coactivators that either repress or activate the receptor, depending on the availability of T3. When T3 is scarce, corepressors are recruited and transcription (gene expression) is repressed; when T3 becomes available, corepressors are released, coactivators are recruited, and transcription is activated.[79] In other words, lack of T3 will cause a corepressor (not rT3) to "block" a receptor's action.

It may be that the "clearing" people experience has something to do with the last step—where enough T3 enters the cells and causes a release of corepressors, so that co-activators can be recruited to activate gene expression in the cell. Reverse T3 is not involved in this process; corepressors in the cell are what silence any gene expression until there's enough T3 available. The T3 receptor, like most hormone receptors, has an extremely high specificity and affinity (attraction) for its own hormone, partially based on its unique physical structure.[80] In other words, it is highly unlikely that anything other than T3 can fit in and activate the T3 receptor.

High rT3 means the D3 enzyme is dominant, converting much T4 to rT3, and T3 to T2. Because little to no T3 is available to the cell, the corepressors on the receptor will have silenced any gene expression. If T3 can somehow make its way into the cell (higher than normal doses of T3 may be one way to achieve this), then the corepressors will be released and replaced by coactivators, and gene expression will be activated. However, if the cause of the high rT3 is not corrected (non-thyroidal illness, severe dieting, high corti-sol, etc.), then a return to normal T3 levels will not be able to overcome the high D3 enzyme levels that should still be present, and the patient would return to their previous hypothyroid state. Reverse T3 is a symptom of a problem, not the actual cause of the problem.

Corepressors may be the body's method of rationing out what little thyroid hormone is available when levels are low. The brain requires oxygen and glucose to stay alive, so the heart and lungs are always rationed a share of the available hormone. But in terms of priorities for sustaining life, normal hair, bowel movements, and skin are not high on the list, and corepressors may be the mechanism the body uses to temporarily "shut off" those energy-draining systems. It would be analogous to trying to heat a whole house with a space heater. It's possible to keep one room warm, but there's less strain on the system if the doors to adjacent rooms are closed.

Hyperthyroid human models (Graves' patients) prove that the concept of rT3 blocking the receptors is flawed. They have extremely high levels of rT3, yet they are hyperthyroid. Therefore, rT3 cannot be said to block the receptor.

In the Absence of T3, Thyroid Receptors Are Kept Inactive by Corepressors

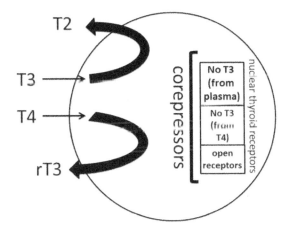

Figure 23-5. Significantly elevated reverse T3 levels (not a low ratio) are a sign of an overactive D3 enzyme, which means little T3 reaches the nuclear receptor. Corepressors silence any gene expression until enough T3 induces a change from corepressors to coactivators.

Optimal thyroid dosing

The reference range for T3 is not based on a normal (bell-shaped) distribution curve. The values are actually negatively skewed, meaning the majority of the values fall in the upper half of the reference range, and the peak (the most common value) is somewhere to the right of the midpoint,[81] and not at the top of the range. If someone's optimal dose is at the 50% mark, but they are dosing to 100-120% of range, then the high reverse T3 could very well be from high T3 levels that are encouraging any T4 to convert to reverse T3 (because T3 levels are already too high). The high T3 levels in Natural Desiccated Thyroid (NDT) may also trigger the D3 enzyme and reverse T3 production in those who may not need as much T3 as NDT provides. Since desiccated thyroid contains reverse T3, lowering the dose also eliminates another source of reverse T3. Splitting the dose so smaller amounts are taken in multiple doses throughout the day may also reduce the reverse T3, by lowering the unnaturally high peaks of T3 that a single dose might cause. Additional T4 could be added to compensate for the loss of T4 from a lower NDT dose, as long as conditions that favor reverse T3 production are not present (such as diabetes, alcoholism, or others mentioned earlier). Here is a little known fact: A normal thyroid gland produces about 100 mcg T4 and 6 mcg T3 daily. Daily T3 secreted may be closer to 10 mcg, because some T4 to T3 conversion occurs in the gland before secretion.[82] Total daily T3 produced by the body averages 30 mcg, but 80% (24 mcg) of this is from conversion, and not directly from thyroid gland manufacture.[83] A 3 grain dose of desiccated thyroid provides 114 mcg T4 and 27 mcg T3, which is fairly close to daily T3 production, but assumes nearly zero conversion. If someone has any T4 to T3 conversion (some do and some do not), T4 would need to be added to a reduced dose of desiccated thyroid to mimic normal thyroid production. The T3 content in 3 grains of NDT is almost three times higher than what a normal human thyroid gland secretes. In fact, even 2 grains of NDT contains almost two times more T3 than a normal thyroid gland. This explains why some (not all) patients start showing an imbalance in their labs by the time they reach 2 grains, with FT3 levels reaching the top of the reference range, while FT4 levels may not even be mid-range. The high rT3 that patients report on higher doses of NDT may simply be the body's way of dealing with the high T3 content of NDT.

Are some people really recovering with T3? Some swear that the T3-only protocol gave them their lives back, because anything with T4 (even desiccated thyroid) simply did not work. And then you have people like me, who went "brain dead" on only slightly elevated doses of T3, and many men who ended up with sexual problems because the high T3 levels affected their testosterone and estradiol levels. Perhaps the people who can tolerate high doses of T3 have either nonthyroidal illness (where the illness itself causes a rise in the D3 enzyme, resulting in high reverse T3 levels and the inactivation of any T3) or genetic differences in the deiodinase enzymes (which would produce drastically different T4 to T3 conversion rates in different people). This is not that far-fetched, with the genetic variations that were referenced earlier.[27] An analogy most are familiar with is lactose intolerance, caused by a deficiency of the lactase enzyme. People with the lactase enzyme can drink a gallon of milk with no problem, but if someone is deficient in that enzyme, that amount of milk could cause some serious gastrointestinal distress! Perhaps the people who can take extremely high doses of T3 have D1 or D2 deficiencies—those are the deiodinase enzymes that convert T4 to T3, both in the plasma, and at the cellular/peripheral level. People who do *not* have these enzyme deficiencies could quickly become overdosed with the high T3 levels recommended in the T3-only protocol.

To accommodate these deiodinase enzyme genetic differences, thyroid dosing should be thought of as a continuum with 100% T4 on one end, 100% T3 on the other end, and combinations of T4/T3 in the middle. If this were a normal distribution curve, most people would need a combination of T3 and T4, with the individual T4/T3 concentrations customized for each patient's biochemistry. Unfortunately, patience is essential in finding this optimal dose, because this is a trial and error process, and changes should only be made every six weeks.

Conclusion

Reverse T3 is produced in a normal thyroid gland and is found in healthy people. Everyone has some Free T3 and some reverse T3, so everyone will have a ratio. It's the equation that says the ratio must be greater than 20 (or 10) that's questionable. It is a contrived number, and like TSH, has prevented some patients from achieving their optimal dose. Just like some doctors lower patients' doses in an effort to keep their TSH in range (which keeps them ill), patients are needlessly chasing an "optimal rT3 ratio" by taking excessive amounts of T3, and some are suffering dangerous side effects from this protocol (dementia, osteoporosis, diabetes, muscle wasting, hair loss, etc.).

Anecdotal testimonies from patients suggest that the T3-only protocol may be the only thing that works for *some* patients. However, other anecdotal testimonies prove that this protocol is a disaster for others. As mentioned earlier, it certainly is not a "natural" protocol, because no living creature produces *only* T3. Our thyroid glands produce mostly T4.

Key points

- High doses of T3 can negatively affect other hormones; it can raise estradiol in both men and women.
- Reverse T3 can become high for different reasons: too much T3 (found in desiccated thyroid), poor conversion, non-thyroidal illness (tumors, infections), strict dieting, surgery, and beta blocker drugs are some of the reasons.
- D3 is the deiodinase enzyme that converts T4 to rT3. This same enzyme also converts T3 to T2. Its purpose is to keep cellular T3 low.
- All thyroid hormones, including T4, have non-genomic effects, which is an effect initiated outside of the nucleus. Healthy hair needs both T4 and T3.
- There are other metabolites that can only be created from T4.
- Optimal brain functions are highly dependent on adequate T4 levels.
- T3 levels that are too high may cause hyperthyroid dementia, or a form of brain-fog from too much T3. Memory and problem solving skills may be impaired.
- Brain size differs between hyperthyroid and hypothyroid patients. Hypothyroid patients have smaller brains, while hyperthyroid patients have larger brains. Fluid in the brain makes up for the difference in size. Brain size correlates with T4 levels, not T3 levels.
- The T3-only protocol may have many side effects: osteoporosis, muscle wasting, insulin resistance, hair loss, and memory loss are just a few that have been reported.
- Reverse T3 is a dynamic condition, and levels can change within days.
- High T3 levels can trigger high reverse T3. Hyperthyroid patients have the highest levels of rT3. How can they be hyperthyroid if their receptors are clogged?
- T3 in the nuclear receptor comes from two sources: T3 converted from T4 within the cell, and T3 that originated in the plasma. Organs that are highly dependent upon freshly converted T3 (the brain) may not function correctly on the T3-only protocol.
- A cell that is deficient in T3 may have a problem with thyroid hormone entering the cell, with T4 being converted to T3 within the cell, or with binding to the nuclear thyroid receptor. If T3 is insufficient within the cell, corepressors would silence any gene expression that would be activated at the receptor.

- High reverse T3 is a symptom of a problem, not the cause of the problem. If the root cause is not addressed, rT3 will increase anytime more T4 is added.
- Based on the distribution curve for T3, most people may feel best when their T3 is 50-100% of the reference range.
- A normal thyroid gland only produces about 6 mcg of T3 daily. The rest (24 mcg) is converted from T4.
- For people with normal conversion, 3 grains of desiccated thyroid may have too much T3, and T4 would need to be added to a reduced dose of desiccated thyroid hormone to mimic normal thyroid gland output.
- To mimic normal thyroid physiology, most people should take some small amount of T3, because that's what a normal thyroid gland produces.

---

[1] Gavin, L., et al. "Extrathyroidal Conversion of Thyroxine to 3, 3′, 5′-Triiodothyronine (Reverse-T3) and to 3, 5, 3′-Triiodothyronine." *Journal of Clinical Endocrinology & Metabolism* 44.4 (1977): 733-742.

[2] Douyon, Liselle, and David E. Schteingart. "Effect of obesity and starvation on thyroid hormone, growth hormone, and cortisol secretion." *Endocrinology and metabolism clinics of North America* 31.1 (2002).

[3] Sander, M., and L. Röcker. "Influence of marathon running on thyroid hormones." *International journal of sports medicine* 9.02 (2008): 123-126.

[4] Kelly, G. S. "Peripheral metabolism of thyroid hormones: a review." *Alternative medicine review: a journal of clinical therapeutic* 5.4 (2000): 306.

[5] Franklyn, Jayne A., et al. "Amiodarone and Thyroid Hormone Action." *Clinical endocrinology* 22.3 (1985): 257-264.

[6] Perrild, H., et al. "Different effects of propranolol, alprenolol, sotalol, atenolol and metoprolol on serum T3 and serum rT3 in hyperthyroidism." *Clinical endocrinology* 18.2 (1983): 139-142.

[7] Westgren, U., et al. "Effects of Dexamethasone, Desoxycorticosterone, and ACTH on Serum Concentrations of Thyroxine, 3, 5, 3′-Triiodothyronine and 3, 3 ', 5′-Triiodothyronine." *Acta Medica Scandinavica* 202.1-6 (1977): 89-92.

[8] Kabadi, Udaya M., Bhartur N. Premachandra, and Morelly Maayan. "Low serum 3, 5, 3′-triiodothyronine (T3) and raised 3, 3′, 5′-triiodothyronine (reverse T3 or RT3) in diabetes mellitus: Normalization on improvement in hyperglycemia." *Acta diabetologia latina* 19.3 (1982): 233-242.

[9] Visser, Theo J. "Role of sulfation in thyroid hormone metabolism." *Chemico-biological interactions* 92.1 (1994): 293-303.

[10] Malik, R., and H. Hodgson. "The relationship between the thyroid gland and the liver." *Qjm* 95.9 (2002): 559-569.

[11] Mohassel, Payam, and Andrew L. Mammen. "The spectrum of statin myopathy." Current opinion in rheumatology 25.6 (2013): 747-752.

[12] Rafeiyan, Sima, et al. "Relative Effects of Enhanced External Counter Pulsation Therapy on Thyroid Hormones in Heart Failure Treatment." *Official Quarterly Publication Of The Iranian Heart Association* (2012): 35.

[13] Casulari, Luiz Augusto, et al. "Nonthyroidal illness syndrome in patients with subarachnoid hemorrhage due to intracranial aneurysm." *Arquivos de neuro-psiquiatria* 62.1 (2004): 26-32.

[14] Eriksson, Kimmo. "The nonsense math effect." *Judgment and decision making* 7 (2012): 746-749.

[15] Banovac, Krešimir, et al. "Decreased ratio of serum T3: rT3 in patients with hyperthyroidism." *Endokrinologie* 71.2 (1978): 159.

[16] Huang, Stephen A. "Physiology and pathophysiology of type 3 deiodinase in humans." *Thyroid* 15.8 (2005): 875-881.

[17] Wajner, Simone Magagnin, et al. "IL-6 promotes nonthyroidal illness syndrome by blocking thyroxine activation while promoting thyroid hormone inactivation in human cells." *The Journal of clinical investigation* 121.5 (2011): 1834.

[18] Bianco, Antonio C., and Brian W. Kim. "Deiodinases: implications of the local control of thyroid hormone action." *Journal of Clinical Investigation* 116.10 (2006): 2571-2579.

[19] Pol, Christine J., et al. "Left-ventricular remodeling after myocardial infarction is associated with a cardiomyocyte-specific hypothyroid condition." *Endocrinology* 152.2 (2011): 669-679.

[20] Sibilio, A., et al. "Deiodination in cancer growth: the role of type III deiodinase." *Minerva endocrinologica* 37.4 (2012): 315-327.

[21] Dentice, Monica, Dario Antonini, and Domenico Salvatore. "Type 3 deiodinase and solid tumors: an intriguing pair." *Expert Opinion on Therapeutic Targets* 0 (2013): 1-11.

[22] Howard, David, et al. "Consumptive hypothyroidism resulting from hepatic vascular tumors in an athyreotic adult." *Journal of Clinical Endocrinology & Metabolism* 96.7 (2011): 1966-1970.

[23] Huang, Stephen A., et al. "A 21-year-old woman with consumptive hypothyroidism due to a vascular tumor expressing type 3 iodothyronine deiodinase." *Journal of Clinical Endocrinology & Metabolism* 87.10 (2002): 4457-4461.

[24] Kester, Monique HA, et al. "Large induction of type III deiodinase expression after partial hepatectomy in the regenerating mouse and rat liver." *Endocrinology* 150.1 (2009): 540-545.

[25] Huang, Stephen A., and Antonio C. Bianco. "Reawakened interest in type III iodothyronine deiodinase in critical illness and injury." *Nature Clinical Practice Endocrinology & Metabolism* 4.3 (2008): 148-155.

[26] Boelen, Anita, et al. "Type 3 deiodinase is highly expressed in infiltrating neutrophilic granulocytes in response to acute bacterial infection." *Thyroid* 18.10 (2008): 1095-1103.

[27] van der Deure, Wendy M., Robin P. Peeters, and Theo J. Visser. "Molecular aspects of thyroid hormone transporters, including MCT8, MCT10, and OATPs, and the effects of genetic variation in these transporters." *Journal of molecular endocrinology* 44.1 (2010): 1-11.

[28] Cheng, Sheue-Yann, Jack L. Leonard, and Paul J. Davis. "Molecular aspects of thyroid hormone actions." *Endocrine reviews* 31.2 (2010): 139-170.

[29] van Beek, Nina, et al. "Thyroid hormones directly alter human hair follicle functions: anagen prolongation and stimulation of both hair matrix keratinocyte proliferation and hair pigmentation." *Journal of Clinical Endocrinology & Metabolism* 93.11 (2008): 4381-4388.

[30] Gunaratnam, Parameswaran. "The effects of thyroxine on hair growth in the dog." *Journal of Small Animal Practice* 27.1 (1986): 17-29.

[31] Davis, Paul J., et al. "Membrane receptor for thyroid hormone: physiologic and pharmacologic implications." *Annual review of pharmacology and toxicology* 51 (2011): 99-115.

[32] Axelband, F., et al. "Nongenomic signaling pathways triggered by thyroid hormones and their metabolite 3-iodothyronamine on the cardiovascular system." *Journal of cellular physiology* 226.1 (2011): 21-28.

[33] Bunevičius, Robertas, and Arthur J. Prange Jr. "Thyroid–Brain Interactions in Neuropsychiatric Disorders." *Neuropsychiatric Disorders*. Springer Japan, 2010. 17-32.

[34] Fukui, Toshiya, Yukihiro Hasegawa, and Hiroki Takenaka. "Hyperthyroid dementia: clinicoradiological findings and response to treatment." *Journal of the neurological sciences* 184.1 (2001): 81-88.

[35] Ii, Yuichiro, et al. "[Transient dementia during hyperthyroidism of painless thyroiditis. A case report]." *Rinsho shinkeigaku= Clinical neurology* 43.6 (2003): 341.

[36] Orford, M. R., et al. "Treatment with triiodothyronine decreases the abundance of the α-subunits of G_i1 and G_i2 in the cerebral cortex." *Journal of the neurological sciences* 112.1 (1992): 34-37.

[37] Grigorova, Miglena, and Barbara B. Sherwin. "Thyroid hormones and cognitive functioning in healthy, euthyroid women: A correlational study." *Hormones and behavior* 61.4 (2012): 617-622.

[38] Botella-Carretero, J. I., et al. "Quality of life and psychometric functionality in patients with differentiated thyroid carcinoma." *Endocrine-related cancer* 10.4 (2003): 601-610.

[39] Trzepacz, Paula T., et al. "A psychiatric and neuropsychological study of patients with untreated Graves' disease." *General hospital psychiatry* 10.1 (1988): 49-55.

[40] Tu, Helen M., et al. "Regional expression of the type 3 iodothyronine deiodinase messenger ribonucleic acid in the rat central nervous system and its regulation by thyroid hormone." *Endocrinology* 140.2 (1999): 784-790.

[41] Santini, Ferruccio, et al. "Evidence for a role of the type III-iodothyronine deiodinase in the regulation of 3, 5, 3'-triiodothyronine content in the human central nervous system." *European journal of endocrinology* 144.6 (2001): 577-583.

[42] Oatridge, Angela, et al. "Changes in brain size with treatment in patients with hyper-or hypothyroidism." *American journal of neuroradiology* 23.9 (2002): 1539-1544.

[43] Crantz, F. R., J. E. Silva, and P. R. Larsen. "An analysis of the sources and quantity of 3, 5, 3'-triiodothyronine specifically bound to nuclear receptors in rat cerebral cortex and cerebellum." *Endocrinology* 110.2 (1982): 367-375.

[44] Pohunkova, D., J. Sulc, and S. Vana. "Influence of thyroid hormone supply on EEG frequency spectrum." *Endocrinologia experimentalis* 23.4 (1989): 251.

[45] Bauer, M., et al. "The Thyroid-Brain Interaction in Thyroid Disorders and Mood Disorders." *Journal of neuroendocrinology* 20.10 (2008): 1101-1114.

[46] Saravanan, Ponnusamy, Theo J. Visser, and Colin M. Dayan. "Psychological well-being correlates with free thyroxine but not free 3, 5, 3'-triiodothyronine levels in patients on thyroid hormone replacement." *Journal of Clinical Endocrinology & Metabolism* 91.9 (2006): 3389-3393.

[47] Dumoulin, Sonia C., et al. "Opposite effects of thyroid hormones on binding proteins for steroid hormones (sex hormone-binding globulin and corticosteroid-binding globulin) in humans." *European journal of endocrinology* 132.5 (1995): 594-598.

[48] Olivo, Jaime, et al. "Estrogen metabolism in hyperthyroidism and in cirrhosis of the liver." *Steroids* 26.1 (1975): 47-56.

[49] Meikle, A. Wayne. "The interrelationships between thyroid dysfunction and hypogonadism in men and boys." *Thyroid* 14.3, Supplement 1 (2004): 17-25.

[50] Carani, Cesare, et al. "Multicenter study on the prevalence of sexual symptoms in male hypo-and hyperthyroid patients." *Journal of Clinical Endocrinology & Metabolism* 90.12 (2005): 6472-6479.

[51] Lormeau, C., et al. "Sex hormone-binding globulin, estradiol, and bone turnover markers in male osteoporosis." *Bone* 34.6 (2004): 933.

52 Caron, P. H., et al. "Effects of hyperthyroidism on binding proteins for steroid hormones." *Clinical endocrinology* 31.2 (1989): 219-224.

53 Krassas, G. E., and P. Perros. "Reproductive function in patients with thyroid diseases." *Hot Thyroidology* 2 (2002).

54 Kazanavicius, G. "New approach in treatment of hyperandrogenism with triiodothyronine." (2004).

55 Shifren, Jan L., et al. "A randomized, open-label, crossover study comparing the effects of oral versus transdermal estrogen therapy on serum androgens, thyroid hormones, and adrenal hormones in naturally menopausal women." *Menopause* 14.6 (2007): 985-994.

56 Brenner, B., J. Fandrey, and W. Jelkmann. "Serum immunoreactive erythropoietin in hyper-and hypothyroidism: Clinical observations related to cell culture studies." *European journal of haematology* 53.1 (1994): 6-10.

57 Smith, Steven R., et al. "Triiodothyronine increases calcium loss in a bed rest antigravity model for space flight." *Metabolism* 57.12 (2008): 1696-1703.

58 Burman, Kenneth D., et al. "The effect of T3 and reverse T3 administration on muscle protein catabolism during fasting as measured by 3-methylhistidine excretion." *Metabolism* 28.8 (1979): 805-813.

59 Simu, Mihaela, Elena Cecilia Rosca, and Daniela Reisz. "Thyroid Myopathy-A Case Study." Timisoara Medical Journal. Number 1-2 Year 2008.

60 Brenta, Gabriela. "Diabetes and thyroid disorders." *The British Journal of Diabetes & Vascular Disease* 10.4 (2010): 172-177.

61 Dimitriadis, G., et al. "Effect of thyroid hormone excess on action, secretion, and metabolism of insulin in humans." *American Journal of Physiology-Endocrinology And Metabolism* 248.5 (1985): E593-E601.

62 Lambadiari, Vaia, et al. "Thyroid hormones are positively associated with insulin resistance early in the development of type 2 diabetes." *Endocrine* 39.1 (2011): 28-32.

63 Kubota, Sumihisa, et al. "Serial changes in liver function tests in patients with thyrotoxicosis induced by Graves' disease and painless thyroiditis." *Thyroid* 18.3 (2008): 283-287.

64 Fukui, Toshiya, Yukihiro Hasegawa, and Hiroki Takenaka. "Hyperthyroid dementia: clinicoradiological findings and response to treatment." *Journal of the neurological sciences* 184.1 (2001): 81-88.

65 Jabłkowska, Karolina, et al. "Working memory and executive functions in hyperthyroid patients with Graves' disease]." *Psychiatria polska* 42.2 (2008): 249.

66 Karl, Michael, et al. "Hypocortisolemia in Graves hyperthyroidism." *Endocrine Practice* 15.3 (2009): 220-224.

67 Schmidt, Ulla, et al. "Peripheral markers of thyroid function: the effect of T4 monotherapy vs T4/T3 combination therapy in hypothyroid subjects in a randomized crossover study." *Endocrine Connections* 2.1 (2013): 55-60.

68 Chopra, Inder J., et al. "Reciprocal changes in serum concentrations of 3, 3′, 5′-triiodothyronine (reverse T3) and 3, 3′ 5-triiodothyronine (T3) in systemic illnesses." *Journal of Clinical Endocrinology & Metabolism* 41.6 (1975): 1043-1049.

69 Lopresti, Jonathan S., David Gray, and John T. Nicoloff. "Influence of fasting and refeeding on 3, 3′, 5′-triiodothyronine metabolism in man." *Journal of Clinical Endocrinology & Metabolism* 72.1 (1991): 130-136.

70 Kaiser, Catherine A., Michel O. Goumaz, and Albert G. Burger. "In vivo inhibition of the 5′-deiodinase type II in brain cortex and pituitary by reverse triiodothyronine." *Endocrinology* 119.2 (1986): 762-770.

71 Chopra, Indie J. "An assessment of daily production and significance of thyroidal secretion of 3, 3′, 5′-triiodothyronine (reverse T3) in man." *Journal of Clinical Investigation* 58.1 (1976): 32.

[72] Okamoto, Ryoji, and Dieter Leibfritz. "Adverse effects of reverse triiodothyronine on cellular metabolism as assessed by 1 H and 31 P NMR spectroscopy." *Research in experimental medicine* 197.4 (1997): 211-217.

[73] Faber, J., et al. "Urinary Excretion of 3, 3′, 5′-Triiodothyronine (Reverse T3)." *Clinical endocrinology* 9.3 (1978): 279-282.

[74] Laurberg, Peter, and Jørgen Weeke. "Radioimmunological determination of reverse triiodothyronine in unextracted serum and serum dialysates." *Scandinavian Journal of Clinical & Laboratory Investigation* 37.8 (1977): 735-739.

[75] Smallridge, Robert C., et al. "Metabolic clearance and production rates of 3, 3′, 5′-triiodothyronine in hyperthyroid, euthyroid, and hypothyroid subjects." *Journal of Clinical Endocrinology & Metabolism* 47.2 (1978): 345-349.

[76] Gereben, Balázs, et al. "Cellular and molecular basis of deiodinase-regulated thyroid hormone signaling." *Endocrine reviews* 29.7 (2008): 898-938.

[77] van der Deure, Wendy M., Robin P. Peeters, and Theo J. Visser. "Molecular aspects of thyroid hormone transporters, including MCT8, MCT10, and OATPs, and the effects of genetic variation in these transporters." *Journal of molecular endocrinology* 44.1 (2010): 1-11.

[78] Dayan, Colin M., and Vijay Panicker. "Novel insights into thyroid hormones from the study of common genetic variation." *Nature Reviews Endocrinology* 5.4 (2009): 211-218.

[79] Astapova, Inna, and Anthony N. Hollenberg. "The *in vivo* Role of Nuclear Receptor Corepressors in Thyroid Hormone Action." *Biochimica et Biophysica Acta (BBA)-General Subjects* (2012).

[80] Polosak, Jacek. "Small-Molecule Hormones: Molecular Mechanisms of Action." *International Journal of Endocrinology* 2013 (2013).

[81] Dr. Williams, clinical pathologist, Director of Quality Assurance for Quest Labs in Florida. Phone interview. Oct. 19, 2010.

[82] Larsen, P. R., and A. M. Zavacki. "Role of the Iodothyronine Deiodinases in the Physiology and Pathophysiology of Thyroid Hormone Action." *European thyroid journal* 1.4 (2012): 232-242.

[83] Bunevičius, Robertas, et al. "Effects of thyroxine as compared with thyroxine plus triiodothyronine in patients with hypothyroidism." *New England Journal of Medicine* 340.6 (1999): 424-429.

24

Thyroid Physiology FAQ: Separating Fact from Fiction

The earth is flat.

—a rational (but erroneous) conclusion drawn from personal observation.

Both doctors and patients dispense a lot of opinions, which are not often grounded in facts. In fact, what is stated as fact is often just misinformation that has been repeated so many times, that it is accepted as fact. Just because the "fact" comes from a fellow patient, book, doctor, internet site, or from someone who moderates a thyroid group, doesn't make it true. Some beliefs have been around for so long that no one even thinks to check if they're really true! When I tried to point out some of these internet myths on various forums, I would be "corrected" with the same misinformation, and was often referred to the source of the misinformation as "proof." Likewise, there are medical myths too, with official medical guidelines as the source, and most doctors do not seem to welcome ideas that are in polar opposition to what they were taught.

The whole point of this book was to find out how thyroid hormone really works—to find the truth. Here then, are the factual answers to some frequently asked questions (FAQ) that may not agree with what readers have "learned" elsewhere.

I feel hypothyroid but don't want to take prescription medication. Are there any supplements or lifestyle changes I can make instead?

Thyroid production can be negatively impacted by diet, lack of sleep, and nutritional deficiencies, so yes, for those who still have thyroid glands, some improvement could be made by lifestyle modifications.

Goitrogens are raw vegetables in the *Brassica* family such as bok choy, broccoli, and cabbage that contain chemicals that interfere with iodine uptake and consequently, thyroid hormone production. A woman who had no thyroid disease history became extremely hypothyroid by consuming copious amounts of raw bok choy.[1] Consumption of these foods in quantities that exceed normal daily portions can lower thyroid function. Cooking tends to inactivate the goitrogenic chemicals; however, most vegetables have health benefits so should not be completely eliminated from the diet, just eaten in moderation. Vegetarians or vegans may be lowering their thyroid function because their diet is deficient in iodine, Vitamin B12, Vitamin A, zinc, and iron; all are involved in thyroid hormone synthesis and are difficult to get in needed amounts without meat consumption. A vegetarian diet is also high in copper and low in zinc, creating more imbalances [see Cofactors, Chapter 10]. If anyone is vegetarian or vegan and feels they don't have the energy they used to, I recommend they google "ex-vegan blog" and do some reading. Some vegans complain about brain fog, fatigue, dental problems, bad skin, depression, and irritability. Those all happen to be hypothyroid symptoms. Apparently, the human body needs a more balanced diet than these diets provide, and supplements don't fill the deficiencies.

Soy protein is often used in place of animal protein, but is highly goitrogenic. Infants that were fed soy formula have become severely hypothyroid and have developed goiters. Discontinuation of the formula resolved the hypothyroidism and goiter. Soy consumption also interferes with levothyroxine absorption, because infants taking high doses of levothyroxine showed low serum levels of thyroid hormone. Once the soy milk was discontinued, thyroid levels rose.[2]

Studies show that we need eight to nine hours of sleep each night, but with busy lifestyles, many get far less. Partial sleep deprivation has been shown to lower Thyroid Stimulating Hormone (TSH), which would lead to lower thyroid levels.[3] People who don't get enough sleep are tired not only because they are sleep deprived, but because lack of sleep is negatively affecting their thyroid production.

Severe low-calorie diets will cause the body to conserve energy; triiodothyronine (T3) levels will decrease and reverse T3 (rT3) levels will increase. A zero carbohydrate diet will also cause T3 levels to fall.[4] While it may seem counterintuitive, it actually makes more sense to eat balanced, small meals more often, rather than go on a strict, low calorie diet.

Excessive exercise will also lower T3 levels as the body tries to conserve energy. When maximum heart rate reached 70% in one study, there was an increase in T3, T4 (thyroxine), and TSH. But when maximum heart rate was pushed to 90%, Free and Total T3 dropped, while TSH continued to rise, as did T4 and FT4.[5] This is why people on strict diets who overexercise usually hit a plateau in weight loss at some point. The body has built-in safety mechanisms to prevent starvation and wasting away—the body lowers its metabolism.

Certain nutrients are essential for normal thyroid hormone production, and these can be obtained from a well-rounded diet or taken as supplements. Iodide enters the thyroid gland through the sodium-iodide symporter, which means sodium is essential; a sodium-restricted diet may negatively affect this process. The enzymes that convert T4 to T3 use selenium, and this is often found in a daily multivitamin. While tyrosine is also a component of thyroid hormone, it is the precursor to adrenaline, so is not recommended as a supplement. It may make people feel wired and anxious instead of energetic.

The liver is the primary site of conversion of T4 to T3, so a healthy liver is important. Alcoholics with cirrhosis or those with hepatitis may have conversion problems, so any lifestyle changes that improve liver health will be beneficial. Alcohol appears to have multiple effects on the hypothalamo-pituitary-thyroid axis and the functioning of the thyroid gland, resulting in lower T3 levels.[6] Likewise, patients with chronic hepatitis C in one study had a higher TSH and lower FT4 and FT3 levels compared to others.[7]

There are numerous "thyroid supplements" marketed, and I don't know that they're worth their cost. Some of the ingredients are common ones found in daily multivitamins, along with some herbs that may help adrenal function. If someone really has adrenal insufficiency and constant, chronic fatigue, they may need more than a few supplements to restore their health. They may have autoimmune thyroid disease and should look into full thyroid testing [see Blood Tests, Chapter 9].

It appears that the lifestyle of the typical modern working woman induces hypothyroidism. Women today are so busy, working and raising families, and many also diet, consuming unknown goitrogens, and overexercise, thinking it is benefiting them. Combine that with limited sleep, and a few alcoholic drinks to relax, and even a healthy thyroid will downregulate its output! This is before even considering that our food supply now has multiple chemicals and preservatives that may also affect the endocrine system. These endocrine-disrupting compounds (EDCs), such as polychlorinated biphenyls (PCBs) affect the hypothalamo-pituitary-thyroid axis and can negatively affect thyroid levels.[8]

Can acupuncture help my thyroid?

Anecdotal stories say yes, and there are studies that show positive results. Acupuncture treatment for one group of female patients with a high TSH but normal thyroid hormone levels (subclinical hypothyroidism) resulted in a significant decrease in number and severity of symptoms, and TSH fell back into the normal range.[9] Acupuncture has also successfully been used to reduce stress,[10] asthma,[11] and improve fertility.[12] I believe acupuncture can be used to alleviate some symptoms, but it will be ineffective if there is no thyroid gland due to radioactive iodine or thyroidectomy. My layman's understanding is that acupuncture opens up "blockages" in the energy flow in the body. But if someone does not have a working thyroid gland, then there will never be any energy coming from it. Some people *must* take prescription thyroid hormone or they simply won't function.

I read that the iodine protocol could restore my thyroid health, and that any reactions I may have are due to bromide detox.

The thyroid gland needs approximately 150 mcg of iodine daily to create thyroid hormone. I cannot recommend high dose iodine supplements because reactions are variable—from hyperthyroidism to hypothyroidism to improved health. Hyperthyroidism is a serious complication, because it can be fatal if untreated. In addition, many report iodine poisoning symptoms on the high dose protocol (acne, dripping sinuses, etc.) and are told it is "bromide detox," where bromide is being purged from the body. It is actually "money detox," where money is being purged from your wallet. Taking high doses of iodine is like playing Russian Roulette: sometimes you win, and sometimes you lose [see Iodine, Chapter 18].

My iron is low and I was told I need to take iron supplements.

Iron is a component of multiple enzymes and should be supplemented if tests show someone is truly deficient. However, it is important that a full iron panel is run before iron supplementation, because low iron does not always mean the person is anemic. In certain disease states, the body purposely shunts iron to ferritin, so supplementing iron can make the person worse [see Cofactors, Chapter 10].

Hemochromatosis is a hereditary iron loading disease that damages the liver and endocrine glands, and hypothyroidism is often the result. This is another reason a full iron panel should be run at least once on everyone [see Ironman, Chapter 4].

My cortisol tested low and I was told I need to take hydrocortisone.

Cortisol is an essential hormone, but hydrocortisone (HC) supplementation has some severe side effects that many are not aware of. Diabetes, osteoporosis, and glaucoma have been reported by patients who innocently followed the advice they were given [see Adrenal Dysfunction, Chapter 6]. Some patients do need HC replacement; however, this is a very difficult hormone to dose, and unsuspecting patients are not warned of the potential serious side effects. For example, a patient must manually provide the necessary amount of HC during periods of high stress (car accident or something traumatic) or the lack of cortisol can be fatal.

Desiccated thyroid is superior because it's natural and bioidentical.

These are two different concepts. Desiccated thyroid is natural because it came from a living source and was not manufactured in a laboratory. Levothyroxine, on the other hand, is synthetic, but it is bioidentical. There is a sodium salt attached to the thyroxine molecule, but it cleaves off in stomach acid. What remains is bioidentical (same molecular structure) to human T4. I personally take both types of hormones to give me both T4 and T3 in a ratio that's suitable for my body [see Prescription Choices, Chapter 20]. Ironically, the same people who believe desiccated thyroid is superior because it's natural have no problem recommending patients take additional T3, which is synthetic!

Desiccated thyroid is superior to all other thyroid medications because it has everything found in a thyroid gland, including T4, T3, T2, T1 and calcitonin.

A normal thyroid gland produces T4 and T3. It does not produce T2 or T1, but it does produce rT3! T2 and T1 are primarily formed from peripheral conversion outside of the thyroid gland, so they would not be found within the gland except in trace amounts. The effect of any calcitonin found in desiccated thyroid may be minimal because it does not absorb well when taken orally. Prescription calcitonin is administered nasally or by injection [see Prescription Choices, Chapter 20]. For those without sufficient stomach acid, desiccated thyroid may be a better source of T4, because no stomach acid is required. Once the pill dissolves, the T4 is available. With levothyroxine sodium, T4 only becomes available after the sodium is cleaved off by stomach acid.

Free T3 and Free T4 are the only valid thyroid hormone tests. Total T3 and Total T4 are useless.

Studies show Free T3 has a far better correlation with symptoms than Total T3, and personal anecdotal experience supports this. However, Total T4 can sometimes be a better barometer of thyroid gland output than Free T4, because medications like aspirin, diuretics, or heparin can artificially inflate FT4 [see Blood Tests, Chapter 9]. The laboratory tests that measure Total T4 are also far more reliable than those for FT4; they are measured using different techniques. People have reported FT4 lab values that were about mid-range, while Total T4 was rock bottom. Total T4 confirmed the true hypothyroid state that the FT4 did not show. In this particular case it was FT4 that was "useless"! In perplexing cases, both lab values should be tested.

My lab tests show I'm truly hypothyroid, with a high TSH and low T3 and T4. My doctor wants to prescribe levothyroxine or T4, but I've read that it's "crap" and I should ask for desiccated thyroid instead.

The average human thyroid gland secretes approximately 100 mcg T4 and 10 mcg T3 daily, which means normal people produce mostly T4. Patients who do not do well on T4 pills may be low in gastric acid, and unable to break the pill form down into the bioavailable T4 [see Prescription Thyroid Choices, Chapter 20]. Others do relatively well on T4 pills, but would probably benefit from some additional T3.

The problem with T4-only treatment is that it does not replicate normal thyroid physiology, because the treatment itself lowers TSH, which reduces T4 to T3 conversion, which results in lower than normal T3 levels. T4 treatment thus creates a lower FT3/FT4 ratio, which is easily remedied by adding some T3, which is exactly what a normal thyroid produces! Patients cannot be dosed by TSH while taking replacement hormone, because the simple act of taking thyroid hormone breaks the normal TSH-FT3 feedback loop [see TSH & T3, Chapter 25].

Some amount of T3 should be taken to replicate normal thyroid physiology. T4 can be combined with synthetic T3 or desiccated thyroid, or desiccated thyroid can be taken alone, or even combined with additional T3; every individual has a different set point ratio in terms of how much T3 and T4 is necessary for them to feel well.

TSH cannot be used to determine the correct dose, but other lab values may indicate when a dose is too high: high sex hormone binding globulin (SHBG), alkaline phosphatase, fasting blood glucose, and calcium may be indicators that a dose is too high. Typical signs of overmedication include a fast heart rate and diarrhea. Signs of overmedication should not be ignored because too much thyroid hormone (not a low TSH) can lead to osteoporosis.

My lab tests show I have high reverse T3 and a low rT3 ratio. I was told I need to take T3-only to clear my blocked receptors.

The reverse T3 *ratio* is a misleading number because it can be low for different reasons. People with high levels of rT3 are hypothyroid because neither T3 nor rT3 is able to get to a cell's receptor. Corepressors are keeping anything from getting through; rT3 is not blocking the receptor [see Reverse T3, Chapter 23]. Some thyroid patient groups say that rT3 "clogs" the receptors for 12 weeks. Even though lab tests will show minimal amounts of rT3 in serum after only a few weeks on the T3-only protocol, rT3 is said to cling tenaciously to the receptors for 12 weeks or more. In 12 weeks (or three months), kids finish their summer break, I get two haircuts, trim my fingernails several times, and a fertilized egg grows into a recognizable, although miniature human. Hormones do not last for 12 weeks—they degrade in a few days, which is why they must be taken daily at a minimum. For those who want to learn the real science behind thyroid hormone receptors, and how the presence or absence of T3 invokes corepressors or coactivators, read http://www.thyroidmanager.org/chapter/cellular-action-of-thyroid-hormone/. [13] There are some excellent charts and diagrams that illustrate the points. It is a detailed, lengthy, technical explanation, but not once is *reverse T3* ever mentioned!

There are basically three causes of a "low rT3 ratio."
1. A high desiccated thyroid dose (too much T3) will raise rT3, because rT3 is the body's safety mechanism to lower excessive T3 levels. Desiccated thyroid also contains rT3, because rT3 is found in a normal thyroid gland; as the dose is increased, T3, T4, and rT3 levels should all rise.
2. A patient who only takes T4 may have unnaturally low T3 levels and rT3 within the reference range. This patient may benefit from adding some T3 to their dose.
3. Levels of rT3 that are hundreds of points over the reference range may indicate a serious, systemic illness such as acute renal failure, heart failure, and metastasized cancer. This is called non-thyroidal illness. The body is purposely trying to keep T3 levels low by converting T4 to rT3 and T3 to T2. High doses of T3 may be necessary to break through the corepressors, but the cause of the illness should also be addressed. Reverse T3 does not *cause* the systemic illness, it is merely a marker of an illness. Trying to eliminate rT3 is analogous to eliminating firemen who show up at a house fire. The firemen didn't *cause* the fire, though they tend to be present in high numbers wherever there is a fire.

T4 is only a prohormone and completely unnecessary. T3 is the active hormone; therefore all we really need is T3. In fact, T3 levels should be kept at the top of the reference range, or even above it.

All hormones, including T4, have non-genomic effects, which means they can have an effect without binding to a nuclear receptor or converting to another hormone. T4 can exert an effect on the cell membrane or in the cytoplasm—not all effects are initiated in the nucleus of the cell. Cells in the body obtain their T3 from two sources: directly from plasma, and by converting T4 at the cell membrane. Therefore, insufficient T4 levels can contribute to low T3 levels. The brain is highly dependent on adequate T4 levels and someone on T3-only, or even on too low a dose of desiccated thyroid, may have a cognitive deficit due to insufficient T4. This may not be apparent without specific testing of brain functions, and the deficits involve memory, math, language, and problem solving. High levels of T3 can also cause anger, irritability, quarrelsomeness, impatience, and sometimes, an explosive rage.[14] Patients who intentionally maintain their Free T3 levels above the reference range have been observed to write and speak in an angry tone if anyone dares to disagree with them.

High levels of T3 can also cause osteoporosis, muscle wasting (the heart is a muscle), insulin resistance, and hyperthyroid dementia [see Reverse T3, Chapter 23].

I'm pregnant, and was told it's ok to stay on the T3-only protocol (or high dose iodine protocol or desiccated thyroid dose of less than 3 grains).

Fetal brain development is highly dependent on adequate levels of T4, not T3. The T4 dose in a pregnant woman usually needs to be increased by around 50%. This means the T4 portion of the dose must exceed 100 mcg, which doesn't happen in desiccated thyroid until the dose approaches 3 grains. That dose may be too much T3 for some women. Obviously, the T3-only protocol supplies zero T4, which may result in cognitive, visual, or hearing deficits in the child. The iodine protocol is dangerous because it can induce hypothyroidism in the newborn [see Reproductive Problems, Chapter 22].

100 mcg T4 = 25 mcg T3 = 1 grain of desiccated thyroid (38 mcg T4 + 9 mcg T3).

T4 and T3 are two completely different hormones, each with different properties and uses by the body; therefore, the above equivalency statement does not make much sense. It's like comparing apples and apple juice. Since apple juice comes from apples, is an exceedingly high amount of apple juice equivalent to one apple? A real apple has crunch and fiber and gives a sense of fullness that the juice does not. If we apply these concepts to the different thyroid hormones, we have an interesting analogy. Since a normal thyroid gland secretes about 100 mcg T4 + 10 mcg T3, we could say that 100 mcg T4 = 1 apple, and 10 mcg T3 = 10 ounces of apple juice, and we could call that normal—a snack of one apple +10 ounces of apple juice. The T4-only analogy gives me one apple but no juice. I'm left thirsty. The T3-only analogy gives me 25 ounces of juice but no apple. That is more than three cups of juice! I might feel full from all that liquid, but it would pass right through me, and I'd feel hungry later without the real apple. With desiccated thyroid I'd only get a little more than a third of an apple, with 9 ounces of juice. I don't think I'd feel satiated. None of these other combinations replicates the "normal snack," in the same way that neither T4-only, T3-only, or desiccated thyroid mimics normal thyroid gland function.

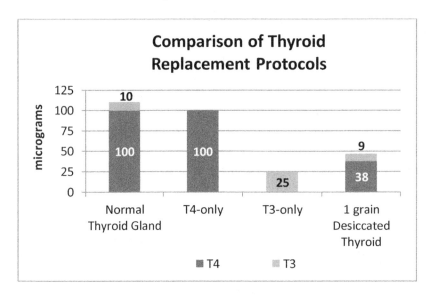

Figure 24-1. A visual depiction of the T4 and T3 content in various protocols shows they are not equivalent in any way.

If someone only takes 100 mcg T4, they will be short on the small amount of T3 produced by the thyroid gland. This protocol does not replicate normal thyroid physiology because it results in a relative T3 deficiency, with a lower FT3/FT4 ratio than found in normal controls [see TSH & T3, Chapter 25]. The common dose recommended on the T3-only protocol is 75-125 mcg T3 and zero T4. This would create an extremely high FT3/FT4 ratio, which does not replicate a normal thyroid gland's output. Desiccated thyroid contains 9 mcg T3 and 38 mcg T4 per grain. The T3/T4 ratio from a normal thyroid gland would be expressed as 10/100 or 0.10; desiccated would be expressed as 9/38 or 0.24. A strictly mathematical comparison shows that desiccated is 2.4 times higher in T3 than T4 when compared to a healthy human thyroid gland. So this does not replicate normal thyroid physiology either.

There are many thyroid patients trying different protocols, and several studies analyzing the benefits, if any, of adding any amount of T3 to T4. But none of these protocols replicated the true physiological ratio, which can only be obtained if some small amount of T3 is added to a dose that is primarily T4. Most of the studies I've read either overdosed the patients with T3, or underdosed them with T4, believing they had to subtract T4 if T3 was added, following the equivalency statement that 100 mcg T4 = 25 mcg T3. They then concluded that combination T3/T4 therapy was not that much better than T4-only treatment.

Because of absorption differences, the interference of diet on absorption, the size difference among people, and the genetic variations in conversion rates, etc., I don't believe everyone's dose should be 100 mcg T4 + 10 mcg T3. Mine isn't. But that number should be used as a guideline, and it's not. Instead, a "normal" TSH is the standard guideline (the TSH rule), and that has left many of us undermedicated for years. Because of the suppressive effect of T3 on TSH, someone could be prescribed 1 grain of desiccated thyroid, which lowers their TSH into range, and a doctor would then declare them "normal." However, if their actual thyroid levels (FT3 and T4) were looked at in terms of where they fell within the reference range, they might find a patient woefully low in T4, who still has quite a few hypothyroid symptoms! Figure 24-1 illustrates the concept.

I read that most people need 3 - 5 grains of desiccated thyroid, but I'm already feeling hyperthyroid on 2 grains.

If the average thyroid gland secretes 100 mcg of T4 and 10 mcg T3, and 3 grains of desiccated thyroid has 114 mcg T4 and 27 mcg T3, then 3 grains has almost 3 times more T3 than a normal thyroid gland secretes. Since T3 is the active thyroid hormone, it does provide immediate energy, and for many people, 3 grains is a serious overdose. For me, other lab values started to rise above the reference range on 2 grains, which means 2 grains was too much *for me*. Fasting blood glucose, ALT (a liver enzyme), and RBC, hemoglobin, and hematocrit were flagged as high on my lab report. Essentially, the high T3 levels were raising my blood sugar, causing liver damage, and speeding up my red blood cell production. Not good. Dropping the dose to 1.5 grains normalized all lab values, but my FT4 was then rock bottom. My optimal dose is somewhere between 1-1.5 grains with 25-75 mcg T4 [see Prescription Choices, Chapter 20].

I'm "only" on 2 grains but feel shaky, anxious, and can't sleep. I was told these are adrenal symptoms and that I need to take hydrocortisone.

As explained in the previous paragraph, 2 grains is not exactly a low dose and has considerably more T3 than some people need. When a person takes too much thyroid hormone, it depletes their cortisol levels, and results in those shaky, anxious feelings. Simply lowering the dose will use up less cortisol, and hydrocortisone may not be needed.

I feel hypothyroid but my doctor said that's impossible because I'm not fat.

I looked anorexic when I was taking only ½ grain of desiccated thyroid and obviously undermedicated. The endocrine system consists of many hormones, and a thyroid hormone deficiency can trigger changes in other hormones. In my particular case, when my thyroid levels were too low, my cortisol also tanked, which meant my biochemistry was then similar to that of an Addison's patient (thin, due to minimal cortisol). Other hypothyroid patients will have their cortisol levels rise, and they will then resemble a Cushing's patient (heavy, due to high cortisol).

Another patient's physical measures never changed: weight, bowel movements, and hair were relatively the same for her whether over or undermedicated. But thyroid hormone levels that were either too high or too low really affected her brain and her ability to think. She used the word "comatose" to describe the feeling.

I started taking desiccated thyroid and now have no TSH, and my doctor is concerned and wants to lower my dose. But the internet thyroid groups I'm on say TSH is useless and not to worry about it.

There are actually two important issues here. Desiccated thyroid will normally suppress TSH because of its T3 content; this does not mean the patient is hyperthyroid. Other symptoms and lab results should be checked to verify that the patient is not hyperthyroid and it's just a lab number on a piece of paper that's low. The doctor is incorrect in wanting to lower the dose based solely on TSH (the TSH rule). However, while TSH cannot be used to gauge the dose of a patient on desiccated thyroid, it is not useless. It stimulates T4 to T3 conversion, so is absolutely essential for someone on T4-only treatment [see TSH & T3, Chapter 25].

My doctor prescribed T4, my lab tests show my TSH, FT3 and FT4 are all normal now, and yet I still feel hypothyroid. My doctor won't raise my dose because my labs are normal.

There are two different issues here. The normal feedback loop of TSH to thyroid levels is broken when someone manually doses their thyroid hormone. T3 may need to be prescribed, in addition to T4, to make the patient feel well and to normalize the FT3/FT4 ratio. Studies show that patients will only reach more normal FT3 levels when TSH is suppressed. The patient may not be hyperthyroid, but just have a suppressed TSH. On T4-only, a normal TSH usually results in a lower than optimal T3 level [see TSH & T3, Chapter 25].

The reference ranges for all three variables are not normal distribution curves. TSH is a right skewed curve, meaning the higher values are questionable as being "normal." FT3 and FT4 are left skewed curves, meaning the lower values are questionable as being "normal." In other words, a high (but normal) TSH combined with low (but normal) FT3 and FT4 levels may be indicators of a hypothyroid state [see Reference Ranges, Chapter 21].

I feel hypothyroid and want to increase my dose, but my doctor said I'll get osteoporosis if I raise it, because my TSH is already low.

Osteoporosis is a real risk factor if someone is overmedicated, meaning they have high T3 and/or T4 levels, not a low TSH. Both T3 and T4 are intimately involved in bone health, and an excess or deficiency of either can result in weak bones. T4 treatment without T3 can cause weak bones, because adequate T3 has a role in bone health too [see Osteoporosis, Chapter 19].

I feel hypothyroid but my TSH is low, even though my FT3 and FT4 are also low. My doctor won't prescribe anything because he said my labs indicate I'm actually hyperthyroid, not hypothyroid.

Some people have damaged pituitary glands, so all their pituitary hormones, including TSH, will always be low. In other words, their TSH will never indicate their true hypothyroid state. Additional pituitary hormones should be tested to confirm whether the patient is hypopituitary [see Peter's Perplexing Pituitary Problem, Chapter 2].

My cholesterol test came back high so my doctor has prescribed statins for me, but I'm having terrible side effects.

High cholesterol is often a symptom of low thyroid function; many with high cholesterol find their levels drop once they start thyroid hormone. In fact, high cholesterol was used to diagnose hypothyroidism a century ago. Today, however, anyone with high cholesterol is prescribed a statin. The knowledge that high cholesterol is a low thyroid symptom seems to have been lost.[15] In addition, giving statins to a hypothyroid person can magnify the side effects, causing muscle aches, cramps, and weakness, also known as statin-induced myopathy.[16] It would be far safer to run complete thyroid tests and treat the hypothyroidism than prescribe statins [see The Woe of Vertigo, Chapter 3].

I have Graves' hyperthyroidism and my doctor said I must have radioactive iodine treatment (RAI).

What form of treatment you choose is completely your decision, and what your doctor finds most convenient should not play a role in the decision. RAI has a lot of documented side effects, some of them irreversible, so thorough research should be done before consenting to this procedure. Anti-thyroid drugs combined with replacement thyroid hormone is a protocol that has worked for some, but is not well-known. Since RAI and thyroidectomies are permanent, all other options should be tried first [see Graves', Chapter 11 and Winning the Battle Against Graves' Disease, Chapter 5].

I'm hypoglycemic (or depressed, or anxious, or have high blood pressure) and my doctor wants to prescribe anti-depressants, anti-anxiety, or blood pressure medications.

Get your thyroid levels tested first [see Blood Tests, Chapter 9]. These can all be signs of low thyroid levels that may disappear or improve with thyroid hormone supplementation [see Hyperthyroid Symptoms, Chapter 16].

I have asthma, eczema, hives, and allergies and my doctor wants to prescribe an inhaler and topical corticosteroids.

Get your thyroid levels tested first [see Blood Tests, Chapter 9]. These can all be signs of low thyroid levels that may disappear or improve with thyroid hormone supplementation [see Asthma, Chapter 7].

I have vertigo and nausea, so my doctor prescribed a motion sickness pill.

Get your thyroid levels tested first [see Blood Tests, Chapter 9]. These can all be signs of low thyroid levels that may disappear or improve with thyroid hormone supplementation [see The Woe of Vertigo, Chapter 3].

My husband and I can't get pregnant. We have some hypothyroid symptoms but all our tests say we're fine.

Both of you should get your thyroid levels tested [see Blood Tests, Chapter 9]. Infertility can be a sign of low thyroid levels that may disappear with thyroid hormone supplementation [see Reproductive Problems, Chapter 22].

I have high blood sugar and my doctor wants to start me on diabetic drugs.

Get your thyroid levels tested first [see Blood Tests, Chapter 9]. High blood sugar can be a sign of low or high thyroid levels that may disappear or improve when thyroid levels normalize [see Insulin Resistance, Chapter 17]. On the other hand, if you are on the T3-only protocol or taking any HC, your high blood sugar may be a direct result of those protocols.

Thyroid physiology – determining an optimum dose

There are four ways I can think of to determine a thyroid dose:

1. TSH – Increase the dose of T4 or desiccated thyroid until the TSH is within the reference range. This doesn't tell where in the reference range TSH should fall and assumes that the TSH feedback loop is 100% operational (it is *not* if thyroid hormone is manually dosed) [see TSH & T3, Chapter 25]. This is probably the most inaccurate way to determine a dose, and leaves most patients under-medicated.

2. Free T3 and Free T4 lab results – Increase the dose of T4 or desiccated thyroid until both FT3 and FT4 are approximately in the middle of the reference range or

higher, which is where most people would fall, because these are left skewed distribution curves [see Reference Ranges, Chapter 21]. This gives better results than dosing by TSH, but still falls short for some patients, because it does not reflect cellular levels, only serum levels.

3. Mimic normal thyroid gland output – A normal thyroid gland secretes approximately 100 mcg T4 + 10 mcg T3 daily; therefore, any dose should be close to this. Assuming a normal distribution curve for these numbers, an average T4 dose could range from 75 – 125 mcg, and T3 from 5 to 15 mcg, *at a minimum*. Doses could theoretically be much higher because of different absorption rates in different people. The only way to approximate these values is to combine prescriptions so that both T4 and T3 are part of the dose; either desiccated thyroid or synthetic T4 + T3 would fill this need.

4. Ignore all labs and just go by "feel" – the only problem is that some hyperthyroid symptoms (like hair loss and fatigue) are identical to hypothyroid symptoms, so it's possible to become grossly overmedicated, thinking that more hormone is needed, when actually less hormone is needed.

In the TSH chapter [Chapter 25], studies showed that the TSH feedback loop does not work the way it normally does when replacement thyroid hormone is taken. Essentially, this means TSH cannot be used to determine the ideal dose, and the TSH rule must be broken. FT3 and FT4 could be used as guidelines, but even knowing that the majority of people have values in the upper half isn't specific enough to say *where* in that upper half of the reference range an individual's values should be. Depending on the person's response, the difference between the middle and top of the reference range may mean adding another ¼ -1 grain or 12.5-50 mcg of T4. That is a huge dose difference.

Other lab values tend to become high and over the reference range when a thyroid dose is too high. These can be used as indicators that the body is being negatively impacted and the dose should be lowered. Values that become too high include: SHBG, fasting blood glucose, red blood cells, hemoglobin, hematocrit, ALT, calcium, and alkaline phosphatase. A high temperature can be a sign of too much thyroid hormone, while a low temperature can be a sign of too little. A low pulse can be a sign of too little thyroid hormone, while a high pulse can be either a hypo or hyper sign. Constipation can be a sign of too little thyroid hormone, while loose stools can be either a hypo or hyper sign, or too much Vitamin C, or too much magnesium.

In the end, these are all just guidelines, and a person's optimal dose is often determined by trial and error. Different prescriptions in different proportions and combinations can be used to custom tailor an individual's dose.

Conclusion

Question everything, no matter who said it, even if it's from a doctor or book. Don't believe everything you think!

[1] Chu, Michael, and Terry F. Seltzer. "Myxedema coma induced by ingestion of raw bok choy." *New England Journal of Medicine* 362.20 (2010): 1945-1946.

[2] Fruzza, Abigail Gelb, Carla Demeterco-Berggren, and Kenneth Lee Jones. "Unawareness of the effects of soy intake on the management of congenital hypothyroidism." *Pediatrics* 130.3 (2012): e699-e702.

[3] Knutson, Kristen L., et al. "The metabolic consequences of sleep deprivation." *Sleep medicine reviews* 11.3 (2007): 163-178.

[4] Spaulding, Stephen W., et al. "Effect of caloric restriction and dietary composition on serum T3 and reverse T3 in man." *Journal of Clinical Endocrinology & Metabolism* 42.1 (1976): 197-200.

[5] Ciloglu, Figen, et al. "Exercise intensity and its effects on thyroid hormones." *Neuroendocrinology Letters* 26.6 (2005): 830-834.

[6] Balhara, Y. P., and K. S. Deb. "Impact of alcohol use on thyroid function." *Indian Journal of Endocrinology and Metabolism* 17.4 (2013): 580.

[7] Antonelli, Alessandro, et al. "Thyroid disorders in chronic hepatitis C." *The American journal of medicine* 117.1 (2004): 10-13.

[8] Schmutzler, Cornelia, et al. "Endocrine disruptors and the thyroid gland—a combined in vitro and in vivo analysis of potential new biomarkers." *Environmental health perspectives* 115.S-1 (2007): 77.

[9] Luzina, K. É., L. L. Luzina, and A. M. Vasilenko. "The influence of acupuncture on the quality of life and the level of thyroid-stimulating hormone in patients presenting with subclinical hypothyroidism]." *Voprosy kurortologii, fizioterapii, i lechebnoĭ fizicheskoĭ kultury* 5 (2011): 29.

[10] Cabıoğlu, Mehmet Tuğrul, et al. "Role of acupuncture in stress management." *Marmara Pharmaceutical Journal* 16 (2012):107-114.

[11] Kim, Ae-Ran, et al. "Acupuncture treatment of a patient with persistent allergic rhinitis complicated by rhinosinusitis and asthma." *Evidence-Based Complementary and Alternative Medicine* 2011 (2011).

[12] Stefan, Dieterle, Neuer Andreas, and Greb Robert. "Acupuncture for infertility: Is it an effective therapy?." *Chinese journal of integrative medicine* 17.5 (2011): 386-395.

[13] Senha, Rohit and Paul Yen. "Cellular Action of Thyroid Hormone." *Thyroid Disease Manager* (2010). http://www.thyroidmanager.org/chapter/cellular-action-of-thyroid-hormone/ accessed 11/14/13.

[14] van der Dennen, Johan MG. "Clinical aggressology: Neuropathology and (violent) aggression." *abstract in Aggressive Behavior* 10.2 (1984): 175.

[15] Rosenman, Ray H., Sanford O. Byers, and Meyer Friedman. "The mechanism responsible for the altered blood cholesterol content in deranged thyroid states." *Journal of Clinical Endocrinology & Metabolism* 12.10 (1952): 1287-1299.

[16] Bar, Simona L., Daniel T. Holmes, and Jiri Frohlich. "Asymptomatic hypothyroidism and statin-induced myopathy." *Canadian family physician* 53.3 (2007): 428-431.

25

The TSH & T3 Dilemma

Your TSH is too low, which means you're hyperthyroid,
so we must reduce your thyroid hormone prescription

> —The TSH rule causes doctors to under-
> medicate thyroid patients, which is how they
> become and remain ill

Thyroid Stimulating Hormone (TSH) levels are used by American endocrinologists to diagnose and treat thyroid problems. The following is from the 2012 Clinical Practice Guidelines For Hypothyroidism In Adults: Cosponsored By The American Association Of Clinical Endocrinologists And The American Thyroid Association:[1]

> *The most reliable therapeutic endpoint for the treatment of primary hypothy-*
> *roidism is the serum TSH value. Confirmatory total T4, free T4, and T3 levels do*
> *not have sufficient specificity to serve as therapeutic endpoints by themselves,*
> *nor do clinical criteria. Moreover, when serum TSH is within the normal range,*
> *free T4 will also be in the normal range. On the other hand, T3 levels may be in*
> *the lower reference range and occasionally mildly subnormal.*

To better analyze the above paragraph, each of the four statements will be examined separately. Thyroxine (T4) and triiodothyronine (T3) are thyroid hormones produced by the thyroid gland. TSH is produced by the pituitary gland. "Free" refers to the unbound part of the hormone that is available to give the body energy.

Statement 1: "The most reliable therapeutic endpoint for the treatment of primary hypothyroidism is the serum TSH value."

This is not logical. TSH is a pituitary hormone, not a thyroid hormone, so TSH is an *implied* measurement of thyroid levels. TSH itself does not give the body any energy, but it stimulates the thyroid gland to produce thyroid hormone that gives the body energy. Those are two different concepts, and if the hypothalamus, pituitary, or thyroid gland are not 100% operational, then a suboptimal amount of TSH will be produced and/or a suboptimal amount of thyroid hormone will be produced. There are too many instances where TSH levels fall below the reference range (which implies hyperthyroidism), when the patient is actually clinically hypothyroid or normal, but certainly *not* hyperthyroid. Many patients have Free and Total T3, and Free and Total T4 levels that are within the reference range with low TSH levels, which contradicts this paradigm (theory). Because of this pseudo-suppression, low TSH levels really should not be used to diagnose hyperthyroidism without confirming the Free T3 and Free and Total T4 levels, nor should low TSH levels alone ever be a reason for decreasing someone's dose. To make dosing decisions based solely on TSH levels (the TSH rule) is a form of paradigm paralysis, which is a fixation on the current paradigm even in the face of overwhelming proof that the paradigm is flawed. This is not much different than people who insisted the earth was flat, because, well, because they said so. Is this flawed paradigm why so many with "normal" TSH levels have so many hypothyroid symptoms?

More from the 2012 Clinical Practice Guidelines For Hypothyroidism In Adults: Cosponsored By The American Association Of Clinical Endocrinologists And The American Thyroid Association:[1]

The normal range for TSH values, with an upper limit of 4.12 mIU/L is largely based on NHANES III data, but it has not been universally accepted. Some have proposed that the upper normal should be either 2.5 or 3.0 mIU/L for a number of reasons:

- *The distribution of TSH values used to establish the normal reference range is skewed to the right by values between 3.1 and 4.12 mIU/L.*

- *The mean and median values of approximately 1.5 mIU/L are much closer to the lower limit of the reported normal reference range than the upper limit.*

- *When risk factors for thyroid disease are excluded, the upper reference limit is somewhat lower.*

Reference ranges are established by testing thousands of people, and then plotting their values on a graph to see how high and low the values range, and where they cluster. A *mean* value is simply the average of all values. The words *distribution* and *skewed to the right* are statistical terms that describe how a particular data set looks. A *normal* distribution is perfectly symmetrical, with an equal number of values to the right and left of the mean. A distribution that is skewed to the right has far more values clustered on the left, with only a trickle of values to the right, or higher end. This means the values to the right are more questionable, and it would even make sense to exclude them and lower the upper end of the reference range. As they state in the second bullet point, the *average* TSH is actually closer to 1.5 mIU/L. The third bullet point says that patients with thyroid disease were included in the sample population and their higher TSH values are the reason the upper limit of the reference range is more than double the average of 1.5 mIU/L. In essence, they are stating that a "normal" TSH in the upper part of the reference range may be an indicator of thyroid disease. This means that TSH, with its current reference ranges, is not a valid diagnostic tool and should *not* be used as such.

Statement 2: "Confirmatory total T4, free T4, and T3 levels do not have sufficient specificity to serve as therapeutic endpoints by themselves, nor do clinical criteria."

Anyone reading any thyroid forum, where thousands of patients share actual lab results, will conclude that a "normal" TSH is really inconclusive, and that actual thyroid hormone levels, especially T3, are much more predictive of thyroid function. *Clinical criteria* refer to observable signs and symptoms in the patient, such as dry skin, thin hair, cold hands, low body temperature, weight problems, etc. The above statement says that physicians should ignore T4, T3 and clinical signs, and instead use the TSH. This makes no sense, when studies indicate that T3 has a much stronger correlation to symptoms than TSH.

Urine Free T3 collected over 24 hours had the highest inverse correlation with clinical symptoms in a study of 832 hypothyroid patients. In other words, the higher the urine Free T3, the fewer the hypothyroid symptoms and vice versa. Urine Free T3 is not influenced by binding globulins and correlated well with the severity of eight clinical hypothyroid symptoms: fatigue, depression, coldness, headache, muscle cramps, constipation, arthritis, and Achilles tendon reflex. Serum T4, Free T4, and TSH often had no correlation to these symptoms.[2]

A study of healthy men in Finland compared thyroid lab results over 14 months to see if there was any correlation with colder temperatures. Only Free T3 showed a statistically significant correlation with severe cold, being lowest in February and highest in August. Serum Total T3, Total T4, Free T4, rT3, and urinary T4 were basically unchanged throughout the year. Urinary T3 displayed an inverse relationship with serum T3, being significantly higher in winter than in summer, which indicates higher clearance or usage of the hormone by the body during colder months. Interestingly, TSH did not show any correlation to the thyroid hormone levels, but did change throughout the year, with a peak in December, when sunlight is lowest.[3]

Patients without clinically obvious coronary heart disease who presented with chest pain were found to have a significant negative correlation of their T3 levels with high-sensitivity cardiac troponin T (hs-cTnT), a measure of damaged heart muscle. The lower the T3 levels, the higher the hs-cTnT. There was no correlation with TSH or FT4.[4]

Another study found FT3 levels were inversely correlated with Coronary Artery Disease (CAD) and mortality. In other words, the lower the FT3 levels, the worse the prognosis. TSH and FT4 showed no correlation with CAD.[5]

Statement 3: "Moreover, when serum TSH is within the normal range, free T4 will also be in the normal range."

Patients may appear "normal" on paper, but if TSH and FT4 have no correlation to symptoms, what's the point to keeping these values in the normal range? T3 is more biologically active than T4, and TSH itself does not give cells energy—T3 does. So why are TSH and FT4 the standard tests that are ordered? Again, it really makes no sense. These tests are analogous to making sure there's oil in a car's engine and water in the radiator, but not checking to see if there's gas in the gas tank. The car won't go anywhere without gas, and the heart won't beat properly without ample T3. T3 is required for normal heart contractions, heart rate, and diastolic blood pressure.[6]

Statement 4: "On the other hand, T3 levels may be in the lower reference range and occasionally mildly subnormal."

And this is ok? The *low T3 syndrome* is associated with severe illness and mortality and has been cited in numerous case studies since the 1970s. A Google Scholar search for *low T3 syndrome* brings up the following studies:

- Low-T3 syndrome a strong prognostic predictor of death in patients with heart disease[7]
- A low T3 syndrome in diabetic ketoacidosis[8]
- Low T3 Syndrome in psychiatric depression[9]
- Low T3 syndrome and chronic inflammatory rheumatism[10]

Summary: From my point of view, none of the four statements in the guidelines makes much sense. Do the people that establish these guidelines live in ivory towers? Have they ever truly examined real thyroid patients? There is a huge disconnect between what these guidelines say, what patients report, and what studies reveal. The rest of this chapter presents study after study that shows how illogical it is to dose someone by TSH.

* * *

Mathematical models question the validity of using TSH as a dosing guideline

Does a normal TSH while taking levothyroxine (T4) replacement mean physiological levels of T3 and T4 have been attained? Not according to several studies. A Japanese study in 2012 compared the TSH, FT3, FT4, and FT3/FT4 ratio in 135 patients at two points in time: before they had a thyroidectomy for papillary thyroid cancer, and after they had been on a stable dose of levothyroxine for at least three months (usually six to twelve months after their thyroidectomy). Their TSH post-surgery (while taking levothyroxine) was significantly lower compared to their TSH pre-surgery. After taking levothyroxine, serum FT4 levels significantly increased and FT3 levels significantly decreased. Only if TSH was suppressed to near 0.1 µIU/ml could FT3 reach pre-thyroidectomy levels. If TSH was kept in the normal range, then serum FT4 was higher and serum FT3 lower than pre-surgery. A physiological (typical) FT3/FT4 ratio could not be maintained on a T4-only regimen. A patient taking levothyroxine may have a relative T3 deficiency, which is not visible if only TSH and FT4 are measured and fall within the normal reference ranges.[11]

An earlier 2002 California study of 53 patients with chronic autoimmune thyroiditis confirmed the exact same relationship between TSH and FT4 and FT3. Patients taking T4 replacement with a normal TSH had a significantly higher FT4 and lower FT3 than normal controls or even patients with chronic autoimmune thyroiditis. The ratio of FT4/FT3 was significantly higher in T4 treated patients, which means that T4 treatment does not replicate normal thyroid physiology.[12]

A 2005 Russian study of 58 hypothyroid women (from autoimmune thyroiditis) duplicated the same findings. T4 treatment resulted in a significantly higher FT4 and significantly lower FT3 compared to normal controls.[13]

A 2013 German study of 1,994 patients used mathematical models to examine the relationship between TSH, FT3, and FT4. To analyze the data, points were plotted and a straight line that best represented the data was drawn between all points. A line going straight up at a 45 degree angle is said to show a positive relationship between the two values that are plotted. Age and height (in children) are an example of a positive relationship: as age increases, height increases. In contrast, a line going down at a 45 degree angle shows an inverse relationship, which means as one value increases the other decreases. TSH should have an inverse relationship to FT4, because normally, as FT4 increases, TSH decreases. Likewise, as FT4 decreases, TSH normally increases. The angle of this line is referred to as a "slope." The slope can be expressed as a mathematical equation. When the slopes of log (a compressed way to depict numbers on a graph) TSH vs. FT3 (or FT4) of T4-treated patients were compared to untreated patients, the correlation slopes were markedly different.[14] This means the relationship of TSH to either FT3 or FT4 is different for someone taking T4, as compared to a normal control. Mathematically, this proves that T4 replacement does not replicate normal thyroid physiology. If it did, the slopes would be identical, or certainly much closer than they are in reality.

In this same study, deiodinase (conversion) activity plotted against TSH showed a positive relationship in untreated subjects. In other words, as TSH rose, the conversion of T4 to T3 also rose. This suggests that TSH aids in conversion. However, in T4-treated patients, as the T4 dose increased, the conversion rate decreased. This relationship confirms the findings of the first study, where T4-treatment resulted in a higher FT4 and lower FT3 than before thyroidectomy. Again, T4-treatment is not replicating normal physiology.

Finally, a 2011 Italian study of 1,811 hypothyroid patients (after thyroidectomy for thyroid cancer) reported the same findings. FT4 was significantly higher and FT3 significantly lower in levothyroxine treated patients with a normal TSH. This resulted in an abnormally low FT3/FT4 ratio, which became even lower as the levothyroxine dose increased.[15] The low ratio was more pronounced in both female and aged patients. For the euthyroid (normal) subjects who were not on replacement, men had a higher FT3/FT4 ratio than women. The euthyroid subjects also displayed an inverse relationship between TSH and FT4. In other words, as FT4 rose, TSH fell. Surprisingly, there was no inverse relationship between TSH and FT3. In other words, even though the euthyroid subjects had a range of TSH levels, they all displayed roughly the same FT3 level, as if the body was designed to produce a specific amount of FT3, regardless of the TSH or T4 level. Since TSH aids T4 to T3 conversion, all three hormones (TSH, T4, T3) could work together to achieve a target T3 level. If T4 drops, then TSH could rise to increase conversion and maintain the target T3. Likewise, if T4 rises, TSH will drop and decrease conversion; target T3 could be maintained by either raising or lowering conversion, depending upon the availability of T4.

Graphs for this study show that the normal relationship of TSH to FT3 is completely lost during T4 treatment; this is illustrated by the vastly different slopes of the two lines. If the line on the graph representing T4 treatment is extrapolated (extended to see the theoretical result), FT3 would only reach the level of euthyroid patients when TSH was closer to 0.1 mU/L, which is below the reference range and considered "hyperthyroid." This is exactly what the first Japanese study concluded. In essence, one cannot have both a normal TSH and a normal FT3 (comparable to a euthyroid control) on T4 treatment. It is an either or scenario on T4 treatment: if TSH is normal, then FT3 will be lower than normal; if FT3 is normal, then TSH must be lower than normal. Given that T3 gives the body energy and TSH does not, which hormone would most patients probably prefer to have more of?

Graphical depictions of the data further illustrate that T4 replacement does not completely replicate normal thyroid physiology. When compared to normal patients, T4 replacement that resulted in a normal TSH caused 7.2% of the patients to have a FT4 that was above the normal reference range. Likewise, 15.2% had a FT3 below the normal reference range. When calculated as a FT3/FT4 ratio, 29.6% fell below the normal reference range. Ratios are a simple mathematical expression used to compare the relationship between two numbers. If the lower number (FT4) is kept constant, then the ratio can be manipulated by simply raising or lowering the top number. Raising the top number (FT3) will raise the ratio. Lowering the top number will lower the ratio. Since the ratio is too low for those on T4 replacement, the way to raise the ratio is to raise FT3. If T3 was prescribed in addition to T4, FT3 should rise and the ratio would rise into the normal range. A physiological ratio could only be attained if both T4 and T3 are taken.

A paper from the United Kingdom uses charts to explain what all the studies above prove—that the desired level of T3 and T4 (taken as replacement hormone) can only be attained when TSH falls below the reference range.[16] The author states that only metabolic measurements such as basal temperature should be used to determine the optimal dose, because those show the actual metabolic effects of thyroid hormone at the cellular level. Serum T3 and T4 levels are an inferred level of thyroid levels because of thyroid hormone resistance at the cellular level. TSH is actually a second level of inference.

Why doesn't T4 replacement result in physiological levels of T3?

A normal thyroid gland secretes about 100 mcg T4 and 10 mcg T3 daily (it produces 6 mcg,[17] and an additional 4 mcg is converted from T4 in the thyroid gland before release). However, doctors typically only prescribe T4, assuming that the body converts T4 to T3 as needed. What has been overlooked is that there are two deiodinase enzymes that convert T4 to T3, and the presence of T3 increases conversion by one enzyme, while the presence of T4 decreases conversion by the other. The D2 enzyme generates the majority of T3 at the cellular level (because it is located inside the cell), while the D1 enzyme generates T3 in the liver, kidneys, and thyroid, and contributes to circulating T3 in the body. Understanding the differences in how these two enzymes work is the key to understanding *why* a T4-only protocol is insufficient replacement. The most important differences, in my opinion, are bolded below.

D1 (type 1 iodothyronine deiodinase)
- D1 is found in the cell plasma membranes of the liver, kidneys, and thyroid
- The half-life of D1 is greater than 12 hours
- T4 concentration does not affect the rate of conversion by D1
- Most of the T3 formed by D1 remains in the cell or exits, but does not enter the nucleus
- TSH increases conversion by D1
- **The presence of T3 will increase D1 gene transcription**

D2 (type 2 iodothyronine deiodinase)
- D2 is found in the endoplasmic reticulum (located inside the cells) in the central nervous system, pituitary, thyroid, bone, brown adipose tissue, cochlea, skeletal muscle, retina, and brain (glial cells, tancytes)[18]
- The half-life of D2 is 20-30 minutes in the presence of T4
- The presence of T3 will decrease D2 gene transcription
- The majority of T3 formed by D2 enters the cell nucleus and binds with thyroid receptors
- T3 from D2 has 2 to 3 times the effect on gene transcription than T3 from D1
- **The more T4 present, the lower the percentage of T4 converted to T3 by D2**

The D2 enzyme is considered the primary source of human T_3 in the euthyroid (normal) state; in fact, about twice as much T3 is produced from D2 (66%) than from D1 in a normal person. In the hypothyroid state, D2 accounts for about 70% of the T3 produced, but in the hyperthyroid state, only about 30%. In other words, D2 conversion is downregulated when T4 or T3 levels are high. When T4 was increased by a factor of 10, T3 formed from D1 also increased by a factor of 10; however, T3 formed from D2 only increased by a factor of 2.5.[19] This downregulation explains why prescribing more T4 often does not result in any improvement in patients. With each incremental increase in T4, there's a significant decrease in the percentage that's converted to T3. This is probably a safety mechanism to protect the body from excess T3 levels, which can be damaging.

In contrast, D1 enzyme conversion increases in the presence of T3, but decreases in the hypothyroid state. This may be why it's so important for someone on replacement thyroid hormone to include some T3 in their dose. Without T3, D1 enzyme activity may be limited. The two enzymes create T3 through different mechanisms, with D1 contributing to circulating T3, and D2 contributing to local T3. Having two different enzymes that both produce T3 may be a redundant system to ensure that some T3 is always available to the cells that need it.

The levels of both T3 and T4 circulating in the body determine the activity of these enzymes. This is the reason that patients must wait 6 weeks between dose changes; the conversion rates change with different levels of T4 and T3, and the body needs time to find a new equilibrium.

While T3 is produced in two different ways by two different enzymes, lab tests only measure circulating levels of T3 in serum (and not levels inside the cell), which means lab tests only show D1 conversion. Patients on T4 replacement would be expected to have lower serum T3 because they lack the direct T3 that stimulates D1 conversion. Those with normal levels of serum T3, yet many hypothyroid symptoms, may lack T3 at the cellular level, due to impaired D2 conversion or other factors. Taking either too much T3 or T4 will repress D2 activity.

TSH levels fluctuate

Hashi's patients have thyroid peroxidase and thyroglobulin antibodies and often cycle from hyper to hypo, which can cause huge fluctuations in TSH levels. Eventually the weakened thyroid stays in a hypothyroid state, so patients generally feel better when placed on enough thyroid hormone to keep their levels stable, which also results in a lower TSH.[20] The lower TSH reduces stimulation to the thyroid, which results in lowered antibodies, and stops the continuous hyper/hypo fluctuations. Levothyroxine treatment lowered the antibodies in one study, which rose when the levothyroxine was discontinued.[21]

TSH displays a seasonal variation in healthy people, with TSH levels lowest in the spring. The variation from the mean TSH (average of 12 monthly TSH values) was 29.1%.[22]

TSH decreases when fasting.[23] Most patients do their lab tests in a fasting state, because it is required for other labs like glucose and cholesterol. But this may result in an artificially low TSH that does not reflect true thyroid levels. In fact, TSH has a circadian rhythm, with a peak around midnight (with much variability between individuals), and a low in the afternoon; fluctuations are normal. The change in TSH from peak to trough is approximately 72%. Free T3 levels also show a similar circadian rhythm (with a smaller amplitude) with a time lag approximately 90 minutes behind the TSH curve. The Free T4 curve does not follow the TSH curve at all.[24] Labs drawn in the morning could be significantly different from labs drawn in the afternoon after lunch, with one TSH in the "normal" range and the other in the hyperthyroid or hypothyroid range. A test with such wide variation cannot be valid and certainly should not be used to make dosing decisions.

A study compared early morning fasting serum TSH levels to late morning non-fasting serum TSH levels in the same patients on the same day. In 97 of 100 subjects, the second test results declined by an average of 26.39% when compared to the first test results. This meant that 6% of patients who would be diagnosed as subclinical hypothyroid (high TSH) after the first test results would be reclassified as "normal" after the second test results. Since time of day and fasting status of the patient can significantly affect serum TSH test results, a diagnosis based solely on TSH, a value that fluctuates, really does not make any sense.[25]

TSH can be suppressed (near zero) when a patient is *not* hyperthyroid

The TSH in people with a dysfunctional hypothalamus or pituitary gland will never accurately reflect their actual thyroid levels.[26] This is common in people who have had head injuries from sports, car accidents, etc. Has anyone *not* bumped their head at some point, ever?

Graves' disease patients who have had radioactive iodine treatment (RAI), a thyroidectomy, or who take anti-thyroid drugs (ATD) should take replacement thyroid hormone to restore their thyroid levels. Each individual may need a different dose, but Graves' patients should *not* be dosed by TSH. Graves' is caused by *TSH* Receptor antibodies, and TSH levels can stay suppressed (near zero) for months or longer, even after treatment brings thyroid hormone levels down into the normal range or even below normal.[27] This is because thyroid ablation (destruction) does not remove the Graves' antibodies from the blood, it merely eliminates the organ (the thyroid) that was under attack. If the antibodies remain high, TSH levels will continue to be suppressed, no matter how low the actual thyroid levels are; the normal TSH feedback loop does not work because Graves' antibodies control the TSH. A broken gas gauge with an empty gas tank is a good analogy. The gauge might read full, but there's really no gas in the tank, and likewise some of these patients are literally "running on fumes." If Graves' patients are unable to get adequate thyroid hormone replacement because of their suppressed TSH levels, they may suffer from their untreated hypothyroid condition. They would fare much better by adjusting their dose to Free T3 and Free and/or Total T4 levels, instead of the TSH. Some Graves' patients suffer greatly because their TSH does not return after their thyroid has been destroyed by RAI or thyroidectomy. This means they have close to zero thyroid function, but because their TSH remains suppressed, doctors refuse to prescribe them any thyroid hormone, thinking they are still hyperthyroid, even though they have no thyroid gland! Their life changes from being hyperthyroid to being profoundly hypothyroid. First person stories on Graves' thyroid forums are absolutely heartbreaking, and their misery is a direct result of the rigid TSH rule that is followed.

Any thyroid medication that contains T3, like Cytomel or desiccated thyroid, will suppress TSH levels.[28] The direct T3 in the blood is sensed by the hypothalamus/pituitary, the body determines that no additional thyroid is needed, so no TSH is released. A normal thyroid secretes only a minimal amount of T3. The majority of the body's T3 is converted from T4 as needed throughout the day, whereas someone taking T3 or desiccated thyroid takes a concentrated dose of T3 all at once in a pill. This may explain the TSH suppression. Surprisingly, patients can have suppressed TSH levels on these replacement hormones but do not exhibit any hyperthyroid symptoms. Dosing a patient who takes any T3 by TSH will usually leave the patient undermedicated with hypothyroid symptoms. The mathematical models discussed earlier showed that it was only possible to attain a normal T3 if TSH was suppressed.

One reason suppressed TSH levels are frowned upon by doctors is because they feel it can lead to pituitary atrophy. However, a study where thyroid hormone was discontinued after long-term use and TSH suppression, showed a return to normal levels within two to five weeks. Serum T4 also returned to normal at least four weeks after hormone withdrawal.[29]

Thyroid cancer patients on TSH suppression therapy did not show hyperthyroid signs and symptoms unless their serum Free T4 was also high. There was no correlation with TSH. The abstract states: "Although the degree of TSH suppression can now be exactly monitored with new third generation TSH assays, hyperthyroidism cannot be defined using TSH concentration . . ."[30]

Non-thyroidal illness (NTIS) is the medical term for acute or chronic illness that causes a fall in TSH, even though both T4 and T3 also decline. The normal feedback loop is not operating correctly, because TSH would normally rise if T4 and T3 decrease. Some causes of NTIS are severe dieting, sepsis (severe infection that affects the whole body), trauma, burns, acute renal (kidney) failure, and glucocorticoid use. Changes within the hypothalamic–pituitary–thyroid (HPT) axis are thought to be the cause of NTIS, rather than damage to the thyroid gland. The illness affects normal thyroid output even though the thyroid gland may still be functional. TSH, T3 and T4 sometimes rise back to normal levels in patients who recover, indicating that NTIS can be a transient condition.[31]

Other conditions that affect TSH

Pregnancy,[32] diabetes,[33] liver disease,[34] and cardiac conditions (heart transplant or bypass)[35] all impact TSH for different reasons and therefore make TSH levels a poor diagnostic tool. In pregnancy, TSH levels decrease due to elevated human chorionic gonadotropin (HCG) levels that cross-react with the TSH receptor. Diabetics tend to have abnormal TSH levels (both high and low) that normalize with treatment for their blood sugar. TSH is increased in liver cirrhosis, probably because Free and Total T3 are usually lower, and the liver is where much systemic conversion from T4 to T3 is performed. In cardiac patients, TSH drops significantly after surgery, which is believed to be a form of NTIS.

Thyroid hormone resistance syndrome is a condition where the body's tissues are resistant to the effects of thyroid hormone. In Generalized Resistance to Thyroid Hormone (GRTH), a patient can have elevated serum thyroid hormone levels but normal or elevated TSH levels, when a suppressed TSH would be expected. These people are usually clinically euthyroid and require no treatment.[36] This is just another example where the TSH cannot and should not be used to make a diagnosis.

Cushing's disease or glucocorticoid administration will lower TSH, which results in lower T3 levels. Dexamethasone in one study significantly lowered TSH, but T4 and FT4 did not change significantly, though T3 and FT3 levels fell.[37] Even physiologic levels of cortisol have a suppressive effect on TSH, and this is seen in the opposite circadian rhythms of TSH and cortisol. TSH rises before midnight and falls through the night, while cortisol is lowest before midnight and rises overnight while we sleep.[38]

Sleep deprivation affects TSH; women who only get 5.5 hours of sleep each night (8.5 hours is preferable) have a lower TSH and FT4. Men are not as affected by limited sleep and did not show a significant change in TSH and FT4. In contrast, total sleep deprivation results in a higher TSH and higher T3 and T4 levels. Many women today with busy lifestyles may only get 5.5 hours of sleep. They may have a working thyroid gland, but lack of sleep is negatively affecting their hypothalamus-pituitary-thyroid axis, making them somewhat hypothyroid.[39]

Does TSH have any value?

A TSH test can sometimes be useful. Low TSH levels (near zero) with hyperthyroid symptoms may be the first indication that someone (who is not taking any thyroid medication) has Graves' disease. Further antibody testing will confirm that diagnosis. When a TSH is greater than 1.0, it *may* indicate some degree of hypothyroidism, and suggests a dose increase may be warranted, or that other factors like iron, cortisol, blood sugar, etc.

need to be addressed. The current TSH reference range includes undiagnosed hypothyroid patients, which means higher TSH values are considered "normal," when they shouldn't be. African-Americans, who have a very low incidence of Hashimoto's thyroiditis, have an average TSH of 1.18. This may be more representative of the true normal mean TSH of a normal population.[40] Another study found increased arterial stiffness (which correlates with heart disease) in subjects whose TSH was 2.01-4.0, which is within the normal range. The authors concluded that "it may be proposed that TSH values between 2.01 and 4.0 µU/ml are rather mildly abnormal and not high-normal and that the definition of the "normal" range for TSH values should probably be reconsidered."[41]

Most doctors say a TSH near zero isn't healthy, because it means the patient is hyperthyroid. Healthy people do not have a TSH that low. There are actually TSH receptors throughout the body,[42] not just on the thyroid, so intuitively, TSH must have a purpose. TSH's role may be to stimulate T4 to T3 conversion at the cellular level, since each organ has its own T3 requirement, which may be higher or lower than that of other tissues. In a lab experiment on isolated rat liver and kidneys, adding TSH had a positive effect on T3 levels. The release of T3, tissue T3 production, net T3 production, and the conversion rate of T4 to T3 in both the rat liver[43] and kidney[44] was significantly higher when perfused with 250 µU/ml TSH, than in the controls that did not have the additional TSH.

If the primary role of TSH is to aid in T4 to T3 conversion at the cellular level, then someone with low TSH may have insufficient T3 levels. In fact, many patients on thyroid forums initially report a low TSH with low T3 levels, but T4 levels close to mid-range. Mathematical models discussed earlier showed this was normal when taking T4 replacement. With desiccated thyroid, a suppressed TSH is a common side effect, because the T3 content in desiccated thyroid suppresses stimulation from both the hypothalamus and pituitary. So anyone taking desiccated thyroid may have limited T4 to T3 conversion due to a lack of TSH. But desiccated thyroid contains T3, so the loss of conversion is compensated for by the same T3 that is suppressing the TSH. In any case, it is possible to live with a suppressed TSH, and many on desiccated thyroid do just that, because they find that keeping their TSH in range means they'll still have hypothyroid symptoms.

Most people on T4 treatment do not have suppressed TSH levels, but most people on desiccated do, probably because desiccated contains T3. Anecdotally, most patients feel better when they take some form of T3, whether it's desiccated thyroid or synthetic T3. Maybe the best of both worlds could be achieved by combining levothyroxine with T3 or desiccated thyroid. Lowering the desiccated dose and splitting it up throughout the day keeps T3 levels more stable. And since desiccated has too high a ratio of T3 to T4 for some people, combining the two would correct that problem too. This obviously would not work for people with conversion or other issues, but it might for some. I know a man who takes a small dose (1/8 grain) of desiccated thyroid every two to three hours, and another woman who doses hourly. They are getting as close as possible to replicating normal thyroid function by giving their bodies small amounts of T3 throughout the day. One study found that reasonably steady levels of T3 could be maintained if T3 was taken three times per day.[45] This evened out the peaks and valleys in once or twice a day dosing.

If I had to prioritize the three hormones (T3, T4, TSH), I would say T3 is absolutely essential, and one could not live without it. In fact, it is preferable to give someone T3 to bring them out of myxedema coma (near-death hypothyroid state), rather than T4. In one study, 50% of the patients presenting with myxedema coma died even though they were given T4.[46] Nearly half of the patients in this particular study were taking diuretics prescribed by their primary care physicians to manage their edema (swelling due to fluid buildup—another hypothyroid symptom). Their hypothyroidism was never diagnosed. In another study, all patients survived, and they were given T3 first, followed by T4.[47] T3 levels did not rise when they were first given T4, indicating poor peripheral conversion of T4 to T3.

In my case, I have to choose between having a "normal" TSH or having asthma, because on desiccated thyroid I have asthma if my TSH is kept in range. Raising my dose by only ¼ grain suppresses my TSH, but completely relieves the asthma. My free and total T3 and T4 levels are not over range with this suppressed TSH. But because breathing is something I do 24/7, I have chosen to overlook the TSH. I've recently switched to a combination of T4 + desiccated, because my labs are very lopsided on desiccated alone, with upper range Free T3 and lower range Free T4. Improvements so far are more hair!

Conclusion

If nothing else, this chapter should make anyone in the medical profession who uses TSH as a dosing guideline rethink that rule. Mathematical models prove that the TSH feedback loop is not the same when thyroid hormone is supplied externally. A German and an Italian study both drew the same conclusions after testing thousands of subjects: the slope depicting the relationship of TSH to FT3 is different when the hormone is naturally produced, versus when it is taken exogenously. In fact, the most important concept in this chapter is that a hypothyroid patient cannot have both a normal TSH and a physiological level of FT3 on T4 treatment. It is an either or scenario: if TSH is normal, then FT3 will be lower than normal; if FT3 is normal, then TSH must be lower than normal. Dosing patients by TSH means they are receiving less than optimal treatment. Optimal treatment can only be obtained if TSH is overlooked. Mathematical models prove that, and patient testimonials further confirm the models. In addition, not taking any T3 creates an abnormally low FT3/FT4 ratio for many patients, which means T4 treatment does not replicate normal thyroid physiology.

A relevant analogy would be the relationship of Adrenocorticotropic Hormone (ACTH) to cortisol. ACTH is the pituitary hormone that stimulates cortisol production, analogous to TSH, which is the pituitary hormone that stimulates thyroid hormone production. If a patient is deficient in cortisol, they would be taking some form of cortisol replacement, which then makes ACTH useless, because of disturbed feedback loops. People with low cortisol do not try to keep their ACTH "in range." They try to reproduce normal cortisol production. Studies about hydrocortisone replacement in Addison's disease patients (no natural cortisol production) discuss the dosage range that patients take, and peak and trough cortisol levels. They compare patient cortisol profiles to healthy controls. They do not compare or even measure ACTH in some of these studies.[48] One study noted there was no reliable and convenient marker to assess glucocorticoid levels; monitoring is based on clinical assessments.[49] Likewise, thyroid patients should try to keep their thyroid levels (T3 and T4) close to those of healthy controls and monitor their symptoms, not keep their TSH "normal."

Doctors need to learn that a suppressed TSH does not mean the patient is hyper-thyroid. In the case study section (Part I in this book), Jane's case is the most dramatic example. One endocrinologist reduced her levothyroxine dose in an attempt to raise her TSH, in spite of the fact that her FT3 was already *below* the reference range. Peter, who had a damaged pituitary gland, is another example of a patient whose TSH prevented him from receiving treatment, because it was always "normal," even though his FT3 and FT4 were at the bottom of the reference range. Tony also had a normal TSH that didn't reflect his hypothyroid condition; iron overload may have damaged his pituitary or thyroid gland or liver (where most conversion occurs). Lucy, who has Graves' disease, has always had very little TSH. This is in spite of the fact that her thyroid levels were sometimes at the bottom of the range because of anti-thyroid drugs used to treat her Graves'. And in my case, I have no TSH because I take T3 in desiccated thyroid. These are just five profiles of real thyroid patients. The thyroid forums are full of hundreds of thousands of patients displaying the same problem—a TSH that is not representative of their thyroid function, at all.

Reliance on TSH is a worldwide problem. There are thyroid forums, websites, and blogs in so many different languages it is mind boggling. Visitors to my Tired Thyroid.com website come from all over the world. Of course, most visitors come from the U.S., but the other countries with the most visitors in 2013 (in descending order) were the UK, Canada, Australia, India, Finland, Germany, Ireland, Sweden and the United Arab Emirates. Hypothyroid patients everywhere are undermedicated, not feeling well, and trying to figure out why by talking to other patients. Their TSH is normal, so why don't they feel well?

Key points

- Studies on thyroid physiology that examine the relationship of TSH to FT3 and FT4 do not support the guidelines of The American Association Of Clinical Endo-crinologists and The American Thyroid Association.
- TSH is a pituitary hormone so can only be an implied measure of thyroid hormone levels.
- The mean and median value of TSH is approximately 1.5 mIU/L. TSH values above 3.0 mIU/L may be due to thyroid disease.
- FT3 has been shown to correlate to symptoms in patients when TSH, Total T4, and FT4 have not shown any correlation.
- Contrary to current medical guidelines, T3 should be measured because low T3 levels are diagnostic of a severe condition called the Low T3 Syndrome.
- Separate studies in Japan, the U.S., Russia, Germany, and Italy all reported that T4 treatment does not replicate normal thyroid physiology because it results in a lower TSH, higher FT4, and lower FT3 than compared to normal euthyroid controls.
- These abnormal labs result in a lower FT3/FT4 ratio than in normal euthyroid controls. One way to normalize this ratio would be to take T3 in addition to T4.
- Mathematical models prove that the TSH-FT3 relationship is different between T4 treated patients and normal euthyroid controls. A T4 treated patient with a

normal TSH will have a lower than normal FT3; likewise, if they have a normal FT3, they will have a lower than normal TSH. It is an either or proposition.

- Mathematical models also prove that the TSH-conversion rate relationship is different between T4 treated patients and normal euthyroid controls. In euthyroid controls, as TSH rises, T4 to T3 conversion also rises. In T4 treated patients, more T4 results in lower TSH, and less T4 to T3 conversion. Therefore, increasing the T4 dose does not result in substantially more T3.

- TSH levels fluctuate in Hashimoto's patients; they vary by season, are affected by fasting, and have a circadian rhythm, being lowest in the afternoon. Such a dynamic variable should not be used as a diagnostic.

- Patients can have suppressed TSH levels even though they are not hyperthyroid. They may have a dysfunctional hypothalamus or pituitary gland, Graves' disease antibodies, non-thyroidal illness, or take T3.

- Pregnancy and heart conditions may decrease TSH, while diabetes and liver disease may raise it. Hydrocortisone supplementation and lack of sleep will also lower TSH.

- A suppressed TSH combined with hyperthyroid symptoms may be the first indicator that someone has Graves' disease. It is a useful indicator in someone who is not taking replacement hormone.

- TSH appears to stimulate T4 to T3 conversion.

- Overreliance on TSH is a worldwide problem.

---

[1] Jeffrey R. Garber, et al. Clinical Practice Guidelines For Hypothyroidism In Adults: Cosponsored By The American Association Of Clinical Endocrinologists And The American Thyroid Association. Endocrine Practice. Vol. 18, No. 6, 988-1028. November/December 2012.

[2] Baisier, W. V., J. Hertoghe, and W. Eeckhaut. "Thyroid insufficiency. Is TSH measurement the only diagnostic tool?" Journal of Nutritional and Environmental Medicine 10.2 (2000): 105-113.

[3] Hassi, Juhani, et al. "The pituitary-thyroid axis in healthy men living under subarctic climatological conditions." Journal of endocrinology 169.1 (2001): 195-203.

[4] Kim, Bo-Bae, et al. "Relation of Triiodothyronine to Subclinical Myocardial Injury in Patients With Chest Pain." The American journal of cardiology (2013).

[5] Coceani, Michele, et al. "Thyroid hormone and coronary artery disease: from clinical correlations to prognostic implications." Clinical cardiology 32.7 (2009): 380-385.

[6] Shojaie, Mohammad, and Ahad Eshraghian. "Primary hypothyroidism presenting with Torsades de pointes type tachycardia: a case report." Cases J 1.1 (2008): 298.

[7] Iervasi, Giorgio, et al. "Low-T3 syndrome a strong prognostic predictor of death in patients with heart disease." Circulation 107.5 (2003): 708-713.

[8] Naeije, Robert, et al. "A low T3 syndrome in diabetic ketoacidosis." Clinical endocrinology 8.6 (1978): 467-472.

[9] Premachandra, B. N., M. A. Kabir, and I. K. Williams. "Low T3 syndrome in psychiatric depression." Journal of endocrinological investigation 29.6 (2006): 568.

[10] Herrmann, F., et al. "[Low T3 syndrome and chronic inflammatory rheumatism]." *Zeitschrift fur die gesamte innere Medizin und ihre Grenzgebiete* 44.17 (1989): 513-518.

[11] Ito, Mitsuru, et al. "TSH-suppressive doses of levothyroxine are required to achieve preoperative native serum triiodothyronine levels in patients who have undergone total thyroidectomy." European Journal of Endocrinology 167.3 (2012): 373-378.

[12] Woeber, K. A. "Levothyroxine therapy and serum free thyroxine and free triiodothyronine concentrations." Journal of endocrinological investigation 25.2 (2002): 106-109.

[13] Fadeyev, Valentin V., et al. "TSH and thyroid hormones concentrations in patients with hypothyroidism receiving replacement therapy with L-thyroxine alone or in combination with L-triiodothyronine." Hormones (Athens) 4.2 (2005): 101-107.

[14] Hoermann, Rudolf, et al. "Is pituitary TSH an adequate measure of thyroid hormone-controlled homoeostasis during thyroxine treatment?" European Journal of Endocrinology 168.2 (2013): 271-280.

[15] Gullo, Damiano, et al. "Levothyroxine monotherapy cannot guarantee euthyroidism in all athyreotic patients." PloS one 6.8 (2011): e22552.

[16] Warmingham, P. "Effect of exogenous thyroid hormone intake on the interpretation of serum TSH test results." Thyroid Science 5.7 (2010): 1-6.

[17] Pilo, Alessandro, et al. "Thyroidal and peripheral production of 3, 5, 3'-triiodothyronine in humans by multicompartmental analysis." *American Journal of Physiology-Endocrinology and Metabolism* 258.4 (1990): E715-E726.

[18] Larsen, P. R., and A. M. Zavacki. "Role of the Iodothyronine Deiodinases in the Physiology and Pathophysiology of Thyroid Hormone Action." *European thyroid journal* 1.4 (2012): 232-242.

[19] Maia, Ana Luiza, et al. "Type 2 iodothyronine deiodinase is the major source of plasma T3 in euthyroid humans." *Journal of Clinical Investigation* 115.9 (2005): 2524-2533.

[20] Aksoy, Duygu Yazgan, et al. "Effects of prophylactic thyroid hormone replacement in euthyroid Hashimoto's thyroiditis." Endocrine journal 52.3 (2005): 337-343.

[21] Rieu, Max, et al. "Effects of thyroid status on thyroid autoimmunity expression in euthyroid and hypothyroid patients with Hashimoto's thyroiditis." Clinical endocrinology 40.4 (1994): 529-535.

[22] Maes, M., et al. "Components of biological variation, including seasonality, in blood concentrations of TSH, TT3, FT4, PRL, cortisol and testosterone in healthy volunteers." Clinical endocrinology 46.5 (1997): 587-598.

[23] Romijn, J. A., et al. "Pulsatile secretion of thyrotropin during fasting: a decrease of thyrotropin pulse amplitude." Journal of Clinical Endocrinology & Metabolism 70.6 (1990): 1631-1636.

[24] Russell, Wanda, et al. "Free triiodothyronine has a distinct circadian rhythm that is delayed but parallels thyrotropin levels." Journal of Clinical Endocrinology & Metabolism 93.6 (2008): 2300-2306.

[25] Scobbo, Ronald R., et al. "Serum TSH variability in normal individuals: the influence of time of sample collection." The West Virginia Medical Journal 100.4 (2003): 138-142.

[26] Lieberman, Steven A., et al. "Prevalence of neuroendocrine dysfunction in patients recovering from traumatic brain injury." Journal of Clinical Endocrinology & Metabolism 86.6 (2001): 2752-2756.

[27] Chung, Yun Jae, et al. "Continued suppression of serum TSH level may be attributed to TSH receptor antibody activity as well as the severity of thyrotoxicosis and the time to recovery of thyroid hormone in treated euthyroid Graves' patients." Thyroid 16.12 (2006): 1251-1257.

[28] Appelhof, Bente C., et al. "Combined therapy with levothyroxine and liothyronine in two ratios, compared with levothyroxine monotherapy in primary hypothyroidism: a double-blind, randomized, controlled clinical trial." Journal of Clinical Endocrinology & Metabolism 90.5 (2005): 2666-2674.

[29] Vagenakis, Apostolos G., et al. "Recovery of pituitary thyrotropic function after withdrawal of prolonged thyroid-suppression therapy." New England Journal of Medicine 293.14 (1975): 681-684.

[30] Taimela, E., et al. "Free thyroid hormones and a third-generation TSH assay in the detection of hyperthyroidism during long-term thyroxine treatment in thyroid carcinoma patients." Scandinavian journal of clinical & laboratory investigation 55.2 (1995): 181-186.

[31] Warner, Maria H., and Geoffrey J. Beckett. "Mechanisms behind the non-thyroidal illness syndrome: an update." Journal of Endocrinology 205.1 (2010): 1-13.

[32] LaFranchi, Stephen. "Thyroid hormone in hypopituitarism, Graves' disease, congenital hypothyroidism, and maternal thyroid disease during pregnancy." Growth hormone & IGF research 16 (2006): 20-24.

[33] Celani, M. F., M. E. Bonati, and N. Stucci. "Prevalence of abnormal thyrotropin concentrations measured by a sensitive assay in patients with type 2 diabetes mellitus." Diabetes research (Edinburgh, Scotland) 27.1 (1994): 15.

[34] Borzio, M., et al. "Thyroid function tests in chronic liver disease: evidence for multiple abnormalities despite clinical euthyroidism." Gut 24.7 (1983): 631-636.

[35] Bayer, Monika F., John A. Macoviak, and I. Ross McDougall. "Diagnostic performance of sensitive measurements of serum thyrotropin during severe nonthyroidal illness: their role in the diagnosis of hyperthyroidism." Clinical chemistry 33.12 (1987): 2178-2184

[36] McDermott, Michael T., and E. Chester Ridgway. "Thyroid hormone resistance syndromes." The American journal of medicine 94.4 (1993): 424-432.

[37] Re, R. N., et al. "The effect of glucocorticoid administration on human pituitary secretion of thyrotropin and prolactin." Journal of Clinical Endocrinology & Metabolism 43.2 (1976): 338-346.

[38] Samuels, M. H. "Effects of metyrapone administration on thyrotropin secretion in healthy subjects—a clinical research center study." Journal of Clinical Endocrinology & Metabolism 85.9 (2000): 3049-3052.

[39] Kessler, Lynn, et al. "Changes in serum TSH and free T4 during human sleep restriction." Sleep 33.8 (2010): 1115.

[40] Wartofsky, Leonard, and Richard A. Dickey. "The evidence for a narrower thyrotropin reference range is compelling." Journal of Clinical Endocrinology & Metabolism 90.9 (2005): 5483-5488.

[41] Dagre, Anna G., et al. "Arterial stiffness is increased in subjects with hypothyroidism." International journal of cardiology 103.1 (2005): 1-6.

[42] Davies, Terry, Russell Marians, and Rauf Latif. "The TSH receptor reveals itself." Journal of Clinical Investigation 110.2 (2002): 161-164.

[43] Ikeda, Tadasu, et al. "Effect of thyrotropin on conversion of T4 to T3 in perfused rat liver." Life sciences 38.20 (1986): 1801-1806.

[44] Ikeda, Tadasu, et al. "Effect of TSH on conversion of T4 to T3 in perfused rat kidney." Metabolism 34.11 (1985): 1057-1060.

[45] Celi, Francesco S., et al. "The pharmacodynamic equivalence of levothyroxine and liothyronine: a randomized, double blind, cross-over study in thyroidectomized patients." Clinical endocrinology 72.5 (2010): 709-715.

[46] Dutta, Pinaki, et al. "Predictors of outcome in myxoedema coma: a study from a tertiary care centre." Critical Care 12.1 (2008): R1.

[47] Pereira, V. G., et al. "Management of myxedema coma: report on three successfully treated cases with nasogastric or intravenous administration of triiodothyronine." Journal of endocrinological investigation 5.5 (1982): 331.

[48] Ross, I. L., et al. "Salivary Cortisol Day Curves in Addison's Disease in Patients on Hydrocortisone Replacement." Hormone and Metabolic Research EFirst 45(01) (2013): 62-68.

[49] Grossman, Ashley, et al. "Therapy Of Endocrine Disease: Perspectives on the management of adrenal insufficiency: clinical insights from across Europe." European Journal of Endocrinology 169.6 (2013): R165-R175.

PART III:

WHERE DO WE GO FROM HERE?

26

The Problem with Current Thyroid Treatment

Just how big does this elephant have to get before we address it?

Current thyroid treatment today leaves much to be desired, primarily because one unreliable blood test, the Thyroid Stimulating Hormone (TSH) test, is dictating whether treatment is even allowed. The TSH test is also used to determine whether a dose can be raised to alleviate a patient's hypothyroid symptoms. In other words, because of "normal" TSH test results, hypothyroid patients are being denied treatment, and suboptimally treated patients cannot get their medication increased [see TSH, Chapter 25]. This rigid TSH rule must change and several other issues need to be addressed before thyroid patients can receive appropriate care.

Compounding this medical testing travesty, the current reference ranges for "normal" are so broad that they include hypothyroid patients. If severely hypothyroid patients test as "normal," what is the point of the test? Shouldn't another test, or combination of tests, be used instead? It would certainly make sense to tighten up all the thyroid reference ranges. Ranges that are known to be skewed to the right or left should certainly be redefined so that they become more symmetrical, like normal distribution curves. The "long tail" (of the distribution curve) should be cut off! [see Reference Ranges, Chapter 21]

Medical treatment in the U.S. today revolves around "Standards of Care," the official guidelines that doctors use to treat certain medical conditions. For suspected thyroid disease, the recommended tests are TSH and Free T4 (FT4). A number of studies have repeatedly shown that TSH and FT4 often have no correlation to symptoms, but Free T3 (FT3) does. Yet FT3 is not even considered part of a standard thyroid panel and must be specifically requested. Sadly, many doctors do not know to test for it. Insurance companies also tend to follow these guidelines, so the Standard of Care for thyroid patients must change.

Doctors are the gatekeepers to all thyroid tests and prescriptions; therefore, they should have comprehensive instruction in thyroid physiology. With recent advances in molecular biology, we now know that deiodinase enzymes are responsible for normal or abnormal T4 to T3 conversion, that T3 provides a synergy that results in better conversion, that T3 is secreted by a normal thyroid gland, and that the normal TSH feedback loop does not work with exogenous thyroid supplementation in the same way as a normal person secreting their own thyroid hormones. Doctors need to learn that it is safe, and in fact, it should be required, that all hypothyroid patients who need it be prescribed some amount of T3 to replicate normal thyroid function.

Most doctors will *only* prescribe T4, and in contrast, there are militant patient groups that insist that desiccated thyroid is the *only* valid form of thyroid replacement. The dogmatic intransigence of both groups has hurt thyroid patients like me, who just need something very close to what a normal thyroid produces—mostly T4 with a little T3. T4-only leaves me deficient in T3, and desiccated leaves me overdosed on T3 and underdosed on T4, because of the higher T3/T4 content in pig thyroid glands. The *only* way around this, for someone like me (and countless others), is to combine the two prescriptions. A fellow patient, upon hearing that I combined the two prescriptions, asked her doctor if she could add ½ grain of desiccated thyroid to her T4 dose. The doctor was absolutely incredulous and said she'd never heard of such a thing. She'd heard that some people take desiccated thyroid, and she knew that most doctors like herself only prescribed T4, but she had never heard of someone combining both prescriptions! It is extremely closed-minded to reject something without even taking the time to learn about it.

Thyroid hormone provides energy to every single cell and organ in the body. Unfortunately, modern medicine breaks down the human body into the study of different organs, so no one is seeing the big picture. The specialist system is dangerously myopic. When I tried to explain to a doctor that the thyroid and adrenal glands were "connected," the doctor shook his head, pointed to his neck, and said, "the thyroid is here," then pointed to his kidney area, and said, "and the adrenals are here." How does one argue with that? He's anatomically correct, but physiologically incorrect. Thyroid function is directly correlated with adrenal function [see Adrenal Dysfunction, Chapter 6].

A cardiologist only studies the heart. There are numerous studies that show that low levels of T3 can cause heart disease. While some cardiologists are aware of this, are general practitioners (GPs), the doctors that patients see first, also aware of this? Are endocrinologists aware of this? Many endocrinologists and GPs will not test T3 levels, only T4 and TSH. As a patient, I can only speculate that maybe insurance regulations or Standards of Care are behind this archaic testing methodology. Patients on thyroid internet support groups often report that when they asked a doctor to test their FT3 levels, they were refused. Why?

What would happen if everyone who had high cholesterol was prescribed thyroid hormone instead of statins? Pharmaceutical sales of statins would certainly decline, and long-term, the cardiologists would lose their future supply of customers. We live in a capitalist society, which means a business model only works if it's profitable. This applies to the medical profession as well—revenue must exceed expenses for the business to be sustainable, and there must be enough customers to sustain the business. This is a huge conflict of interest to our health. It means that Standards of Care may be designed with profits in mind, not our health.

Unfortunately, thyroid patients are often seen as easy scam victims, and there appear to be numerous bogus supplements and "thyroid treatment centers," all willing to exploit thyroid patients for profit. Anecdotally, I have heard of "thyroid treatment programs" that want over $10,000 up front for their programs. This is for "natural healing" using herbs and supplements (conveniently sold by the treatment center), because these practitioners are not physicians and are not licensed to prescribe any real thyroid hormones. Sadly, I have also heard that these places are booked and it takes months to get an appointment, because patients are desperate. They would all be out of business if patients could just get the correct amount of prescription hormone they need!

There are other clinics where doctors market themselves as experts, and patients are led to believe that their exorbitant fees are therefore warranted, because they possess healing secrets that will cure us. Of course, few of these types of doctors accept insurance, and many push their own expensive supplements or prescription formulas. For someone who has already made the mainstream medical rounds and is still on suboptimal thyroid treatment because of their TSH, the hope of being cured can be very alluring. Unfortunately, these experts may not know much more than a local physician, and the patient's condition doesn't really improve, though their wallet certainly becomes lighter. Some patients have spent tens of thousands of dollars seeing various "experts." As a male thyroid patient, age 51 said:

> *The lesson I have learned is that the patient must play an integral role in their own healing, and not rely on doctors to direct their efforts to get well. The best doctors are the compassionate ones, the doctors that will listen to the patient and be open minded enough to work with the patient. Fancy offices, websites and reputations (and the associated large medical bills) don't get patients well.*

We live in a litigious society, which means everyone is afraid of being sued; therefore, doctors will strictly adhere to the Standards of Care, even if it's quite clear the patient is hypothyroid or undermedicated. Their hands are tied due to an erroneous paradigm!

Patients afflicted with other diseases work hard on raising visibility for their cause, so that more research and better treatments can be found for their condition. Yet there are already numerous studies on thyroid physiology showing that T3 is an essential thyroid hormone, and T3 types of medications already exist. But few doctors will prescribe any form of T3 to a patient. How ironic is that?

Many disease states are caused by a lack of thyroid hormone. Patients are often referred to different specialists, when their problems might resolve if they were just treated with thyroid hormone. Here are just a few examples:

- Allergy and Immunology
  Hypothyroid patients have longer mucociliary clearance times than normal controls. This refers to the ability of mucosal surfaces in the lungs to remove foreign particles and keep the mucosal surfaces moist and fresh. This makes hypothyroid patients more susceptible to lower and upper respiratory tract infections.[1] I can personally say that I was constantly plagued with colds that often turned into bronchitis before I added some T3 to my dose.

- Cardiology:
  Thyroid hormone, especially T3, is essential to normal heart function. Lack of T3 or the "Low T3 syndrome" is associated with heart failure and cardiovascular disease.[2] High cholesterol is often caused by low thyroid levels and drops when thyroid hormone is prescribed.[3] My blood pressure was 170/100 when I was only

taking ½ grain of desiccated thyroid and undermedicated. Raising my thyroid dose brought the blood pressure down.

- Dermatology
Dry skin, hair loss, and itching are common complaints of hypothyroid patients. Other diseases associated with hypothyroidism include alopecia areata (hair loss in round patches), chronic urticaria (hives), vitiligo (white patches on the skin) and scleroderma (connective tissue disease that thickens the skin).[4] I know that I only developed vitiligo when my thyroid dose was too low, and after I raised my dose, no new spots formed. This suggests that optimizing thyroid levels may lessen the severity of these diseases. I also had chronic hives at one point, and eczema for most of my life, but I haven't been bothered by those since eliminating yellow #5 food color from my diet and adding T3 to my thyroid dose.

- Dentistry
Delayed permanent teeth eruption,[5] root resorption during orthodontia,[6] and decreased saliva flow (which can contribute to cavities)[7] are signs of hypothyroidism that dentists should notice. I notice that my gums bleed and are tender when my thyroid dose is too low. My teeth also tended to stain when I was only taking desiccated thyroid and my FT4 was at the bottom of the reference range. After adding T4 to a lower desiccated thyroid dose, the staining diminished considerably, as if T4 somehow hardens the teeth.

- Endocrinology
Thyroid and other hormone disorders should be recognized and properly treated by endocrinologists, but they are not, or there would be no need to write this book. Endocrinologists seem to believe that when pituitary hormones (TSH, ACTH, LH, and FSH) fall into the normal reference range, then everything is "fine." Peter's story (Chapter 2) shows how difficult it is to get a diagnosis of pituitary dysfunction, because his pituitary secreted just enough hormone that he always tested in the normal range, even though his pituitary was damaged. He hardly had any thyroid, adrenal, or sex hormones and spent most of his life in a state of fatigue, yet his endocrinologist had declared him fine! Are endocrinologists aware that lack of thyroid hormone affects the adrenal gland [see Adrenal Dysfunction, Chapter 6], the ovaries and testicles [see Reproductive Problems, Chapter 22], and may cause insulin resistance [see Insulin Resistance, Chapter 17] and osteoporosis [see Osteoporosis, Chapter 19]? Are they aware that a normal thyroid gland secretes T3? Why are they so reluctant to prescribe enough of a key hormone that could give people their lives back?

- Gastroenterology
Thyroid hormone appears to be involved in the development, progression, and prevention of cancers of the alimentary tract (esophagus, stomach, pancreas, colorectal) and liver.[8] Most thyroid patients are familiar with constipation, a typical hypothyroid symptom. Delayed gastroesophageal motility (slow movement of food through the digestive tract) is a confirmed feature of hypothyroid-

ism with reduced stomach, small intestine, and colon activity. Patients often report a feeling of indigestion.[9] Overt hypothyroidism is also associated with small intestinal bacterial overgrowth (SIBO), which displays as abdominal discomfort, bloating, and flatulence.[10] People start changing their diets to deal with their symptoms, when really, they are probably just deficient in thyroid hormone.

- Hematology
  Hypothyroid patients have higher IgE (Immunoglobulin E) levels and tend to be anemic (lower hemoglobin, red blood cell count, and hematocrit) compared to normal controls. Increased IgE levels are often seen in patients with allergic diseases.[11] How many people are prescribed iron for anemia, when they really need thyroid hormone instead? I have had allergies my entire life, and display the opposite of anemia, or erythrocytosis (high hemoglobin, red blood cell count, and hematocrit) when my thyroid dose is too high. A hematologist tested me for a rare genetic mutation (which was negative) and even suggested I go to Shands Hospital for further testing, because he couldn't figure out *why* I had erythrocytosis. He was completely unaware of the effects of thyroid hormone on blood parameters, even though he was highly credentialed and displayed equally high levels of arrogance.

- Nephrology
  Low thyroid levels can cause nephrotic syndrome, a form of kidney disease where plasma proteins are lost in the urine.[12] Hypothyroidism also contributes to a lower estimated glomerular filtration rate (eGFR), especially in chronic kidney disease patients. Thyroid hormone replacement therapy raises eGFR in these patients.[13] Acute renal failure in other patients has also significantly improved with thyroid hormone replacement; however, other unnecessary diagnostic procedures were usually performed first.[14] Again, this myopic view results in testing of the kidney, when the cause of the problem is a lack of thyroid hormone.

- Obstetrics and Gynecology
  Low thyroid levels contribute to dysfunctional reproductive cycles in women, with periods that are either sporadic or too far apart. This contributes to infertility in some women. Many women undergo multiple *in vitro* fertilization cycles without success because the underlying cause, hypothyroidism, is never addressed. Fetal brain development is also affected if the mother's thyroid hormone levels, specifically T4, are too low. Men's fertility is also affected, and sperm may be abnormal [see Reproductive Problems, Chapter 22]. My periods were as far as six weeks apart before I was prescribed thyroid hormone.

- Otolaryngology
  Hearing loss may be caused by hypothyroidism, and may occur alone, or in conjunction with vertigo and tinnitus. In one study, there was no significant association between audiometric thresholds (the lowest sound that can be heard by an individual) and serum TSH and FT4, but more hypothyroid patients had

higher audiometric thresholds. Abnormal audiometric tests were also observed in patients with "normal" FT4 levels.[15] Again, both FT4 and TSH are not good diagnostics for hypothyroidism.

- Pediatrics
  Congenital hypothyroidism appears to be increasing, and replacement thyroid hormone must be given to these infants shortly after birth, or they can develop mental retardation.[16] Soy formula can induce hypothyroidism in a newborn because soy is a goitrogen.[17] Insufficient thyroid hormone limits bone growth, and untreated patients will be shorter than peers their age. In severe cases, growth can halt.[18]

- Pulmonary Disease
  Hypothyroidism and obstructive sleep apnea are associated with pulmonary hypertension. The hypothyroidism may contribute to the severity of the pulmonary hypertension.[19] Thyroid levels also affect lung function and central respiratory drive, or breathing.[20] Many hypothyroid patients complain of "air hunger," or a feeling that they can't breathe. I developed asthma when my thyroid dose was too low, and it cleared up when my dose was raised.

- Psychiatry
  Thyroid hormone plays a huge role in normal brain function, and thyroid levels that are either too high or too low can cause mental disturbances. Because this is not recognized by many physicians, anti-depressants, anti-anxiety, and other pharmaceuticals are often prescribed for mood disorders. If actual thyroid levels (FT3 and T4) were tested, they might show levels that are too high or too low. Correcting thyroid levels is certainly preferable to taking addictive pharmaceuticals with dangerous side effects. Searching Google Scholar for "thyroid psychiatry" brings up articles on the following mood disturbances that are associated with abnormal thyroid function: suicidal behavior in depressed patients,[21] postpartum psychosis,[22] bipolar affective disorder,[23] chronic schizophrenia,[24] oppositional defiant disorder,[25] and autism.[26] Depression is mentioned often on thyroid internet support groups, and I've heard people say that taking just a little bit of T3 eliminated their depression. "Brain fog" is another common complaint.

- Rheumatology
  Hypothyroidism is a known cause of aches and pains: myalgia (muscle pain), muscle cramps, stiffness, low back pain, arthralgia (joint pain), adhesive capsulitis (frozen shoulder), limited joint mobility, myopathy (muscle weakness), carpal tunnel syndrome, trigger finger, Dupuytren's contracture (thickening of the fibrous tissue layer underneath the skin of the palm and fingers) and tarsal tunnel syndrome (compression of the tibial nerve in the foot). Rheumatologic disorders associated with hypothyroidism are: osteoarthritis, mild inflammatory arthritis involving hand joints, rheumatoid arthritis, systemic lupus erythematosus (SLE), fibromyalgia, Raynaud's phenomenon, and mixed connective tissue disease. Other autoimmune disorders associated with hypothyroidism are viti-

ligo, lichen planus, recurrent aphthous stomatitis, and alopecia areata. Laboratory abnormalities detected were thyroid autoantibody (anti-TPO), elevated creatine phosphokinase (CPK) enzyme, rheumatoid factor, and antinuclear antibodies (ANA).[27]

Jane [The Woe of Vertigo, Chapter 3] is a perfect example of someone with symptoms (vertigo and vomiting) caused by low T3 levels that no one connected to her hypothyroid condition. Even though lab tests flagged her Free T3 levels as below the reference range, she was not prescribed any T3, but was referred to multiple doctors: a rheumatologist, the ER, pathologist, gastroenterologist, surgeon, cardiologist, radiologist, ophthalmologist, otolaryngologist, endocrinologist, primary care physician, hospital outpatient services, audiologist, gerontologist, and physical therapist. Procedures performed on Jane included an upper GI endoscopy biopsy, upper GI contrast x-ray, drain joint/bursa, EKG, brain CT, brain MRI, ear microscopy exam, hearing test, echo exam of abdomen, and EKG with Doppler. None of these medical tests resulted in a change in her thyroid treatment. She was only able to try some T3 because she begged her endocrinologist for it, and lo and behold, the vertigo and vomiting stopped! The rationale for adding T3 was already there, in a simple blood test that had been performed before any of these additional tests were ordered. Is it any wonder that medical costs are so high?

---

[1] Uysal, İsmail Önder, et al. "Evaluation of nasal mucociliary activity in iatrogenic hypothyroidism." *European Archives of Oto-Rhino-Laryngology* (2013): 1-4.

[2] Iervasi, Giorgio, and Giuseppina Nicolini. "Thyroid hormone and cardiovascular system: from basic concepts to clinical application." *Internal and emergency medicine* (2013): 1-4.

[3] Teixeira, Patrícia De Fátima Dos Santos, et al. "Lipid profile in different degrees of hypothyroidism and effects of levothyroxine replacement in mild thyroid failure." *Translational Research* 151.4 (2008): 224-231.

[4] Keen, Mohammad Abid, Iffat Hassan, and Mohammad Hayat Bhat. "A clinical study of the cutaneous manifestations of hypothyroidism in kashmir valley." *Indian journal of dermatology* 58.4 (2013): 326.

[5] Chandna, Shalu, and Manish Bathla. "Oral manifestations of thyroid disorders and its management." *Indian journal of endocrinology and metabolism* 15.Suppl2 (2011): S113.

[6] Marques, Leandro Silva, et al. "Root Resorption in Orthodontics: An Evidence-Based Approach." *Orthodontics-Basic aspects and Clinical considerations. InTech* (2012).

[7] Muralidharan, Dhanya, et al. "Qualitative and quantitative changes in saliva among patients with thyroid dysfunction prior to and following the treatment of the dysfunction." *Oral surgery, oral medicine, oral pathology and oral radiology* (2013).

[8] Brown, Adam R., Rosalia Simmen, and Frank A. Simmen. "The Role of Thyroid Hormone Signaling in the Prevention of Digestive System Cancers." *International journal of molecular sciences* 14.8 (2013): 16240-16257.

[9] Yaylali, Olga, et al. "Does hypothyroidism affect gastrointestinal motility?" *Gastroenterology research and practice* 2009 (2010).

[10] Lauritano, Ernesto Cristiano, et al. "Association between hypothyroidism and small intestinal bacterial overgrowth." *Journal of Clinical Endocrinology & Metabolism* 92.11 (2007): 4180-4184.

[11] Jafarzadeh, Abdollah, et al. "Immunological and hematological changes in patients with hyperthyroidism or hypothyroidism." *Clinical & Investigative Medicine* 33.5 (2010): E271-E279.

[12] Uddin, Md Julhash, et al. "Hypothyroidism and Nephrotic Syndrome-A Rare Association." *Journal of Medicine* 10.1 (2009): 34-35.

[13] Hataya, Yuji, et al. "Thyroid hormone replacement therapy for primary hypothyroidism leads to significant improvement of renal function in chronic kidney disease patients." *Clinical and experimental nephrology* (2012): 1-7.

[14] Liakopoulos, Vassilios, et al. "Acute renal failure: a rare presentation of hypothyroidism." *Renal failure* 31.4 (2009): 323-326.

[15] Santos, Karlos Thiago Pinheiro dos, et al. "Audiologic evaluation in patients with acquired hypothyroidism." *Brazilian journal of otorhinolaryngology* 76.4 (2010): 478-484.

[16] Ford, George, and Stephen H. LaFranchi. "Screening for congenital hypothyroidism: A worldwide view of strategies." *Best Practice & Research Clinical Endocrinology & Metabolism* (2013).

[17] Fruzza, Abigail Gelb, Carla Demeterco-Berggren, and Kenneth Lee Jones. "Unawareness of the effects of soy intake on the management of congenital hypothyroidism." *Pediatrics* 130.3 (2012): e699-e702.

[18] Soliman, Ashraf T., Vincenzo De Sanctis, and M. A. El Said. "Congenital Hypothyroidism: Effects on Linear Growth, Catch-Up Growth, GH-IGF-I Axis and Bones." (2013).

[19] Araz, O., et al. "The incidence and severity of pulmonary hypertension in obstructive sleep apnea with hypothyroidism." *Medical science monitor: international medical journal of experimental and clinical research* 19 (2013): 883.

[20] Milla, Carlos E., and Jacquelyn Zirbes. "Pulmonary complications of endocrine and metabolic disorders." *Paediatric Respiratory Reviews* 13.1 (2012): 23-28.

[21] Duval, F., et al. "2566–Chronobiological thyroid axis activity and suicidal behavior in depressed patients." *European Psychiatry* 28 (2013): 1.

[22] Bergink, Veerle, et al. "Prevalence of autoimmune thyroid dysfunction in postpartum psychosis." *The British Journal of Psychiatry* 198.4 (2011): 264-268.

[23] Krishna, Vinay Narasimha, et al. "Association between bipolar affective disorder and thyroid dysfunction." *Asian journal of psychiatry* (2012).

[24] Themeli, Y., I. Aliko, and A. Hashorva. "P03-345-Thyroid dysfunction in chronic schizophrenia in albania." *European Psychiatry* 26 (2011): 1515.

[25] Cakaloz, Burcu, et al. "Thyroid Function and Oppositional Defiant Disorder: More Than a Coincidence in Prepubertal Boys With Attention-Deficit Hyperactivity Disorder?" *The Journal of Neuropsychiatry and Clinical Neurosciences* 23.2 (2011): E9-E10.

[26] Hoshiko, Sumi, et al. "Are thyroid hormone concentrations at birth associated with subsequent autism diagnosis?" *Autism Research* 4.6 (2011): 456-463.

[27] Kole, Alakes Kumar, Rammohan Roy, and Dalia Chanda Kole. "Rheumatic manifestations in primary hypothyroidism." *Indian Journal of Rheumatology* (2013).

27

Recommendations to Improve Thyroid Treatment

> Me: *You cannot base your dose on your TSH--it just doesn't work. Besides, you have no TSH! You need to get your Free T3 tested, and if it's low, you have to add some T3 to your prescription if you want to feel well.*
>
> Jane: *How come doctors don't know this?*
>
> —the reason I wrote this book

Any thyroid patient who has battled with doctors to get the prescription thyroid hormone they need will agree that we need change. But exactly what changes are needed and how do we accomplish that?

Educate practicing doctors

Doctors must better understand thyroid physiology because they are the gatekeepers of all lab tests and prescriptions. If I were a doctor, I would want to see proof that TSH (Thyroid Stimulating Hormone) is *not* the best indicator of optimal thyroid levels, and that T3 (triiodothyronine) is not dangerous, before prescribing it. Chapter 25, the TSH and T3 Dilemma, presents that information with multiple references, and it should be required reading for practicing doctors. That is the core paradigm that needs to change.

In addition, I have presented five case studies, and over a dozen other chapters that illustrate thyroid hormone's wide-ranging effect on the body, from insulin resistance to osteoporosis. This should be required reading for anyone in the medical profession.

Educate doctors in training

The real problem lies in medical school training, which really doesn't cover thyroid physiology, because treating hypothyroidism is considered "simple." After all, a prescription for levothyroxine will bring the patient's TSH into the normal range, which means they're now "normal." Readers of this book know that last statement is pure sarcasm, because a normal TSH level rarely reflects the patient's true thyroid status. This dogmatic rule, that if TSH is normal then the patient is fine, must be overturned. The information in Chapter 25, the TSH and T3 Dilemma, needs to be incorporated into medical school curriculums, or offered as Continuing Medical Education (CME) conference topics to those who are now out of medical school. Education is the key to change.

A quick glance at medical school curriculums around the country reveals that endocrinology is just one of many topics taught within just one semester; in other words, thyroid physiology may not amount to more than a few days' of instruction when lumped in with other endocrinology topics such as infertility, diabetes, parathyroids, adrenal diseases like Addison's and Cushing's, obesity, pituitary dysfunction, growth problems, menopause, and tumors in the endocrine system. I have limited my own research to thyroid physiology and related hormones, and have already logged over six years of study. It would be impossible for a medical student to devote six years of study to each organ—they would never graduate! That means the knowledge that doctors obtain from the first four years of medical school is really just an overview. That fact needs to be acknowledged.

After completing medical school, endocrinologists have a three year residency followed by a two year fellowship, which means they have five additional years of training. And yet, from the stories that patients share on thyroid internet groups, many endocrinologists do not consider anything but a TSH test. They pay little attention to any of the patient's symptoms, many will not consider adding any form of T3 to a dose, some are militant about T4 (levothyroxine) being sufficient replacement, and many frown on patient input of any kind, sometimes in a very condescending manner. I respect anyone who successfully completes nine additional years of school after the typical four years of college, but there is obviously something terribly wrong here.

It may be that endocrinology depends heavily on statistical analysis, because everyone has hormones, but it's only when hormone levels are too high or too low that they become problematic. Statistics allow us to determine what is high and what is low, because most people will cluster around some average value for any measurement. Endocrinologists may place far too much emphasis on numbers, which causes them to be blind to the human element. Perhaps patients are thought of as data points on a chart, which is fine if they fall into the normal reference range. But what endocrinologists fail to recognize is that people outside of the reference range aren't just "outliers" (a statistical term referring to points outside of the normal range), but real people. In the science classes I took, outliers were ignored as anomalies, and conclusions were drawn based on the majority of the data points. However, a person that takes desiccated thyroid hormone who then has a suppressed TSH is not an anomaly, but the norm. And there are logical explanations for that, as I have detailed in this book. It would certainly help patients if doctors understood that it is nearly impossible to have a "normal" TSH when taking any form of T3. The patient is not overmedicated; the TSH is simply not an accurate yardstick of thyroid health when thyroid hormone is manually dosed. Enforcing a faulty paradigm by under medicating thyroid patients is inhumane.

Create a new standard "thyroid panel" of tests

TSH and Free T4 (FT4) are two lab tests that have little correlation with hypothyroid patient symptoms, yet those are the two lab tests that are routinely ordered. This is not only a waste of time, but a waste of lab resources and medical insurance premiums. A comprehensive list of recommended lab tests is found in Blood Tests, Chapter 9, and at a bare minimum, Total T4 and Free T3 (FT3) should be run. Ideally, the entire list of lab tests would be run, because each test contributes clues as to what may be wrong. For example, antibody tests will confirm whether or not an autoimmune disease is affecting the thyroid. Graves' and Hashimoto's are both autoimmune thyroid diseases, but a Graves' patient has specific antibodies and should be tested for them. Sadly, many doctors do not know which antibody tests to run for Graves' patients, and often just run the Hashimoto's antibody tests.

Modify the reference ranges so they are more like normal distribution curves

When a reference range is left or right skewed, the excess "tail" should be cut off so the remaining datapoints form a more normal distribution curve [Chapter 21, Reference Ranges]. Anecdotal reports suggest that the higher TSH levels and lower T4 and T3 levels (found in the "tail") are really hypothyroid numbers. It really makes no sense that reference ranges are so broad that they include people who are "half dead" (Peter's words, Chapter 2).

T3 should be prescribed, as needed, to patients who need thyroid hormone replacement

A normal thyroid secretes a small amount of T3 along with T4. Therefore, a small amount of T3 should be prescribed to thyroid patients, along with T4. A normal thyroid gland's T3 and T4 output could be expressed as a ratio of T3/T4. When doctors prescribe zero T3 and only T4, they are creating a ratio of zero/T4, which is hardly "normal." Anecdotal stories from numerous patients say doctors are extremely reluctant to prescribe T3. I can only assume this is due to Standards of Care or insurance guidelines that mandate that only T4 be prescribed. If this is the case, then both the Standards of Care and the insurance guidelines must change. If anything, insurance companies should be some of the most vocal advocates for overturning these rigid guidelines. As shown in the previous chapter, lack of thyroid hormone causes a cascade of other medical conditions to develop. If the cause were properly treated, then there would be less demand on the medical system for numerous specialists, including cardiologists, gastroenterologists, obgyns, etc. Thyroid hormone is relatively inexpensive compared to statins, cardiac procedures, *in vitro* fertilization, and other medical procedures that treat low thyroid hormone conditions.

There are only two options for prescription T3: synthetic liothyronine or natural desiccated thyroid. Both are valid options and doctors should be able to freely prescribe either one to thyroid patients. Doctors should not be constrained by the current erroneous Standards of Care and insurance guidelines that only "allow" T4 prescriptions. Insurance should cover desiccated thyroid since it is a valid prescription that has been used for over a century.

Manufacturers of T3 should offer a smaller 2.5 mcg size pill

T3 pills are available in 5, 25, and 50 mcg (microgram) size. It would be ideal if a 2.5 mcg size were available, because most people need just a little bit of T3, and cutting the pills in half is sometimes difficult. I remember when I tried to cut a 5 mcg pill it just crumbled.

Thyroid patients should be involved in their thyroid dosing, the way diabetics are involved in their insulin dosing

Most people take medication in an attempt to feel better, not worse. Patients who have been both hyper and hypothyroid state that hyper is worse, because of the racing, over-anxious feeling that accompanies that state. Anyone who reaches that state by manual thyroid hormone dosing will automatically cut back their dose for relief. The problem is that doctors are cutting patients' doses prematurely, before they reach that hyperthyroid state, based solely on their disappearing TSH, which simply does not reflect their thyroid state. The TSH feedback loop is altered in manual dosing, and a normal TSH and optimal FT3 are mutually exclusive goals [Chapter 25, the TSH and T3 Dilemma]. A patient that is manually dosed can either have a normal TSH *or* optimized FT3, but not both. In other words, when a doctor keeps a patient's TSH "normal," they condemn the patient to a hypothyroid state.

Patients don't need to see lab reports to confirm what they can already feel. They feel hypothyroid, yet their TSH is suppressed, or close to zero, so their doctor refuses to prescribe any more thyroid hormone. And therein lies the crux of the problem today. Doctors bound by erroneous dogma create angry patients. It doesn't have to be this way!

Diabetics are low in the hormone insulin, and are responsible for dosing it themselves, though a doctor prescribes the insulin. They learn, through symptoms and how they feel, what their optimal dose is. There are consequences from taking either too much insulin (hypoglycemia) or too little (hyperglycemia). Diabetic patients are aware of this. Is there any reason that thyroid patients could not be trusted to have similar input on their own daily doses? As stated earlier, no one will purposely overdose themselves, because it feels awful. The sad fact is that patients today can sit in front of a doctor, complain about being cold, fatigued, constipated, brainfogged, with thin hair, dry skin, and a pulse in the 50s, and a doctor will look at their TSH and pronounce them "fine." There is obviously a huge disconnect here, and it makes no sense to blame the patient for their symptoms. That can only mean that the TSH does not always accurately reflect a patient's thyroid health. Therefore, the TSH rule must be overturned and replaced with a new diagnostic approach that includes, at a minimum, testing of Free T3, iron and ferritin, cortisol, thyroid antibodies, and acknowledgment of the patient's symptoms.

This book was conceived,
researched, written,
illustrated, formatted,
and published by someone
with no TSH . . .
who broke the TSH rule!

ABOUT THE AUTHOR

Barbara Lougheed was born and raised in Honolulu, Hawaii, where she earned a Bachelor's of Business Administration in Marketing from the University of Hawaii at Manoa. She moved to Florida for the warmer, calmer weather, and has now lived through multiple freezes and hurricanes.

She worked as a database map analyst at a major newspaper before her early retirement. She loves analyzing data and looking for patterns, and this trait has served her well as a thyroid researcher. This knack for medical research led her to write TiredThyroid.com and to publish the book *Tired Thyroid: From Hyper to Hypo to Healing--Breaking the TSH Rule*. Her love of travel, photography, and food then led her to write WhereWeVacation.com and two travel ebooks, *A Hawaiian Family Vacation: Oahu*, and *A Hawaiian Family Vacation: Maui*. She also wrote a children's book with her husband, *It's Okay to be Different Thorina-Bina*, about their unique cat. The book's animal characters teach children about differences, self-acceptance, and tolerance. Read more about her books on BarbaraLougheed.com.

* * *

If you liked this book and found it helpful, please write a review on amazon. Thank you!

Made in the USA
Middletown, DE
22 January 2019